Pathology

The Mammographically Directed Biopsy

Guest Editors:

James L. Bennington, M.D.
Michael D. Lagios, M.D.
Department of Anatomic Pathology
   and Clinical Laboratories
California Pacific Medical Center,
   California Campus
San Francisco, California

Official Publication of the
CALIFORNIA SOCIETY OF PATHOLOGISTS

STATE OF THE ART REVIEWS

Volume 1/Number 1   1992
HANLEY & BELFUS, INC.   Philadelphia

Publisher: HANLEY & BELFUS, INC.
 210 South 13th Street
 Philadelphia, PA 19107
 (215) 546-7293
 FAX (215) 790-9330

Authorization to photocopy items for internal or personal use, or the internal or personal use of specific clients, is granted by Hanley & Belfus, Inc. for libraries and other users registered with the Copyright Clearance Center (CCC) Transaction Reporting Service, provided that the base fee of $1.00 per copy plus $0.25 per page is paid directly to the CCC, 21 Congress St., Salem, MA 01970. Identify this publication by including with your payment the fee code, 1041-3480/92 $1.00 + .25.

PATHOLOGY: State of the Art Reviews   **(ISSN 1041-3480)**
Volume 1, Number 1   **(ISBN 1-56053-079-0)**

© 1992 by Hanley & Belfus, Inc. under the International Copyright Union. All rights reserved. No part of this book may be reproduced, reused, republished, or transmitted in any form or by any means without written permission of the publisher.

PATHOLOGY: State of the Art Reviews is published quarterly by Hanley & Belfus, Inc., 210 South 13th Street, Philadelphia, Pennsylvania 19107.

POSTMASTER: Send address changes to PATHOLOGY: State of the Art Reviews, Hanley & Belfus, Inc., 210 South 13th Street, Philadelphia, PA 19107.

Contents

Needle Localization Guided Excisional Biopsy for Mammographically Identified Nonpalpable Breast Lesions 1
Frederick R. Margolin

> The capability of high-quality mammography to discover early, preclinical breast cancer has demanded the development of a new relationship between radiologists, surgeons, and pathologists. It is only through mutual understanding and appreciation of the technical requirements and interpretive difficulties involved in the successful identification, preoperative localization, and excision of these lesions that the full benefits of this method of early cancer detection can be brought to all patients.

Impact of Mammographic Screening on the Size and the Relative Frequency of Invasion in Breast Cancers Seen in a Community Hospital from 1975-1988 11
James L. Bennington, Michael D. Lagios, and Frederick R. Margolin

> This report documents a significant reduction in the average size of invasive breast cancers and an increase in the frequency of in situ, relative to invasive, breast cancers observed at California Pacific Medical Center/California Campus (CPMC) during the years following the introduction of routine screening mammography in 1975. The implications of early discovery of in situ duct and relatively small invasive duct carcinomas are for improved patient survival through: (1) preventing progression from in situ to invasive carcinoma, and (2) the removal of invasive duct cancers before reaching a size where there is a high risk of metastasis.

Protocol for the Pathologic Examination and Tissue Processing of the Mammographically Directed Breast Biopsy 23
Michael D. Lagios and James L. Bennington

> Achieving the maximum yield of breast cancers detected by mammography has required certain changes in tissue handling and examination of the mammographically directed breast biopsy. This new radiographic technique, increased use of breast-conserving surgical approaches for the treatment of breast cancer, more enlightened and demanding patients, and increasing medical-legal exposure have all contributed to changes in the way surgical pathologists should process and sample breast biopsy specimens.

Handling the Mammographically Directed Biopsy: Another Approach 47
Mahendra Ranchod

> Because of cost and manpower considerations, the approach to handling the mammographically directed biopsy in the author's hospital is a modification of the approach described in the previous article. The differences in approach are described.

Processing the Small Invasive Carcinoma Detected in the Mammographically Directed Breast Biopsy 51
James L. Bennington

> During the next few years pathologists can expect to be called upon with increasing frequency to extract data on a number of cell cycle, biochemical, and genetic features of breast cancers as a routine part of the specimen examination. Obtaining this information without compromising the histologic diagnosis or losing morphologic-based prognostic information is challenging, particularly with small invasive breast cancers, but is a service pathologists should be able to provide.

In Situ Proliferative Epithelial Lesions of the Breast 65
Onsi W. Kamel, Richard L. Kempson, and Michael R. Hendrickson

> Considerable progress has been made over the last several years toward understanding the significance of noninvasive epithelial changes in the breast. This progress, in essence, is the result of categorizing in situ alterations according to their clinical significance, or more specifically, according to the risk that such lesions carry to the patient for development of a subsequent invasive carcinoma. This article summarizes the histopathological criteria that are currently used to define morphologic categories and, perhaps more importantly, it reviews the clinical implications of the diagnoses that result from this categorization.

Steroid Receptors in Surgical Pathology—With Special Reference to Small Mammographically Detected Breast Lesions 103
Jon C. Ross, Scott Binder, Mark C. Rounsaville, and Klaus Lewin

> The cellular receptors for estrogen, progesterone, and other steroid hormones appear in the cytosol fraction of homogenated specimens of hormonal target tissues. These receptors have traditionally been detected and quantitated by biochemical techniques that involve binding tritium-labelled marker steroids to the receptor proteins. An important recent development has been the creation of various monoclonal antibody reagents that specifically recognize antigenic determinants on receptor molecules.

Significance of DNA Content and Proliferative Rate of the Invasive Carcinoma Found in the Mammographically Directed Breast Biopsy 137
James L. Bennington

> During the last few years considerable effort has been made to find genetic and biochemical markers that could be used to predict the behavior of cancers with greater accuracy than that obtained by histologic grading or the assessment of other established morphologic features. Because there is considerable evidence that malignant neoplasms have cytogenetic abnormalities, and because atypical features of the nucleus such as pleomorphism and hyperchromasia are known to be prognostically unfavorable findings, quantitative analysis of nuclear DNA was a prime candidate for evaluation. Also, the rate at which malignant tumor cells replicate, and the fraction of tumor cells participating in the proliferative process, are of considerable interest to oncologists for use in assessing patient prognosis and for guiding decisions on the use of various endocrine and cytotoxic agents for adjuvant endocrine and chemotherapy.

Breast Biopsies: The Content of the Surgical Pathology Report **161**
Onsi W. Kamel, Michael R. Hendrickson, and Richard L. Kempson

> In the context of recent developments, the role of the surgical pathologist in evaluating and reporting breast cancer specimens has become more important. The pathologist must not only diagnose carcinoma in a given patient, but must also document a set of morphologic features that have been shown to be important in determining prognosis and guiding therapy.

Index **183**

Contributors

James L. Bennington, M.D.
Clinical Professor of Pathology, Stanford University School of Medicine, Stanford, California; Chairman, Department of Anatomic Pathology and Clinical Laboratories, California Pacific Medical Center/California Campus, San Francisco, California

Scott Binder, M.D.
Department of Dermatopathology, Scripps Clinic and Research Foundation, LaJolla, California

Michael Roger Hendrickson, M.D.
Associate Professor of Pathology, Stanford University School of Medicine; Associate Director, Laboratory of Surgical Pathology, Stanford University Hospital, Stanford, California

Onsi W. Kamel, M.D.
Fellow in Surgical Pathology, Department of Pathology, Stanford University Hospital, Stanford, California

Richard L. Kempson, M.D.
Professor of Pathology, Stanford University School of Medicine; Co-Director, Laboratory of Surgical Pathology, Stanford University Hospital, Stanford, California

Michael D. Lagios, M.D.
Senior Surgical Pathologist, Department of Anatomic Pathology and Clinical Laboratories, California Pacific Medical Center/California Campus, San Francisco, California

Klaus J. Lewin, M.D., F.R.C.Path.
Professor of Pathology and Medicine, Departments of Pathology and Medicine, UCLA School of Medicine, Los Angeles, California

Frederick R. Margolin, M.D.
Clincial Professor of Radiology, University of California, San Francisco; Chairman, Department of Radiology, California Pacific Medical Center/California Campus, San Francisco, California

Mahendra Ranchod, M.B.Ch.B., M.Med.
Clinical Professor of Pathology, Department of Pathology, Stanford University Hospital; Pathologist, Good Samaritan Hospital, San Jose, California

Mark C. Rounsaville, M.D.
Department of Radiation Oncology, California Pacific Medical Center/California Campus, San Francisco, California

Jon C. Ross, M.D.
Clinical Assistant Professor of Pathology, Stanford University Medical Center, Stanford, California; Pathologist, California Pacific Medical Center/California Campus, San Francisco, California

Pathology: State of the Art Reviews

Forthcoming Issue

SURFACE EPITHELIAL TUMORS OF THE OVARY

Edited by

Michael Roger Hendrickson, M.D.
Associate Professor of Pathology, Stanford University School of Medicine; Associate Director, Laboratory of Surgical Pathology, Stanford University Hospital, Stanford, California

Future Issues

NEW DIAGNOSTIC METHODS IN PATHOLOGY

DIAGNOSIS OF LOW GRADE LYMPHOMAS

SOFT TISSUE SARCOMAS: A PRACTICAL APPROACH TO DIAGNOSIS

BIOPSY DIAGNOSIS OF ESOPHAGEAL AND GASTRIC DISEASE

PATHOLOGY: State of the Art Reviews is an official publication of the California Society of Pathologists. The Executive Director is Mr. Robert Achermann. The CSP Executive Office is at 1303 J Street, Suite 250, Sacramento, CA 95814. Telephone: 916-446-6601.

Ordering information:
Issues in PATHOLOGY: STARs are priced individually. Please contact the publisher to order current or back issues.

Hanley & Belfus, Inc., 210 South 13th Street, Philadelphia, PA 19107.
Telephone (215) 546-7293; (800) 962-1892; FAX (215) 790-9330.

Foreword

The *PATHOLOGY: State of the Art Reviews* monograph series, sponsored by the California Society of Pathologists, is designed to explore in depth subjects of current interest in diagnostic pathology. The aim of each issue is to provide an up-to-date review and critical evaluation for practicing pathologists. Contributions to the series will be by invitation only. The Editorial Board of the California Society of Pathologists will select focal subjects as titles for publication in the series and will invite an expert in the field as the Guest Editor for each monograph. The Guest Editor will be responsible for the content and topics to be covered, and will select the authors to write the individual articles for the issue.

The Editorial Board feels that there is a need for an authoritative series of reviews on emerging and controversial subjects in diagnostic pathology to serve as timely and definitive reference sources. The creation of *PATHOLOGY: State of the Art Reviews* also will provide a unique opportunity for the California Society of Pathologists to promote the contributions of California pathologists to the field of diagnostic pathology.

As so aptly stated by Anthony and MacSween,* "Histopathology is an art to some, a craft to others, and should be a science to all who engage in it." This view is just as applicable to clinical pathology as it is to anatomic pathology. The Editorial Board hopes to provide in the *State of the Art Reviews* a balance of content that will offer articles of interest and value to a diverse audience of pathologists. To help in achieving this goal, the editors and Editorial Board welcome and encourage feedback from the readers.

---

* Anthony PP, MacSween RNM: Recent Advances in Histopathology, No. 11. London, Churchill Livingstone, 1981, p. v.

James L. Bennington, M.D.
SERIES EDITOR

California Society of Pathologists
Editorial Board

James L. Bennington, M.D. San Francisco	Edward Howes, M.D. San Francisco	Mahendra Ranchod, M.D. San Jose
Jerome S. Burke, M.D. Berkeley	Richard L. Kempson, M.D. Stanford	Jon C. Ross, M.D. San Francisco
Walter F. Coulson, M.D. Los Angeles	Eileen B. King, M.D. Larkspur	George S. Smith, M.D. Los Angeles
Seth L. Haber, M.D. Santa Clara	Klaus J. Lewin, M.D. Los Angeles	Daniel P. Stites, M.D. San Francisco
Michael R. Hendrickson, M.D. Stanford	Joseph M. Mirra, M.D. Los Angeles	Nancy E. Warner, M.D. Los Angeles

Preface

The effectiveness of mammography in detecting clinically silent but radiographically suspicious lesions of the breast with a high probability of representing in situ or small invasive carcinomas is well established. The impact of this diagnostic procedure on reducing morbidity and mortality from breast cancer is covered in detail in Chapter 1 by Dr. Margolin and in Chapter 2 (p. 11) by Drs. Bennington, Lagios, and Margolin.

The development of mammography as a diagnostic procedure capable of identifying lesions of the breast too small to be palpable but requiring complete excisional biopsy has placed new demands on the radiologist, surgeon, and pathologist. Maximizing the potential of the mammographically directed biopsy requires a team approach to establishing a diagnosis and demands a high degree of cooperation and mutual understanding of the technical problems inherent in the procedures performed by each specialist.

For the radiologist, adequate localization of the suspicious breast lesion may be time-consuming, beset with problems of paralax and triangulation, and performed under less than ideal circumstances. Newer models of mammographic equipment are equipped with state-of-the-art electronic guidance systems providing accurate stereotactic needle placement to help localize suspicious lesions.

For the surgeon, the challenge is primarily to find and biopsy the region of the breast containing the soft tissue density or cluster of microcalcifications seen on the mammogram directing the biopsy. Without landmarks or a palpable lesion, the surgeon must rely on the accuracy of the needle localization provided by the radiologist in attempting to define the correct X, Y, Z coordinates to biopsy in a soft, pliable, three-dimensional structure of nonrigid shape. The problem is compounded by the patient being in the supine position for biopsy but standing for the localization mammogram. Once the biopsy has been performed, the surgeon must depend on the radiologist or pathologist to provide assurance that the suspicious lesion has been adequately sampled and removed.

The challenges to the pathologist presented by the mammographically directed biopsy are numerous and varied. They are the subject matter of the remaining chapters of this monograph.

In Chapters 3 (p. 23) and 5 (p. 51) Drs. Lagios and Bennington have detailed the procedures for pathologic examination of the mammographically directed biopsy used at California Pacific Medical Center. These discussions include recommendations on intraoperative interpretation of the specimen radiogram, limitations on the use of frozen section, routine specimen processing, specimen sampling for steroid receptor assay, nuclear DNA analysis and proliferative rate, and reporting of pathologic findings. Sources of interpretative error and suggested solutions to may of the more common problems encountered by the pathologist are also covered. In Chapter 4 (p. 47) Dr. Ranchod presents the approach for handling the mammographically directed biopsy used by the Pathology Department at Good Samaritan Hospital. Differences in the approaches used by the two institutions are largely related to the role of the pathologist in the intraoperative interpretation of the specimen radiogram and the extent to which the mammographic biopsy is sampled for histologic examination. The content of the surgical pathology report of the breast biopsy and its importance for directing the management of patient care by the surgeon, oncologist, and radiotherapist are expanded upon by Drs. Kamel, Hendrickson, and Kempson in Chapter 6 (p. 65).

In addition to the problems inherent in routine processing of biopsy specimens for histologic examination, pathologists are increasingly called upon to reserve material for steroid receptor protein assay, nuclear DNA analysis, and proliferative rate assessments, and to interpret and integrate the result of these studies with gross and microscopic findings.

Drs. Ross and Lewin and their associates have provided in Chapter 7 (p. 103) a comprehensive review on the subject of steroid receptor proteins in surgical pathology, with a special emphasis on their importance in breast cancers found in the mammographically directed biopsy. This discussion includes a number of important topics, including guidelines for the pathologist on reserving tumor for ER/PR protein assay. The role of ER/PR receptor protein levels in guiding the management of patients with invasive breast cancer (including T1 N0 tumors), correlation of steroid receptor protein levels with other pathologic features of invasive breast cancer, reproducibility of assay results, evaluation of receptor status over time and with treatment, advantages and disadvantages of various laboratory and immunocytochemical methods for ER/PR determination, and use of steroid receptor protein levels in the differential histopathologic diagnosis of cancer are discussed.

Chapter 8 (p. 137) by Dr. Bennington is a detailed review of our current knowledge of nuclear DNA content and cell proliferative rate as prognostic indicators for breast cancer patients. This topic is particularly relevant to the subject of the mammographically directed biopsy, because many invasive cancers detected by mammography are small and the patient's lymph node-negative. Currently, oncologists are increasingly using adjuvant chemotherapy for the treatment of all breast cancer patients irrespective of lymph node status. Cancer cell nuclear DNA content and rates of cell proliferation may well serve as important discriminants needed to spare those patients who have a low probability of metastasis from unneeded treatment. Also covered are a discussion of nuclear DNA content and rates of cell proliferation as prognostic indicators (individually and in combination), correlation of these two features with established prognostic indicators, and the response of breast cancers to endocrine and chemotherapy in relation to tumor ploidy and cell proliferative rate.

The majority of this monograph on the mammographically directed biopsy focuses on issues related to invasive breast cancers. However, although invasion in breast cancer is the proximate cause of morbidity and mortality, there is a spectrum of noninvasive epithelial changes that are important because of their association with increased risk of progressing to invasive breast cancer. With the introduction of mammography, pathologists increasingly are encountering these proliferative epithelial changes, which must be correctly diagnosed and their clinical significance interpreted to the surgeon and other therapists. In Chapter 9 (p. 161), Drs. Kamel, Hendrickson and Kempson summarize the histopathologic criteria currently used to define the various important proliferative lesions of the breast and review in detail the clinical implications of their diagnosis.

Unfortunately, time and space do not permit covering all of the subjects that might well be included in a review of the subject of the mammographically directed biopsy. It would have been nice to have included discussions on such topics as the possible uses and limitations of the fine needle aspiration biopsy in mammographically directed lesions, approaches to differentiating invasion from pseudoinvasive breast cancers, and cost-benefit analysis of various diagnostic procedures employed in association with the workup of the breast biopsy. Perhaps another time . . . .

Finally, a number of differences of opinion are expressed in this monograph, particularly with respect to the value of total embedding of biopsy material for histologic examination and the utility of ploidy and cell proliferative rate analysis for assessing patient prognosis. This is not a function of editorial laxness or oversight, but rather represents editorial encouragement of opposing but well-reasoned views on important issues. It is hoped that open discussion will speed the resolution of these differences.

James L. Bennington, M.D.
Michael D. Lagios, M.D.
GUEST EDITORS

Needle Localization Guided Excisional Biopsy for Mammographically Identified Nonpalpable Breast Lesions

FREDERICK R. MARGOLIN, M.D.

From the Department of
  Radiology
California Pacific Medical
  Center, California Campus,
  and
Department of Radiology
University of California, San
  Francisco
San Francisco, California

Reprint requests to:
Frederick R. Margolin, M.D.
Department of Radiology
California Pacific Medical
  Center, California Campus
3700 California Street
San Francisco, CA 94118

The demonstrated ability of breast radiography to identify early, nonpalpable breast cancer has prompted the major growth and development of mammography during the past three decades. A steadily increasing proportion of mammographic examinations are now performed on asymptomatic women in an effort to detect early, nonpalpable, and potentially curable breast cancer. In our institution[3] more than 60% of breast cancers are now discovered by mammography alone. In 1974, prior to the development of mammography services at our hospital, the average size of the breast cancer removed at surgery was 40 mm. In 1988, the average breast cancer size was 13.7 mm. The incidence of axillary nodal metastases among our patients with mammographically detected carcinomas is 13%. This contrasts with a 43% rate of positive axillary nodes in those patients whose breast carcinomas were detected clinically. During the 16 years since the introduction of mammography at our hospital, there has been a sixfold increase in frequency of diagnosis of breast carcinoma in situ. Similar results have been reported from other hospitals and clinics in which an active mammography program has been successful in the detection of preclinical breast cancer.

The effect of early detection on mortality reduction has now been documented in several controlled patient population studies in the United States, Sweden, and the Netherlands. A 30% to 50% reduction in overall mortality from breast cancer was found in these studies in women whose lesions were discovered mammographically. The increasing frequency with which early breast malignancy is now diagnosed has changed the pattern of surgical practice for breast carcinoma in many institutions. In our hospital, in 1976, subtotal mastectomy was performed for only 12.5% of breast cancer patients. At the end of one decade, in 1986, subtotal mastectomy comprised 53.4% of all surgical procedures for breast cancer.

The success of any program to identify and appropriately treat early breast cancer requires a cooperative effort and clear communication among radiologists, surgeons, and pathologists. This requires a full understanding of both the technical and interpretive problems that may arise in the identification, localization, excision, and pathologic evaluation of suspected early breast cancer.

MAMMOGRAPHIC TECHNIQUE

Mammography is a method of soft tissue radiography of the breast. Low energy x-rays of limited penetration are passed through the breast creating a latent image on a film or xerographic receptor, which is then developed to provide an image of the soft tissues of the breast. Each link in the this image-production chain is critically important in order to obtain a final mammogram with optimal contrast, resolution, detail, and diagnostic information.

Nearly all mammography in the United States is now performed with dedicated mammographic equipment featuring microfocal spot tubes, which produce the clearest and sharpest image by minimizing geometric unsharpness and blurring. Breasts must be adequately compressed to a uniform thickness for optimal image quality. Finally, whether the image is ultimately recorded on x-ray film or a selenium-coated (xerographic) plate, carefully controlled processing of the final image is critical to produce the most diagnostic mammogram. With highly skilled and experienced mammographic technologists, carefully chosen and well-maintained, dedicated mammographic equipment and optimal processing of the final image, the accuracy of mammographic interpretation improves.

FEATURES OF CLINICALLY OCCULT MAMMOGRAPHICALLY IDENTIFIED BREAST CANCER

The final mammographic image depicts shadows of the internal structures of the breast. This largely reflects fibrous, fatty, and glandular tissue. Fibrous and glandular tissue, as well as fluid-filled spaces, exhibit a uniform radiographic density identical with that of water. Fat exhibits a diminished radiographic density and is relatively translucent. The larger the amount of fat within the breasts, the more sharply defined and clearly delineated will be normal mammary tissue, as well as any other abnormal tissue of water density.

The accuracy of mammographic diagnosis is, therefore, roughly proportional to the amount of fat within the breasts. In many women, the presence of little or no breast fat results in a nearly homogeneously dense mammogram in which the absence of low-density contrasting fat effectively precludes the identification of all but the largest masses.

Calcium deposits within the breast produce mammographic shadows of higher density than either fat or other breast soft tissues. Although the vast majority of calcium deposits within the breast occurs as a result of benign processes—such as fat necrosis, vascular calcification, milk of calcium within breast microcysts, dermal calcifications, plasma cell mastitis, secretory disease, fibroadenomata, and sclerosing adneosis—there is a frequent association between calcium deposition and malignant disease. Approximately 30% to 50% of primary breast cancers have mammographically detectable calcifications.[6] Far more commonly, calcifications within breast cancers can be demonstrated on specimen radiography and on microscopic examination, but are too faint or small to be demonstrated mammographically. In a recent series of patients, microscopic calcifications were found in 41% of 27 consecutive clinically occult noncalcified breast cancers identified mammographically.[8]

Calcifications associated with comedocarcinoma present relatively distinctive radiographic features exhibiting linear, Y, and branching configurations as they follow the course of the ductal lumen. Some clustered calcifications reflect a lobular distribution. Clusters of more than 5 calcifications in 1 cm^2, particularly those exhibiting variation in size, density, and configuration of individual calcific particles, are usually deemed suspicious enough to warrant excisional biopsy.

Masses are most easily identified within fat-containing breasts. Many of these commonly represent intramammary lymph nodes, fibroadenomata, or cysts. Some mammographically identified masses, however, represent circumscribed malignancies. These are usually ductal in type, but medullary or colloid carcinomas may present this appearance. The borders of any mammographically defined mass should be carefully examined, preferably using magnification technique. Any irregularity or indistinctness of border outline raises the level of suspicion for malignancy.

Hyalinized degeneration in a fibroadenoma results in the deposition of dense coarse calcium deposits within a mammographically distinct mass. These present relatively typical mammographic features and, even if palpable, the biopsy of such characteristic lesions can be avoided. The presence of any atypical calcifications within a mass, however, should raise the level of suspicion for malignancy.

Areas of architectural distortion represent an additional mammographic feature of occult malignancy. Suspicious areas of architectural change most commonly appear as stellate densities with spokelike rays extending into surrounding breast tissue. This appearance is associated with the desmoplastic reaction elicited by some infiltrating carcinomas. Similar mammographic features can be produced by postoperative scarring, fat necrosis, and by the sclerosing benign process that has been described as "radical scar."

Less common mammographic features of occult malignancy include solitary prominent ducts, areas of mammographic asymmetry, and focal skin thickening or retraction. Sickles has recently described the mammographic features of 300 cases of occult malignancy.[7] Of these cancers 42% were mammographically detected by the presence of clustered calcifications, but only half of these calcifications were of the linear or branching types characteristic of malignancy; 39% of these cancers presented as mammographically dominant masses, with fewer than half of these demonstrating the marginal irregularities that are associated with malignant masses. Indirect mammographic signs of malignancy, such as focal architectural distortion, asymmetry, dilated ducts, and densities developing between mammographic examinations, were responsible for the detection of nearly 20% of cancers in this series.

POSITIVE PREDICTIVE VALUE OF MAMMOGRAPHY

With what frequency does a biopsy directed by a mammographically identified abnormality yield a pathologic diagnosis of breast cancer? This correlation represents the positive predictive value of mammography and ranges from 20% to 30% in most reported experience in the United States.[1,4,5]

At our hospital, 835 needle localization procedures were performed for nonpalpable mammographically identified lesions from 1974 through mid-1987. The positive predictive value in our experience was 30%. Table 1 indicates the frequency with which each of the mammographically suspicious abnormalities prompting a biopsy recommendation was associated with microscopically demonstrated, clinically occult malignancy.

PREOPERATIVE NEEDLE LOCALIZATION OF MAMMOGRAPHICALLY SUSPICIOUS LESIONS

In order to guide the surgeon to an accurate, complete, and low-volume excision of a mammographically identified suspicious lesion, a variety of preoperative localization techniques have been developed.[2] The most successful and commonly employed of these techniques requires the insertion of a needle in to the breast using the preoperative mammograms to guide the depth and direction of needle insertion. Alternatively, ultrasound may be used to guide needle placement if the suspect lesion is readily identifiable on breast sonograms.

TABLE 1. Needle Localization of 835 Nonpalpable Lesions

Abnormality	Lesions Localized	Malignant Number	Percent (%)
Suspicious calcifications	525	169	32
Discrete mass without calcifications	157	45	29
Suspicious area without calcifications	153	37	24

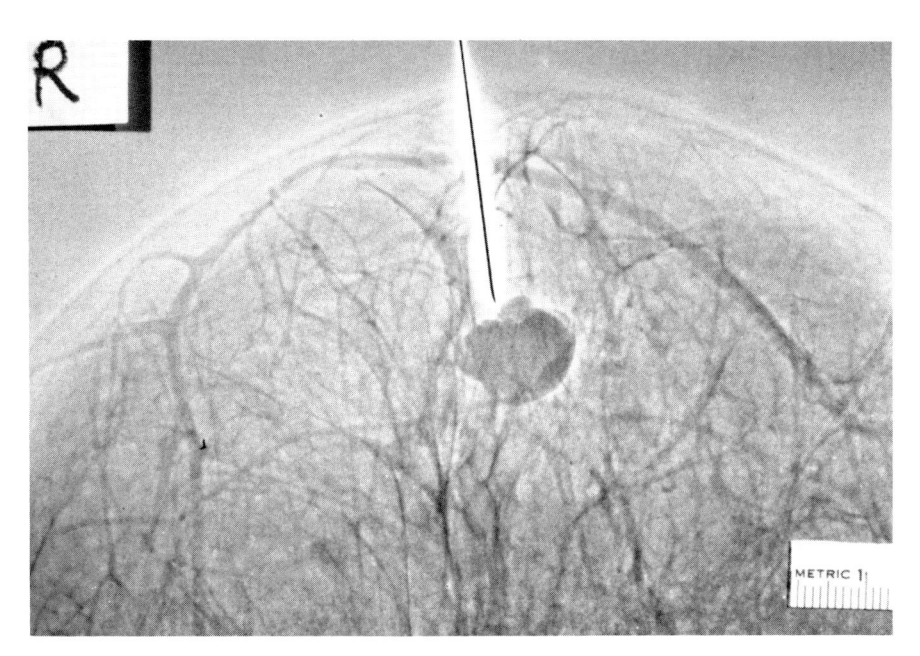

FIGURE 1. Nonpalpable retroareolar mass on xeromammogram localized by insertion of a single 25-gauge needle.

Ideally, the localization needle should pass through or be directly adjacent to the lesion. Final acceptable needle position requires the needle tip to lie within 5 to 10 mm of the target lesion (Fig. 1). At this point, methylene blue can be injected through the needle, staining the tissue for ease of identification by the operating surgeon. A hooked, barbed, or curved end wire may be inserted through the localization needle and is anchored within the breast tissue at this point (Fig. 2). Occasionally, contrast material is injected through the needle so that the needle tip position can be documented on subsequent mammograms.

Some operators prefer the injection of methylene blue as the needle is withdrawn from the breast, staining the needle tract for the operating surgeon. The most commonly employed methods, however, leave a thin hook wire in place. The patient is thus transferred to surgery for excisional biopsy. At this point communication between the radiologist and operating surgeon is essential, because appreciable change in the geometry of the breast occurs between the patient's sitting position in the mammography suite and her recumbent position on the operating table. The radiologist should annotate the final localization mammograms for the operating surgeon, indicating the suspect lesion, the position of blue dye if inserted, the position of the nipple, and the superior, inferior, medial, and lateral sides of the breast, as well as the distance and direction of the needle tip and dye deposit from the lesion to be excised (Fig. 3).

In our practice 25-gauge standard hypodermic needles are used, and the shortest distance and most direct route between the skin and underlying breast

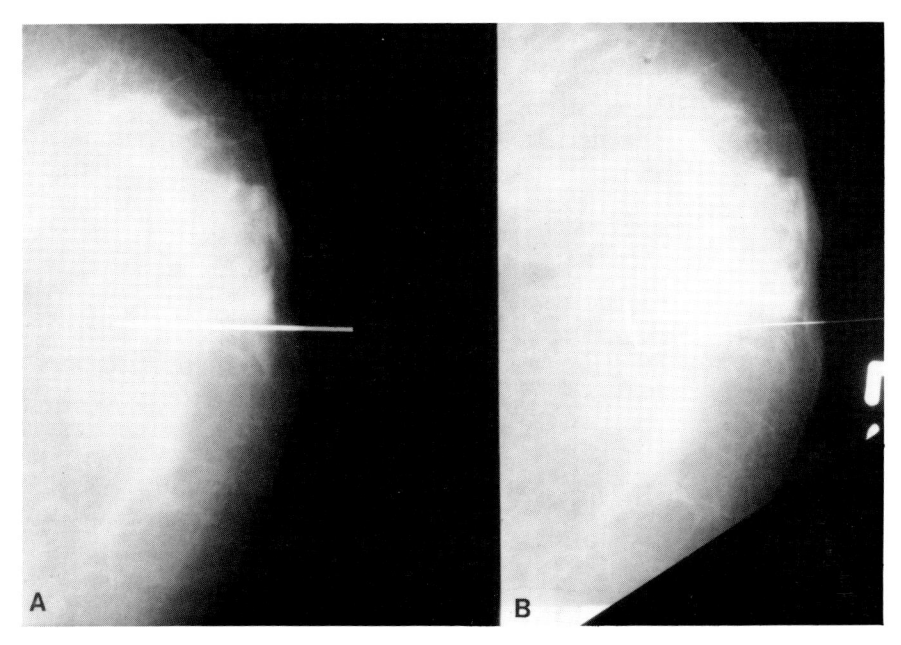

FIGURE 2. *A* and *B*, Faint cluster of calcification on screen film mammograms. Localization by hook wire (Kopans). The 20-gauge localizing needle is inserted to the point of calcifications *(A)*. The thin hook wire is then inserted through the needle and anchored within the breast tissue at the target site. The needle is then withdrawn and the hook wire left in place *(B)*.

lesion are chosen. After final injection of methylene blue, the needle is left in place, allowing the surgeon the option of incising along the shaft of the needle or choosing a more cosmetically acceptable incision site and dissecting toward the palpable rigid needle until the methylene blue stained area is encountered. Bending the needle shaft 90 degrees so that the hub lies flat on the skin surface and securely taping the needle hub to the skin prevents accidental dislodgement during patient transport and preoperative skin preparation (Fig. 4). This localization method has been successfully employed in more than 1200 patients in our practice.

The surgical pathology reports of 93 consecutive patients undergoing excisional biopsy of 100 mammographically suspicious areas of calcification were recently reviewed to assess the accuracy of our needle localization technique. Among 100 biopsied specimens, the target calcification was contained within the first surgical specimen obtained in 83%, and within the second specimen in 12%. In only two cases were more than two tissue excisions required before the specimen radiograph confirmed removal of the target calcifications. In three patients, no calcifications were reported in the specimen radiograph. In one of these, on subsequent review, the calcifications were in the skin, and in another they could not be identified in postoperative mammograms. The average size of the specimen containing the calcific lesion

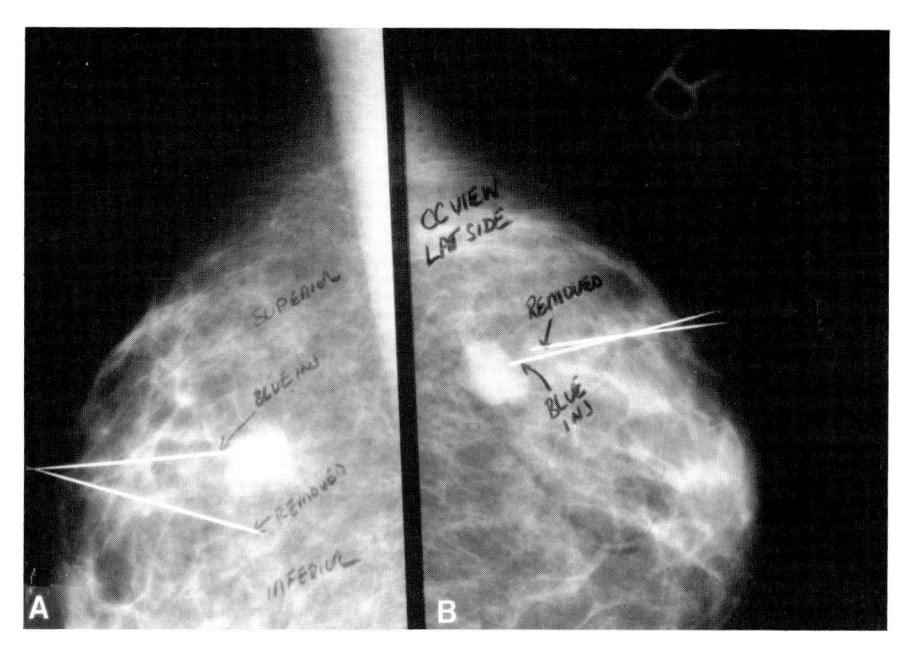

FIGURE 3. *A,* Mediolateral, and *B,* craniocaudal projections of the left breast, illustrating final annotated mammograms following localization procedure using two 25-gauge needles. Needle most remote from target lesion is removed. Position of methylene blue injection is indicated, and superior, lateral, and medial sides of the breast are indicated for the operating surgeon.

was 16.2 cm^3. This corresponds to a cube of tissue approximately 2.5 × 2.5 × 2.5 cm. Methylene blue staining of the tissue fragment containing the target calcification ws described in 76% of excised specimens.

In 1986, a questionnaire was sent to all surgeons performing breast biopsy following needle localization at our hospital. The procedure was considered accurate and reliable in more than 98% of cases reported by those responding to the survey. The addition of methylene blue was considered most helpful in defining the volume of tissue to be excised.

PROBLEMS AND PITFALLS IN NEEDLE LOCALIZATION

Accurate needle localization requires the confident identification of the target lesion in two mammographic views obtained 90 degrees apart. If this prerequisite is not fulfilled, needle localization should not be attempted and further diagnostic mammography performed to exclude the possibility of a pseudodensity produced by the superimposition of benign breast tissue. The failure to confidently identify a suspicious abnormality in two views is probably the most common cause for failure of the needle localization procedure. Various triangulation and parallax techniques have been used to localize those rare lesions that are seen in only one view. Occasionally, ultrasound or CT guidance may be needed to resolve the location of a particularly difficult and elusive abnormality.

Dermal calcifications in the breast are common, and these can be projected so they apparently lie within the deep tissues of the breast. Unless specific tangential views are obtained to demonstrate their true location, needle localization of dermal calcifications will frequently be unsuccessful.

Both rigid needles and hook wires can migrate from their original position or be inadvertently dislodged during preparation of the skin of the breast prior to surgery. There have been rare reports of migration of localizing wires into the pectoralis muscle and occasionally more deeply into the mediastinum. On rare occasion, pneumothorax has been reported. If a fine hook wire is used, it can be inadvertently transected by the surgeon, who may then be unable to locate the two wire fragments. Wires left in the breast have migrated to remote locations in the soft tissues. Methylene blue has been reported to diffuse within the tissues of the breast if biopsy is delayed following a localization procedure. In our practice, a small amount of Xylocaine with epinephrine is mixed with the methylene blue, which both renders the injection painless and prevents the diffusion of blue dye within breast tissue.

RADIOGRAPHY OF THE EXCISED SPECIMEN

Confirmation that the mammographically identified suspicious abnormality is contained within the biopsy specimen is of vital importance. Radiography of the excised specimen can be performed in the mammography department using diagnostic mammographic equipment or, alternatively, in the surgical suite or pathology department using dedicated specimen radiography units. In either instance, the preoperative mammograms must be available for comparison with the specimen radiograph. Unless a mammographically identified, clinically nonpalpable mass is palpable at operation, specimen radiography is necessary, whether the biopsy was prompted by calcifications, architectural abnormalities, or a mass that remains nonpalpable at surgery.

The diagnostic quality of the specimen radiograph should exceed that of the preoperative mammogram, because the tissue is thinner and no motion unsharpness is present. Some form of compression of the excised specimen should be used to optimize the detectability of masses and architectural changes. Efforts should be made to image the specimen in at least two projections in order to accurately localize the excised lesion with respect to the margin of the operative specimen. If mammographically suspicious calcifications are determined to extend to the margin of the excised specimen, the surgeon should be instructed to reexcise tissue so that a complete excision of the lesion is accomplished.

FIGURE 4 *(opposite page).* A, 25-gauge needle in place after methylene blue injection is taped securely to the skin and bent 90 degrees at the skin surface to prevent migration or dislodgement. This rigid needle is easily palpable within the breast tissue and guides the surgeon to the methylene blue deposit (B) at the site of this nonpalpable, 9-mm infiltrating carcinoma.

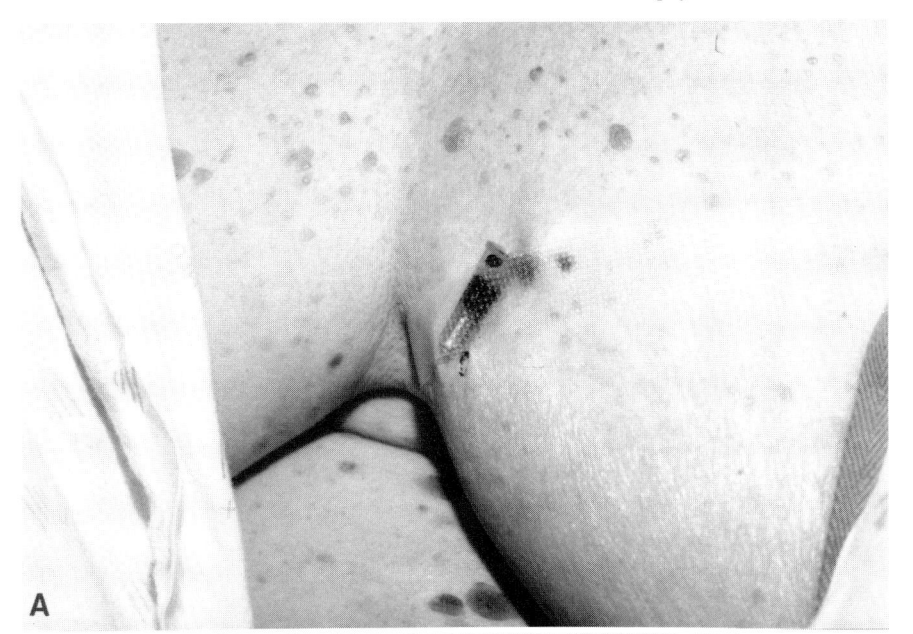

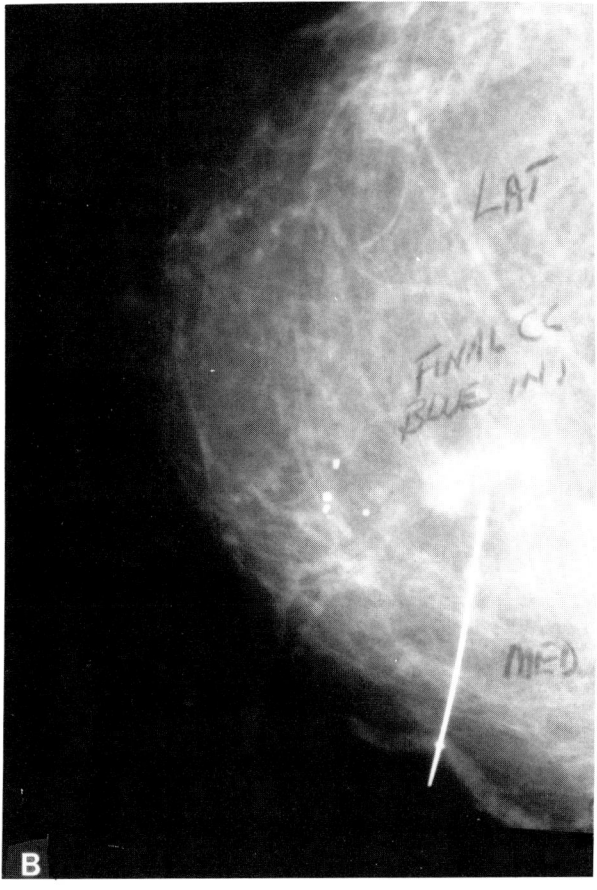

Needle Localization Guided Excisional Biopsy

SUMMARY AND CONCLUSIONS

The capability of high-quality mammography to discover early, preclinical breast cancer has demanded the development of a new relationship between radiologists, surgeons, and pathologists. It is only through mutual understanding and appreciation of the technical requirements and interpretive difficulties involved in the successful identification, preoperative localization, and excision of these lesions that the full benefits of this method of early cancer detection can be brought to all of our patients.

References

1. Gisvold JJ, Martin JK: Prebiopsy localization of nonpalpable breast lesions. Am J Roentgenol 143:477, 1984.
2. Kopans DB, Swann CA: Preoperative imaging-guided needle placement and localization of clinically occult breast lesions. Am J Roentgenol 152:1, 1989.
3. Margolin FR, Lagios MD: Development of mammography and breast services in a community hospital. Rad Clin North Am 25:973, 1987.
4. Meyer JE, Kopans DB, Stomper PC, et al: Occult breast abnormalities: Percutaneous preoperative needle localization. Radiology 150:335, 1984.
5. Rosenberg AL, Schwartz GF, Feig SA, et al: Clinically occult breast lesions: Localization and significance. Radiology 162:167, 1987.
6. Sickles EA: Mammographic detectability of breast microcalcifications. Am J Roentgenol 139:913, 1982.
7. Sickles EA: Mammographic features of 300 consecutive nonpalpable breast cancers. Am J Roentgenol 146:661, 1986.
8. Stemper PC, Davis SP, Weidner N, et al: Clinically occult, noncalcified breast cancer: Serial radiologic-pathologic correlation in 27 cases. Radiology 169:621, 1988.

Impact of Mammographic Screening on the Size and the Relative Frequency of Invasion in Breast Cancers Seen in a Community Hospital from 1975–1988

JAMES L. BENNINGTON, M.D.
MICHAEL D. LAGIOS, M.D.
FREDERICK R. MARGOLIN, M.D.

From the Department of
 Anatomic Pathology and
 Clinical Laboratories and
The Department of Radiology
California Pacific Medical
 Center, California Campus
San Francisco, California

Reprint requests to:
James L. Bennington, M.D.
Department of Anatomic
 Pathology and Clinical
 Laboratories
California Pacific Medical
 Center, California Campus
P.O. Box 3805
San Francisco, CA 94119

In a number of large, closed population studies, mammographic screening has been shown to reduce mortality from breast cancer.[1-4] Although this favorable outcome logically has been assumed to result from earlier detection of breast cancers than is possible by physical examination alone, very little has been published on the effects of mammographic screening, as measured in terms of the size and the relative frequencies of in situ and invasive breast cancers detected. We are aware of only one study where the morphology of breast cancers detected in a mammographically screened population was compared with that detected in an unscreened population.[5]

This report documents a significant reduction in the average size of invasive breast cancers and an increase in the frequency of in situ, relative to invasive, breast cancers observed at California Pacific Medical Center, California Campus (CPMC) during the years following the introduction of routine screening mammography in 1975.

MATERIALS AND METHODS

The adoption of a mammographic screening program at CPMC began with the testing of the diagnostic potential of this technique by the Department of Radiology in 1974. By 1975, the utility of mammography for the detection of occult breast cancers was confirmed and the technique put into routine use.

Subsequently, a monthly radiology-pathology conference was instituted for the correlation of pathologic and mammographic findings on breast specimens obtained from mammographically directed biopsies. To support this ongoing review program, Lagios et al.[6] developed a detailed protocol for the examination and documentation of pathologic findings on all breast biopsies and mastectomy specimens received in our department of pathology (see *"Protocol for the pathologic examination and tissue processing of the mammographically directed breast biopsy,"* this issue).

The data collected according to this protocol have provided the basis for a number of studies on various aspects of the pathology of breast cancer as reported by Lagios et al.[7-12] However, a detailed analysis of the impact of mammographic screening on the number, size, and frequency of in situ and invasive breast cancers at CPMC has not been published prior to this report.

RESULTS

During the 15 years from 1974 (1 year before mammography was introduced as a routine screening procedure) to 1988, a total of 1,746 breast cancers were processed in the department of pathology at CPMC. Of these, 1,281 were invasive and 465 were in situ. For this period, a breakdown of the numbers into in situ and invasive cancers is available for each year (Fig. 1). A further breakdown of the numbers of invasive cancers by histologic types and numbers of in situ cancers into duct (DCIS) and lobular (LCIS) is available for the years 1976 to 1988. During the period from 1976 to 1988, 1,546 breast cancers were examined. Of these, 1,099 (71%) were invasive (998 duct, 111 lobular), and 447 (29%) were in situ (349 DCIS and 98 LCIS).

The maximum diameter of each invasive breast cancer was recorded routinely as part of the pathologic examination, beginning in 1975. A plot of the average tumor diameter for each year from 1975 through 1988 is shown in Figure 2.

Impact of Mammography on the Numbers of Breast Cancers Treated Surgically at CPMC

The annual numbers of breast cancers treated surgically at CPMC nearly tripled during the 14-year period from 1974 to 1988 (Fig. 1). A portion of the volume growth resulted from expansion of the surgical service; however, most of the volume growth was due to increased numbers of in situ and small, clinically occult, invasive cancers, biopsied as a result of detection by mammography (Fig. 3).

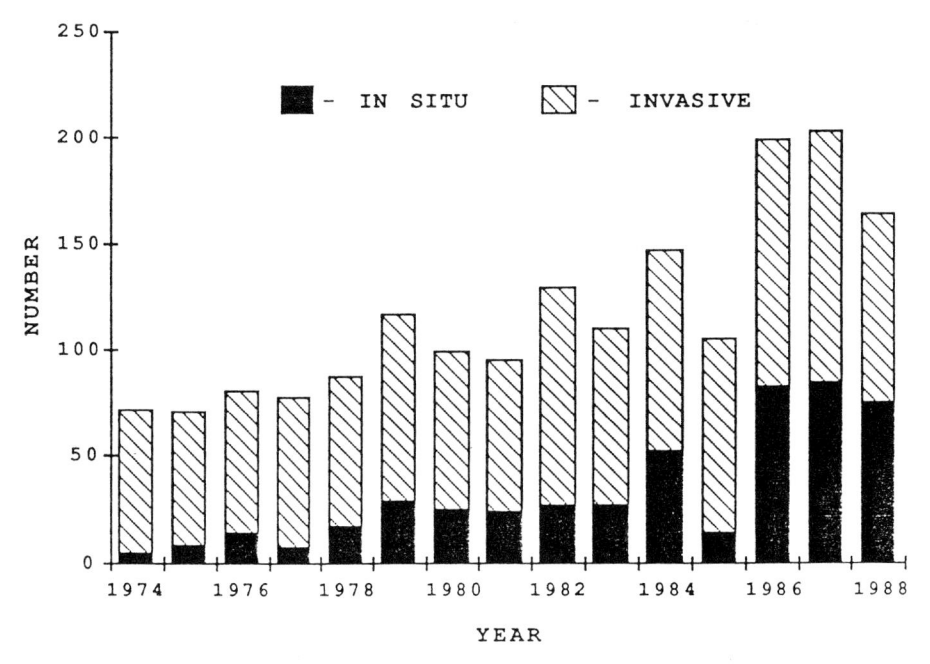

FIGURE 1. Annual numbers of in situ and invasive breast cancers at CPMC for the years 1974–1988.

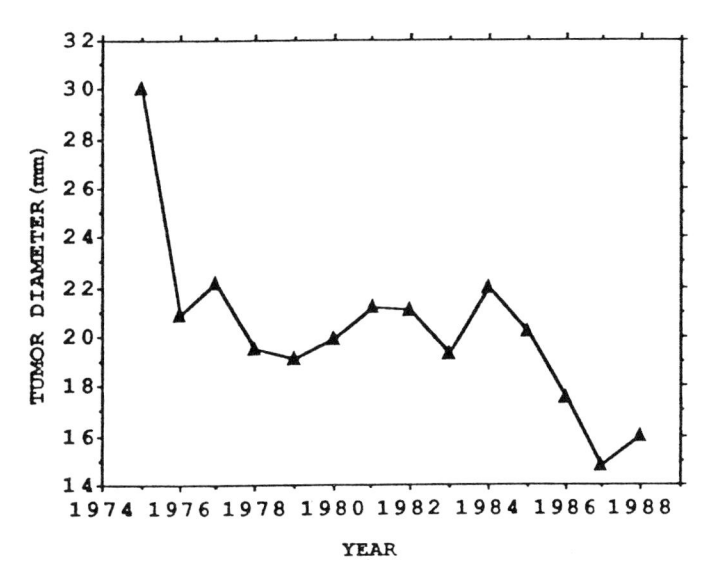

FIGURE 2. CPMC annual mean diameter of all invasive breast cancers combined (1975–1988).

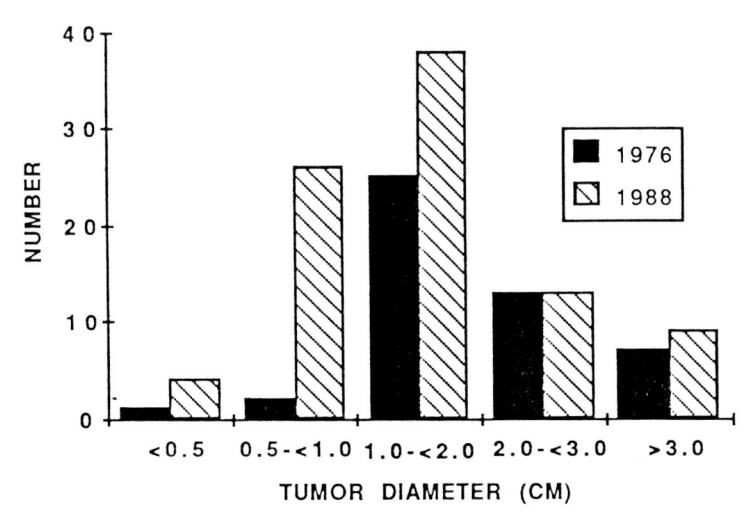

FIGURE 3. Numbers of invasive breast cancers, by size, at CPMC for the years 1976 and 1988.

Impact of Mammography on the Relative Frequencies of In Situ and Invasive Breast Cancers

Although mammography was originally developed as a means of finding asymptomatic invasive breast cancers, the majority of the clinically silent breast cancers detected with its use are in situ rather than invasive. The percentage of all breast cancers diagnosed at CPMC that were in situ increased from 4% in 1974, to a 10-year average of 22% (1976-1985), then increased again with the introduction of high-resolution mammographic film to 45% during the last 3 years covered by this report ((1985-1988); an overall tenfold increase (Fig. 4).

During the period 1975 to 1988 in which mammographic screening has been in use at CPMC, the overall percentages of in situ breast cancers detected were: duct carcinoma in situ (DCIS), 78%; and lobular carcinoma in situ (LCIS), 22%. The year-to-year variation in the relative frequencies of these two histologic types of in situ breast cancers appears to be random. The percentages ranged from: 92.3% DCIS and 7.7% LCIS, to 52.2% DCIS and 47.8% LCIS. No pattern was seen in the percentage distribution of the two types of in situ breast cancer in relation to experience with the use of mammography.

Impact of Mammography on the Average Size of Invasive Breast Cancers Treated Surgically

During the last 6 months of 1975, prior to any substantial impact of mammography on the size of invasive breast cancers, the average diameter of invasive breast cancers detected at CPMC was 30 mm (Fig. 1). Other authors[13,15] have published similar figures.

Impact of Mammographic Screening in a Community Hospital, 1975–1988   15

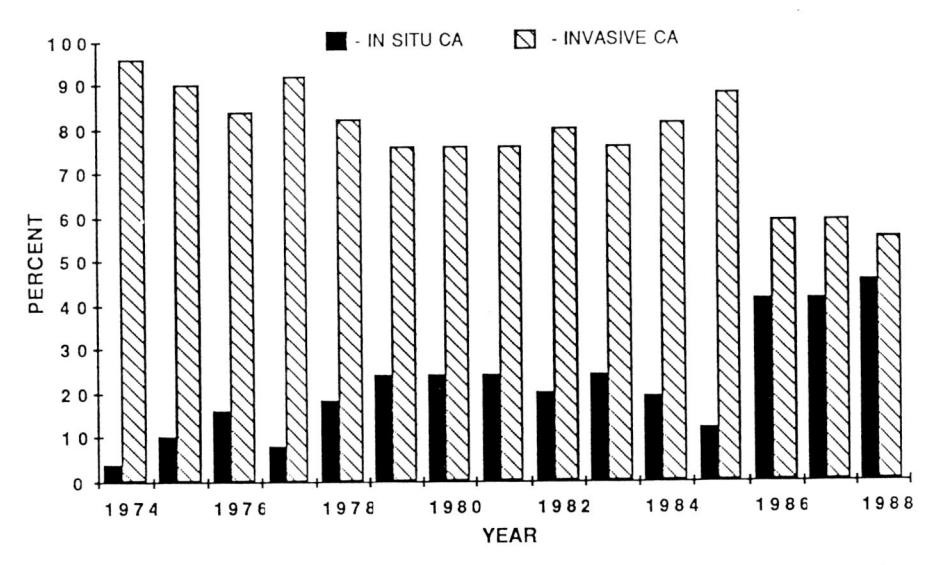

FIGURE 4. Annual percent of in situ and invasive breast cancers at CPMC for the years 1974–1988.

In 1976, the first full year after screening mammography was put into routine use, the average diameter of invasive breast cancers at CPMC fell from 30 mm to 21 mm, and with slight year-to-year variation remained at that level until 1985 (Fig. 1). After high-resolution mammographic film became available, the average diameter of invasive breast cancers fell further, reaching a low of 14.8 mm in 1987 (Fig. 1).

The contribution of mammography to reducing the average diameter of invasive breast cancers in a screened population is largely limited to duct carcinomas. Invasive lobular carcinomas, in contrast to invasive duct carcinomas, are usually not associated with microcalcifications and therefore are not likely to be detected by mammography.

There were 11 invasive lobular carcinomas removed surgically at CPMC from 1975 to 1988. The majority were not detected by mammography, and many were relatively large by the time they were discovered clinically. As would be expected, a plot of invasive lobular carcinoma diameters for the years 1975 to 1988 reveals no apparent trend of change in tumor size (Fig. 5).

Although mammography does not appear to influence the size of invasive lobular carcinomas, it does have a substantial impact on the size of invasive duct carcinomas detected in a heavily screened population. This is fortunate, because duct carcinomas represent the vast majority of all invasive breast cancers; approximately 90% in our hospital. A plot of the average diameters of invasive duct carcinomas seen at CPMC for the years 1976 to 1988 (Fig. 6) reveals a progressive reduction in tumor size following the introduction of mammography. This downward trend in tumor size is much more pronounced than it is for all invasive breast cancers combined, where data for invasive lobular carcinomas are included (Fig. 6).

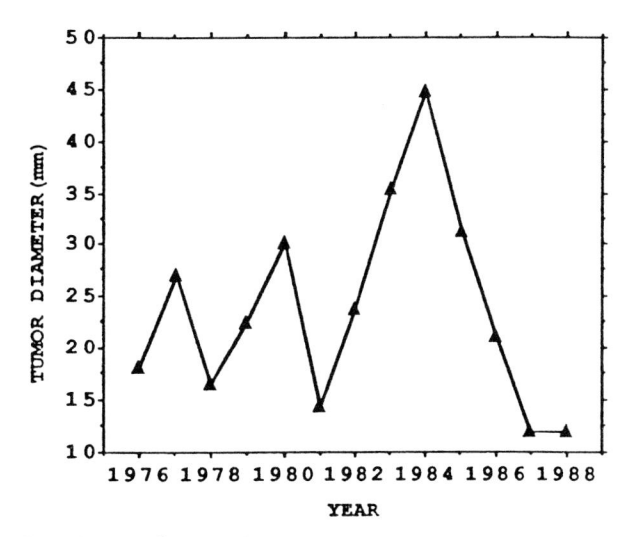

FIGURE 5. CPMC annual mean diameter of invasive lobular breast cancers (1976–1988).

DISCUSSION

Impact of Mammographic Screening on Patient Outcome

Large-scale longitudinal studies on closed patient populations in the United States, Great Britain, and Scandinavia have demonstrated that routine screening mammography is effective in reducing the mortality of women from invasive breast cancer by as much as 20–30%.[1-4] The benefits of mammography measured in terms of a reduction in mortality are derived from the early detection of occult breast cancers. The theoretical advantages of such early diagnosis are that: (1) in situ duct carcinomas can be removed before they became invasive, and (2) invasive breast cancers can be removed before reaching a size where there is a substantial risk of metastasis.

Removal of In Situ Cancer

Trying to assess the impact of early detection and removal of in situ breast cancers is both complicated and somewhat conjectural. On the surface, it would seem obvious that a cancer detected and completely excised while in the in situ stage is a cancer that cannot become invasive. This is usually, but not always, the case for duct carcinomas in situ and is generally not the case for lobular carcinomas in situ.

Lobular Carcinoma In Situ. LCIS, which represents approximately 10% of the in situ breast cancers found in our series, is thought to be only a marker for increased risk of subsequently developing an invasive breast cancer, not a precursor lesion. Both invasive duct and invasive lobular carcinomas occur with increased frequency in patients who have had a diagnosis of LCIS. The reported frequency of invasive cancer occurring after biopsy-proven LCIS ranges from 13.5 to 33%, approximately 1% per follow-up year.[16-19]

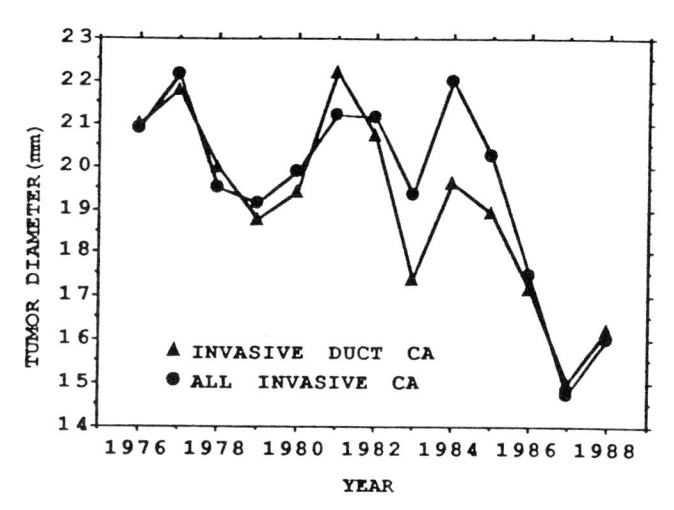

FIGURE 6. CPMC annual mean diameters of invasive breast cancers (1976–1988).

Rosen[16] found that the relative frequencies of the histologic types of invasive cancers arising following a biopsy-proven diagnosis of LCIS were: Invasive lobular (29%), mixed invasive lobular and duct (13%), invasive duct (52%), and other (6%). The invasive cancer may arise in the same breast where the LCIS was found, in the opposite breast, or in both breasts. In Rosen's series of 31 patients with invasive breast cancer that developed after an initial diagnosis of LCIS, 39% occurred in the ipsilateral breast, 39% in the contralateral breast, and 22% in both breasts.[16]

The proper treatment for patient with biopsy-proven LCIS is a much debated but unresolved issue. For patients concerned about the increased risk of developing an invasive breast cancer, bilateral total mastectomy is an effective, albeit extreme, preventative. Excisional biopsy of the focus of LCIS is ineffective in preventing a subsequent invasive cancer. Unilateral total mastectomy would be expected to have the potential for preventing only 50% of subsequent invasive cancers.

Duct Carcinoma In Situ. Unlike LCIS, when a focus of biopsy-proven DCIS is not completely removed, an invasive cancer all too frequently develops. An invasive breast cancer that follows a diagnosis of DCIS is almost invariably a duct carcinoma, usually is found in the biopsied breast, generally near the original biopsy site, and presumably arises in residual DCIS. The overall risk of DCIS not verified by biopsy progressing to invasive duct carcinoma cannot be determined directly. However, data are available that permit estimates of the risk of DCIS progressing to invasive duct carcinoma when the DCIS has been biopsied but has not been completely excised.

With attempted complete excision of DCIS, the frequency of subsequent development of invasive duct carcinoma is substantially lower than it is for patients with incompletely excised DCIS discovered retrospectively who have had no additional treatment. The frequencies of invasive duct carcinoma arising after attempted complete excision of DCIS have been reported by Lagios as 5%[12] and by Fisher as 13.6%[20] (average of the two studies is 5.7%).

There are three well-documented studies on the frequency with which invasive duct carcinoma arises in patients who have had breast biopsies initially interpreted as benign and when DCIS was found on retrospective review of the original biopsy. The frequencies of subsequent development of invasive duct carcinoma in the absence of additional surgery or irradiation therapy among the patients in these three studies were reported as 10.7% by Eusebi et al.,[21] as 25% by Page,[22] and as 53% by Rosen.[16] The average on long-term follow-up for these three studies was 25.4%.

In addition to completeness of excision, the size of the DCIS component is the most important factor in determining the likelihood of subsequent development of invasive breast cancer. The risk of progression to invasion also appears to depend on the presence or absence of microinvasion, multicentricity, Paget's disease, and on the morphologic type (grade) of DCIS.[12] Lagios[12] found no recurrence among 36 patients who had a focus of DCIS less than 40 mm in diameter. However, invasive duct carcinomas subsequently occurred in 3 (18%) of 17 patients with a focus of DCIS greater than 40 mm. The patients with a DCIS less than 40 mm had lesions that were characterized by: a unicentric focus of DCIS, negative axillary lymph nodes, and absence of Paget's disease of the nipple. Only 1 of the 36 (3%) in situ duct cancers had occult invasion. In contrast, among the 17 patients with DCIS > 40 mm, there was occult invasion associated with the DCIS in 6 (35%), multicentricity in 14 (82%), Paget's disease in 5 (29%), and positive axillary lymph nodes in 1 (6%) patient.

If an invasive duct carcinoma subsequently arises in 25% of patients with DCIS when no treatment is received, and in only 6% of patients when complete surgical removal of the DCIS is attempted, then one can infer that at least 19% of the invasive duct carcinomas preceded by DCIS can be prevented. In 1988, there were 61 patients treated surgically for DCIS at CPMC. Based on the estimate that 19% of such patients are spared the subsequent development of an invasive duct carcinoma, one can surmise that the impact of complete surgical removal of DCIS from 61 patients at CPMC in 1988 prevented 12 cases of invasive duct carcinoma. This compares with 2 cases of invasive duct carcinoma prevented by mammographic detection and surgical removal of 12 DCIS in 1976.

The implication for those patients originally destined to develop an invasive duct carcinoma and whose invasion was prevented is that the additional medical costs of treatment, and the potential morbidity and mortality associated with invasive breast cancer, are avoided. We have made no attempt to translate these numbers into projections of patient survival, because such an exercise would be highly speculative.

Invasive Cancer

For patients with nonsystemic invasive breast cancer, primary tumor size is second in importance only to the patient's axillary lymph node status as a morphologic predictor of survival. Carter et al.[23] have shown that although tumor size shows a linear relation to the frequency of axillary lymph node metastases, tumor size and lymph node status are, nevertheless, important independent prognostic variables. In their study, patient survival declined with: (1) increasing tumor size, when the nodal status was held constant; and (2) increasing numbers of metastases to axillary lymph nodes, when tumor size was held constant.

Mammographic screening has substantially increased the numbers and reduced the average size of invasive breast cancers seen at CPMC (Fig. 3). The observed reduction in average tumor size is primarily due to an increase in the numbers of relatively small, preclinical cancers detected with mammography. However, there is also some evidence to suggest that long-term screening of our semi-closed patient population may have contributed to an absolute reduction in the number of larger invasive breast cancers in the population as well. A shift in the relative frequencies of invasive breast cancers of different size ranges from 1976 and 1988 is evident in the plot of the percent distribution of invasive breast cancers by size shown in Figure 7.

Whatever the mechanism producing the observed change in the percent distribution of tumor sizes, the results, in terms of patient survival, should be favorable. Using the survival figures reported by Carter et al.[23] for patients with invasive breast cancers of various size categories, the impact of reducing the size of invasive breast cancers in a population can be estimated. In Table 1, the numbers of invasive breast cancers by sizes seen at CPMC for the years 1976, and 1976 normalized to 1988, are compared to 1988. The relative increase in the frequency of small invasive breast cancers in 1988 compared to 1976 translates into increasing numbers of surviving patients. The calculated net effect of detecting relatively more small invasive breast cancers in 1988 than 1976 is a 6% increase in the numbers of patients surviving 10 years.

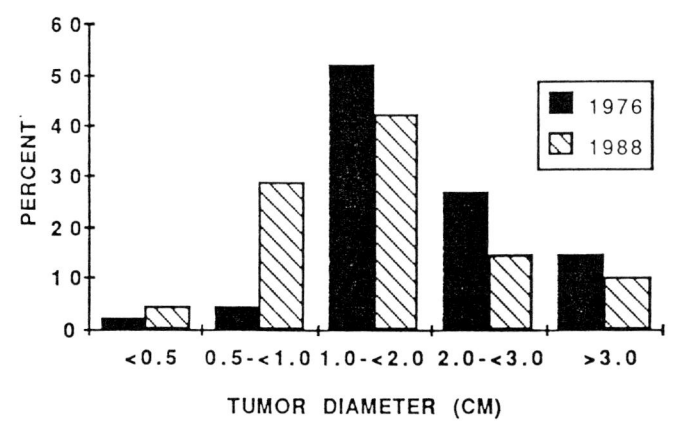

FIGURE 7. Percent distribution of invasive breast cancers, by size, at CPMC for the years 1976 and 1988.

The impact of mammography in terms of estimated improvement in the survival of patients with invasive breast cancer would be considerably more dramatic if detailed data on the sizes of invasive breast cancers seen at CPMC were available for the years prior to 1976 (before the introduction of mammographic screening). By 1976, which is the base year available to us for this comparison, relatively small invasive breast cancers were already being detected routinely by mammography in our hospital. Nevertheless, the comparison convincingly illustrates the potential for improving patient survival through mammographic detection of clinically silent, occult invasive breast cancers.

SUMMARY

At CPMC routine mammographic screening was introduced in late 1975. The total volume of breast cancers, other than outside consultations, seen in the department increased from 71 in 1975 to 164 by 1988, an increase of 230%. This expansion in volume was due largely to surgical removal of mammographically detected occult, in situ duct and relatively small invasive duct carcinomas.

In 1974, prior to routine mammographic screening, in situ carcinomas represented only 4% of all breast cancers seen in the Department of Pathology at CPMC. However, after the introduction of mammographic screening, the proportion of in situ cancers increased steadily. By 1988, 45% of all breast cancers seen in our hospital were found by mammography.

While data on the size distribution of invasive breast cancers are not available at our hospital prior to 1976, an appreciable effect of mammography is still evident when the numbers of relatively small invasive cancers detected in 1976 are compared with those detected in 1988. Invasive breast cancers 10 mm in diameter or less represented only 6% of all cancers in our series in 1976, but 33% in 1988. These findings confirm observations made by Gibbs[7] on the pathology of breast cancers found in mammographically screened and unscreened populations.

The detection of increasing numbers of relatively small invasive duct carcinomas produced an overall reduction in the average diameters of invasive cancers seen at CPMC. The average dropped from 30 mm in 1975 to a low of 14.8 mm in 1987. Mammography did not appear to be effective in the early detection of invasive lobular cancers and had no impact on reducing their size.

The implications of early discovery of in situ duct and relatively small invasive duct carcinomas are for improved patient survival through: (1) preventing progression of in situ duct to invasive duct cancers, and (2) the removal of invasive duct cancers before reaching a size where there is a high risk of metastasis.

References

1. Shapiro S, Venet W, Strax P, et al: Ten to fourteen-year effect of screening on breast cancer mortality. J Natl Cancer Inst 69:349-355, 1982.
2. UK Trial of Early Detection of Breast Cancer Group: First results on mortality reduction in the UK trial of early detection of breast cancer. Lancet ii:411-416, 1988.
3. Tabar L, Gad A, Holmberg LH, et al: Reduction in mortality from breast cancer after mass screening with mammography. Randomized trial from the British Cancer Screening Working Group of the Swedish National Board of Health and Welfare. Lancet i:829-832, 1985.
4. Anderson I, Aspergren R, Janzon L, et al: Mammographic screening and mortality from breast cancer: The Malmo mammographic screening trial. Br Med J 297:943-948, 1988.
5. Gibbs NM: Comparative study of the histopathology of breast cancer in a screened and unscreened population investigated by mammography. Histopathology 9:1307-1318, 1985.
6. Lagios MD: Multicentricity of breast carcinoma demonstrated by routine correlated serial subgross and radiographic examination. Cancer 40:1726-1734, 1977.
7. Lagios MD, Gates EA, Westdahl PR, et al: A guide to the frequency of nipple involvement in breast cancer based on a study of 149 consecutive mastectomies studied in serial subgross and correlated radiographic technique. Am J Surg 138:135-142, 1979.
8. Lagios MD, Rose MR, Margolin FR: Tubular carcinoma of the breast. Association with multicentricity, bilaterality and family history of breast carcinoma. Am J Clin Pathol 73:25-30, 1980.
9. Lagios MD, Westdahl PR, Margolin FR, Rose MR: Duct carcinoma in situ. Relationship of extent of noninvasive disease to the frequency of occult invasion, multicentricity, lymph node metastases, and short term treatment failures. Cancer 50:1309-1314, 1982.
10. Lagios MD: Human breast precancer: Current status. Cancer Surveys 2:383-401, 1983.
11. Margolin FR, Lagios MD: Mammographic detection of early breast cancer. Ten year experience in a community hospital. West J Med 144:46-48, 1986.
12. Lagios MD, Margolin FR, Westdahl PR, Rose MR: Mammmographically detected duct carcinoma in situ. Frequency of local recurrence following tylectomy and prognostic effect of nuclear grade on local recurrence. Cancer 63:618-624, 1989.
13. Kern WH, Mikkelsen WP: Small carcinomas of the breast. Cancer 28:948-955, 1971.
14. Baak JPA, van Dop H, Kurver HJ, Hermans J: The value of morphometry to classic prognosticators in breast cancer. Cancer 56:374-382, 1985.
15. Say CC, Donegan WL: Invasive carcinoma of the breast: Prognostic significance of tumor size and involved axillary lymph nodes. Cancer 34:468-471, 1974.
16. Rosen PP, Lieberman PH, Braun DW, et al: Lobular carcinoma in situ of the breast. Detailed analysis of 99 patients with average follow-up of 24 years. Am J Surg Pathol 2:225-251, 1978.
17. Haagensen CD, Lane N, Lattes R, Bodian C: Lobular neoplasia (so-called lobular carcinoma in situ) of the breast. Cancer 42:737-769, 1978.
18. Hutter RVT, Foote FW Jr: Lobular carcinoma in situ. Long-term follow-up. Cancer 24:1081-1085, 1969.
19. Wheeler JE, Enterline HT, Roseman JM, et al: Lobular carcinoma in situ of the breast. Long-term follow-up. Cancer 34:554-563, 1974.
20. Fisher ER, Sass R, Fisher B, Wickerham, et al: Pathologic findings from the National Surgical Adjuvant Breast Project (Protocol G): I. Intraductal carcinoma (DCIS). Cancer 57:197-208, 1986.
21. Eusebi V, Fosehini MP, Cook MG, et al: Long-term follow-up of in situ carcinoma of the breast with special emphasis on clinging carcinoma. Semin Diag Pathol 6:165-173, 1989.
22. Page DL, Dupont WD, Rogers LW, et al: Intraductal carcinoma of the breast: Follow-up after biopsy only. Cancer 49:751-758, 1982.
23. Carter CL, Allen C, Henson DE: Relation of tumor size, lymph node status, and survival in 24,740 breast cancer cases. Cancer 63:181-187, 1989.

Protocol for the Pathologic Examination and Tissue Processing of the Mammographically Directed Breast Biopsy

MICHAEL D. LAGIOS, M.D.
JAMES L. BENNINGTON, M.D.

From the Department of
  Anatomic Pathology and
  Clinical Laboratories
California Pacific Medical
  Center, California Campus
San Francisco, California

Reprint requests to:
Michael D. Lagios, M.D.
Department of Anatomic
  Pathology and Clinical
  Laboratories
California Pacific Medical
  Center, California Campus
P.O. Box 3805
San Francisco, CA 94119

Mammographic screening for "early" breast cancer has had a profound effect on reducing the size and stage of breast cancers now being detected in the United States,[1,2] United Kingdom,[3,4] and Scandinavia[5] (see also Bennington, et al, *"Impact of mammographic screening on the size and the relative frequency of invasion in breast cancers seen in a community hospital from 1975-1988,"* pp 11-21, this issue). Achieving the maximum yield of breast cancers detected by mammography has required certain changes in tissue handling and examination of the mammographically directed breast biopsy. This new radiographic technique, increased use of breast-conserving surgical approaches for the treatment of breast cancer, more enlightened and demanding patients, and increasing medical-legal exposure have all contributed to changes in the way surgical pathologists process and sample breast biopsy specimens.

Many pathologists in practice today can recall the time 10 to 15 years ago when the biopsy of a breast lesion thought to be benign was sampled in one cassette, and when mastectomy specimens were routinely processed with as few as four slides—one representative section of the breast cancer, one section of the nipple, and one section of each axillary lymph node. Subsequently, a number of studies have shown the importance of systematic and extensive sampling of conventional breast biopsies and mastectomy specimens to establish the correct diagnosis, the size of any tumors, the presence or absence of multicentricity, and completeness of excision.[6-11] However, the adequacy of specimen sampling and examination is as important for the mammographically directed biopsy specimen as it is for the mastectomy specimen.

Proper pathologic examination of a mammographically directed biopsy should provide: (1) identification of the lesion or lesions present—both those associated with the mammographic abnormality and any incidental to it; (2) documentation of the completeness of excision or any atypical hyperplastic or neoplastic lesion present; and (3) an unambiguous record of the significant biopsy findings easily understood by other pathologists and therapists (oncologists, radiation therapists, etc.).

RECOMMENDED PROCEDURES FOR PATHOLOGIC EXAMINATION OF MAMMOGRAPHICALLY DIRECTED BREAST BIOPSIES

Mammographically directed breast biopsies are performed after stereotactic localization of radiographic abnormalities of the breast not associated with other clinical findings. These abnormalities may include: (1) focal areas of microcalcification identifiable by their specific number, distribution, and configuration in the mammogram (Fig. 1); (2) a soft tissue density or densities without accompanying microcalcifications (Fig. 2); and (3) microcalcifications associated with a soft tissue density (Fig. 3).

In our opinion, specimen radiography is best performed by the pathologist on dedicated radiographic equipment, ideally a self-contained x-ray unit, e.g., Faxitron or similar device. Such units have the advantage of being small enough to be housed in or near the operating theater. Access to a self-contained x-ray unit speeds up the intraoperative interpretation of the adequacy of the mammographically directed biopsy, and eliminates the inconvenience and personnel time involved in transporting biopsy specimens from Surgery to the Radiology Department for radiographic examination. It also helps to reduce disruption of the flow of patient studies in Radiology.

In our hospital, a Faxitron industrial x-ray unit and an automatic film developer are both available in the same dark room located within the surgical suite. This arrangement permits a pathologist to pick up a breast biopsy specimen in an operating room, talk to the surgeon, review the mammograms, leave the operating room to radiograph the specimen and develop the film, and then return to the operating room with the results of specimen radiography within less than 7 minutes.

Visualization of microcalcifications is generally enhanced in specimen radiograms as compared to preoperative mammograms, even magnification views. The majority of our specimen radiography is performed on automatic mode at KVPs of 18 to 25 with exposure times of 1.2 to 2.5 minutes. Some compression of thick specimens helps to enhance the image resolution and reduce artifacts related to uneven specimen thickness. Although a number of expensive devices have been developed for this purpose, we have found that sandwiching the specimen in a folded sheet of ordinary wax paper or plastic wrap accompanied by gentle pressure helps to flatten the specimen and reduce these artifacts substantially.

Interpretation of the Intraoperative Breast Biopsy Specimen Radiogram

Ideally intraoperative evaluation of the mammographically directed biopsy specimen is performed by the pathologist, who provides the surgeon with the following information intraoperatively:

- Whether or not the intraoperative specimen radiogram demonstrates the mammographically identified lesion, all or in part.
- Whether or not the intraoperative specimen radiogram permits assessment of the surgical margins of the biopsy specimen.
- Whether or not the biopsy has been removed in a manner that permits correlation of the intraoperative specimen radiogram with the preoperative mammogram, i.e., as an intact, well-oriented specimen rather than in multiple fragments.

Method of Correlation. In order to properly interpret the intraoperative specimen radiogram, the pathologist also must have immediately available the appropriate preoperative mammograms for side-by-side comparison. The needle localization procedure often produces an artifact on the localization film that masks small clusters of microcalcification or small soft tissue densities. Therefore, it is strongly recommended that during the intraoperative consultation the pathologist review the mammograms that initially prompted the biopsy as well as the films used for localization of the lesion.

Assessment of Localization. In addition to documenting the extent to which a mammographic lesion has been sampled, the pathologist should, in relation to specific mammographic findings, provide the following information:

Microcalcific lesions. Completeness of excision should be noted. If only a portion of the microcalcifications have been removed, the pathologist should urge the surgeon to sample more of the breast adjacent to the biopsy site (Fig. 4). The pathologist should also inform the surgeon when microcalcifications appear to lie at the edge of the specimen in the radiogram, suggesting an inadequate margin around the region marked by the microcalcifications (Fig. 5).

Soft tissue abnormalities. The size and the configuration of soft tissue lesions (e.g., circumscribed, stellate, irregular contour, cystic) should be noted. Specimen radiography may provide an immediate definitive diagnosis (e.g., cyst, fibroadenoma, papilloma, etc.) or it may only document that the lesion seen on the preoperative mammogram has been partially or incompletely sampled.

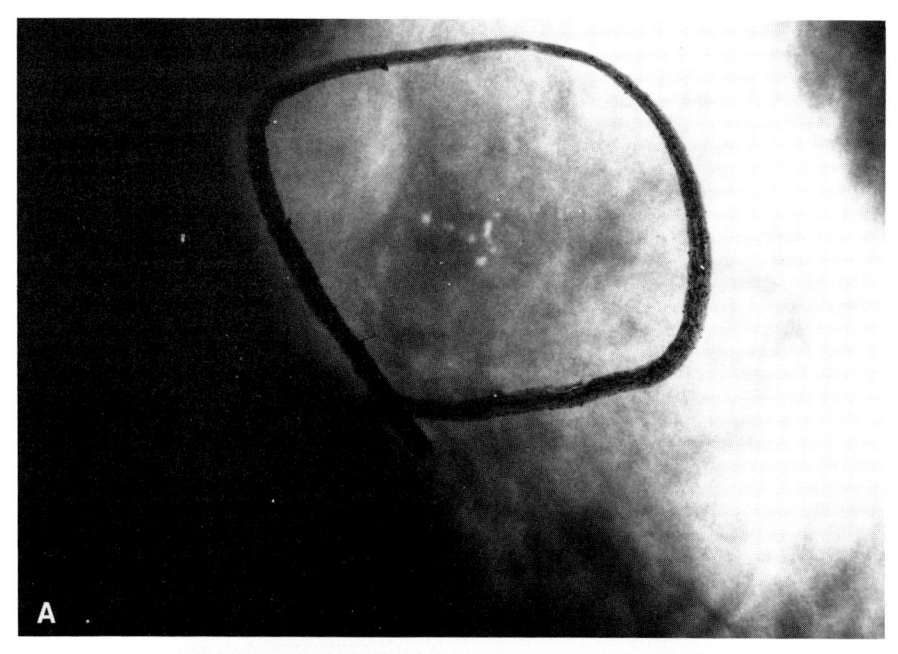

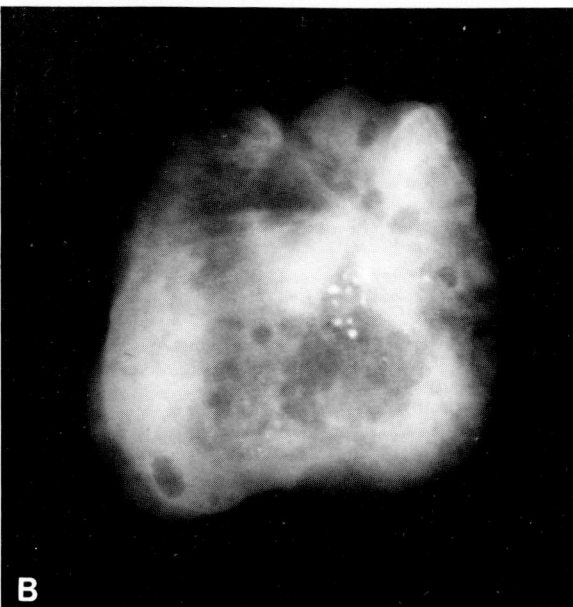

FIGURE 1. *A*, Preoperative mammogram from a 54-year-old woman containing a solitary cluster of suspicious microcalcifications that prompted breast biopsy. *B*, The same distinctive cluster of microcalcifications present in the preoperative mammogram also is seen in the specimen radiogram. No microcalcifications were present at the surgical margins of the biopsy. *(Figure continued on opposite page.)*

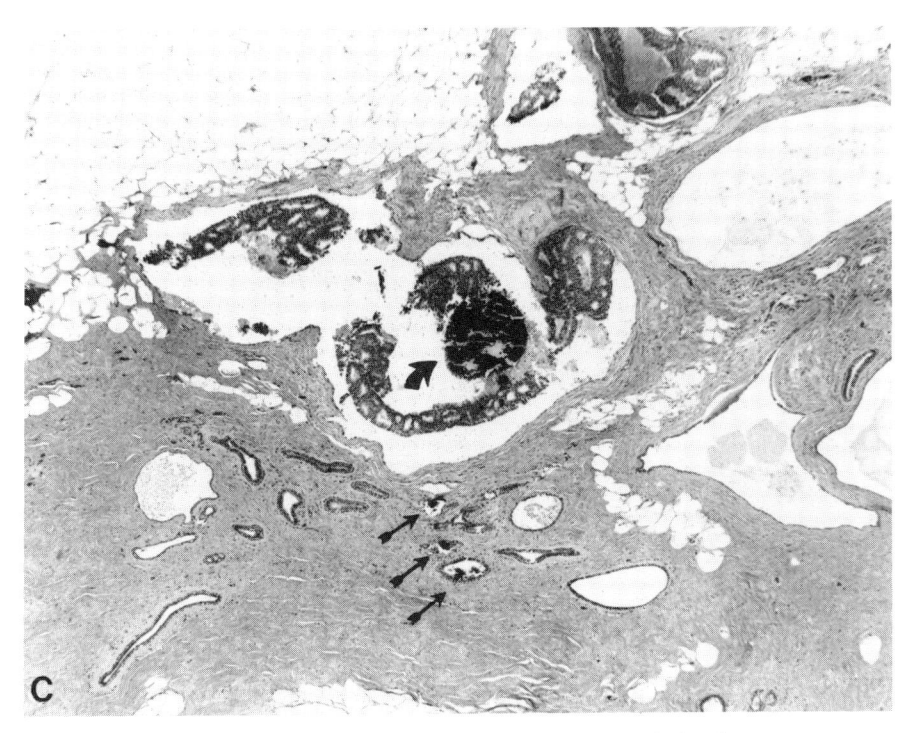

FIGURE 1 *(Continued).* C, Low-power photomicrograph of the biopsy specimen demonstrating coarse microcalcifications in intraluminal necrotic debris of duct carcinoma in situ (large arrow), and fine microcalcifications in tubular lumens in an adjacent focus of adenosis (small arrows).

Documenting the Pathologist's Interpretation of the Intraoperative Specimen Radiogram. The pathologist should document the significant findings of the intraoperative consultation in the patient's chart or on the pathology report, just as one would the results of a frozen section. This description should include:

- A statement describing the *preoperative mammogram(s)*. This should include a description of any microcalcifications and/or soft tissue density and the approximate size of the lesion. For example: *The mammogram contains a soft tissue density 11 mm in maximum dimension with irregular borders.*
- A statement describing the *specimen radiogram(s)*. This should include a description of the presence or absence of microcalcifications and/or soft tissue density, the approximate size and configuration of the lesion seen in the radiogram, and the adequacy of removal. It should also include the pathologist's interpretation. For example: *The specimen radiogram contains a soft tissue density 11 mm in maximum diameter that is identical with the density seen in the preoperative mammogram. The soft tissue density appears completely excised.*

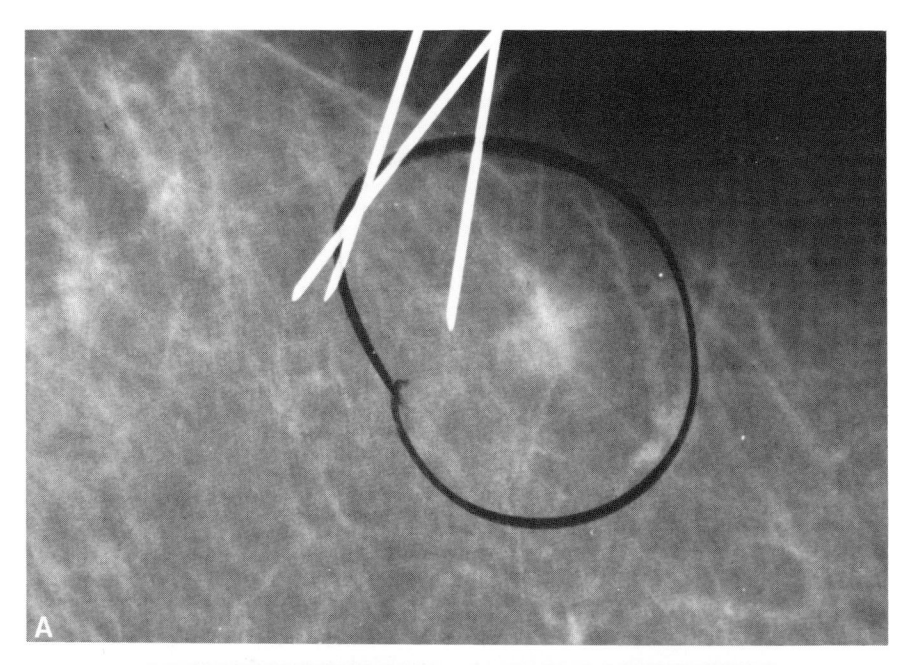

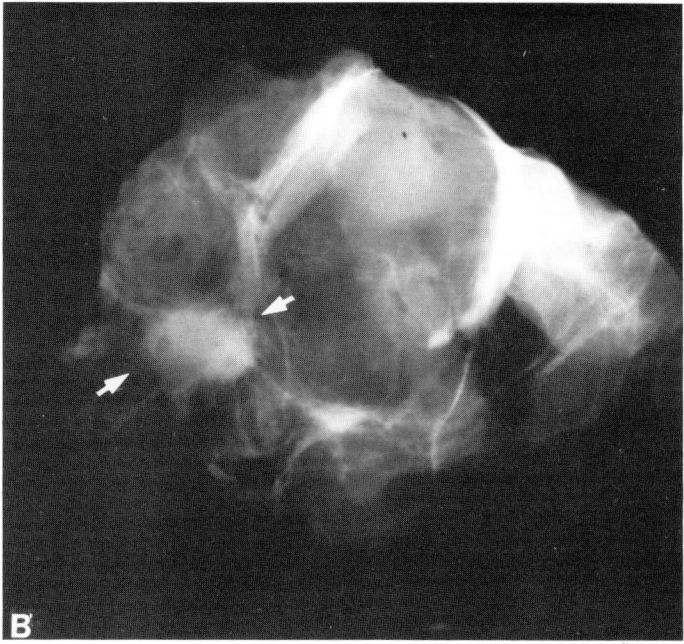

FIGURE 2. *A*, Needle localization film of a soft-tissue density with no associated microcalcifications obtained on a 65-year-old woman. *B*, The specimen radiogram of the breast biopsy demonstrates a well-circumscribed soft tissue density (arrows) situated at one margin of the surgical specimen. *(Figure continued on opposite page.)*

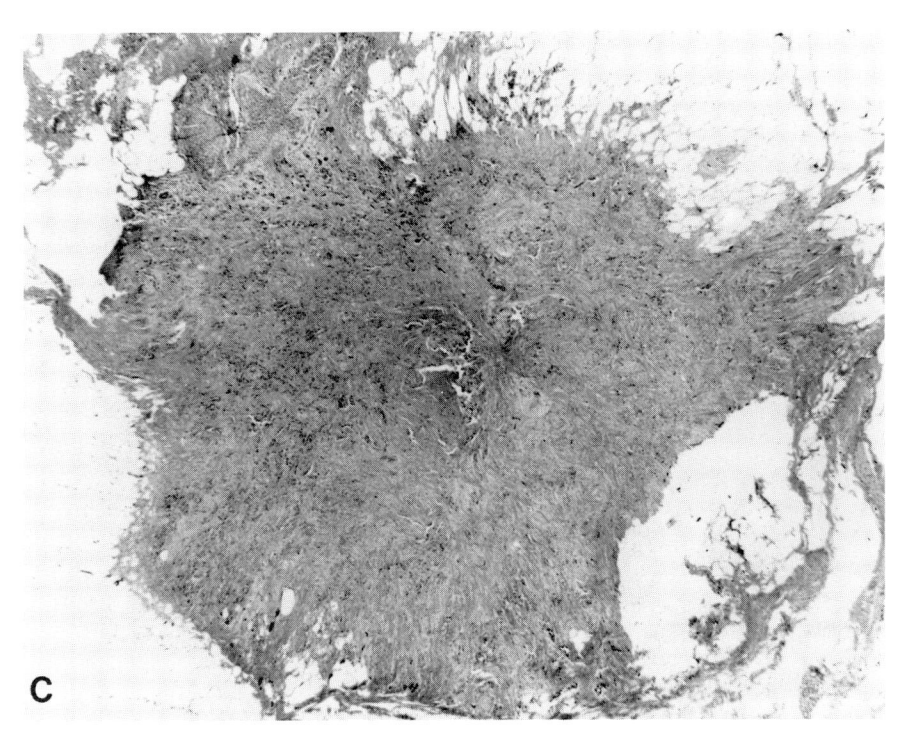

FIGURE 2 *(Continued).* C, Low-power photomicrograph of the lesion that produced the soft-tissue density. The tumor was a 5-mm infiltrating duct carcinoma with marked desmoplasia.

Frozen Section Examination

The pathologist may elect to perform a frozen section on a palpable mass if the mammographically directed biopsy specimen is sufficiently large that permanent section diagnosis will not be compromised by the study, and if the information obtained will be used to make an immediate therapeutic decision. Frozen section of biopsies containing nonpalpable foci of microcalcifications is never appropriate, since small foci of in situ or microinvasive carcinoma may be lost or distorted in the processing. Furthermore, freeze artifact in the remainder of the tissue used for frozen section may limit subsequent interpretation.

Specimen Sampling for Steroid Hormone Receptor Assay

Random sampling of a breast biopsy for estrogen receptor assay without an established diagnosis of invasive breast carcinoma is also inappropriate. Such sampling may severely limit the ability of the pathologist to establish a diagnosis of in situ or microinvasive carcinoma (Fig. 6). Estrogen and progesterone receptor protein levels in in situ breast cancer have not been shown to have diagnostic or prognostic utility. Most in situ breast cancers are

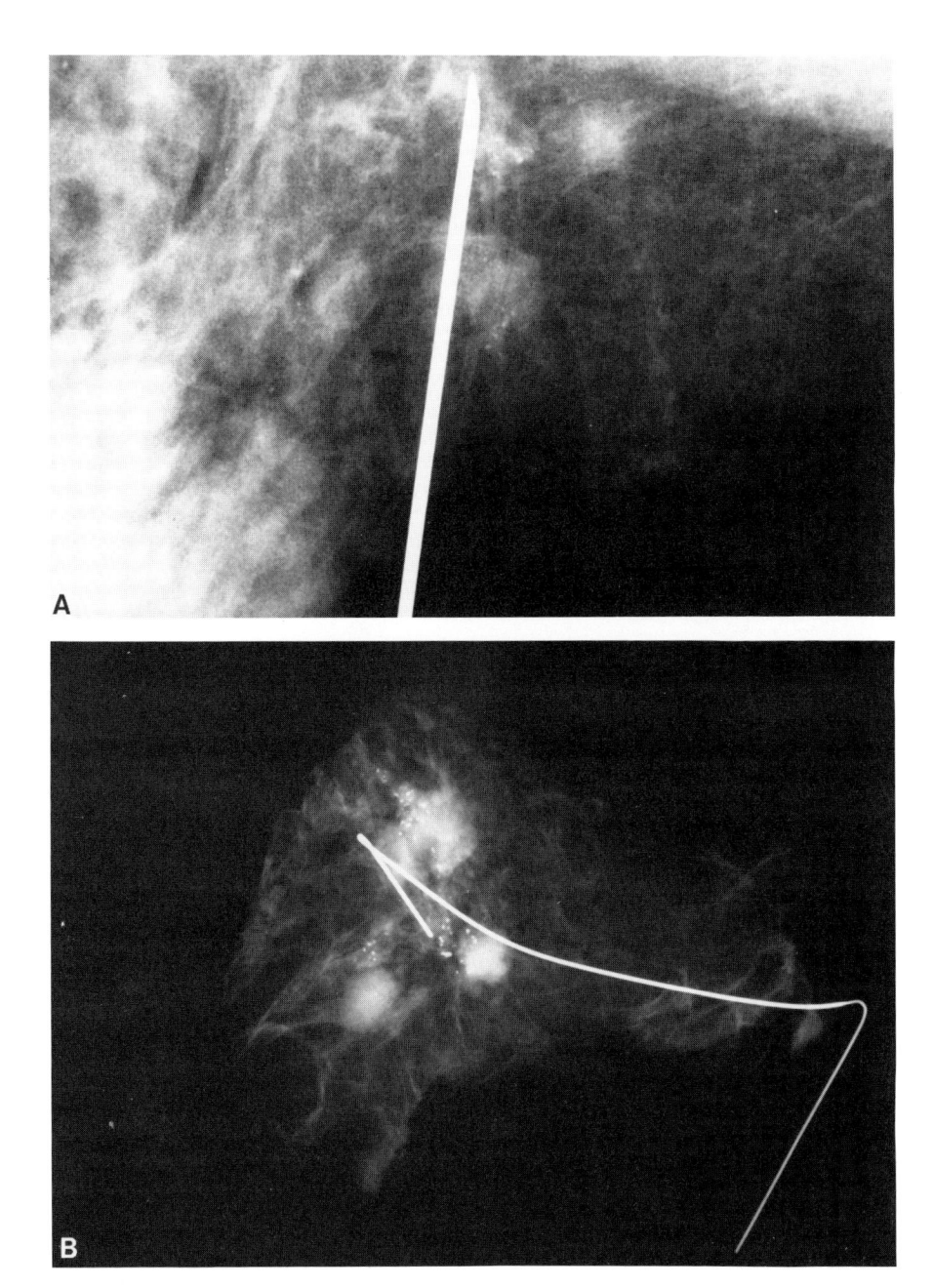

FIGURE 3. *A,* Needle localization film from a 77-year-old woman with three distinct soft-tissue breast densities, each associated with multiple microcalcifications. *B,* Specimen radiogram of the mammographically directed biopsy documenting removal of the three soft-tissue densities and the microcalcifications identified in the preoperative mammogram. *(Figure continued on opposite page.)*

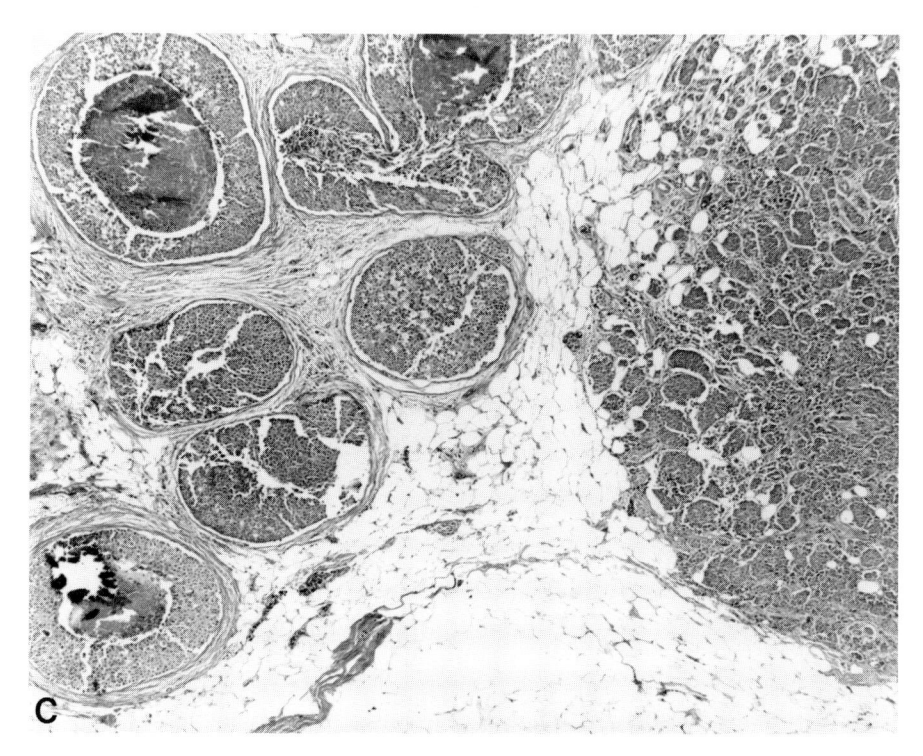

FIGURE 3 *(Continued).* C, Low-power photomicrograph of a focus of invasive duct carcinoma corresponding to one of the soft-tissue densities seen in the radiograms. Microcalcifications are present in an adjacent focus of in situ duct carcinoma.

microscopic and sparsely cellular, and as such cannot provide sufficient tumor for steroid hormone receptor assay.

Processing the Specimen

Sampling. Processing of the biopsy depends on the mammographic as well as the gross pathologic features of the specimen at the time of examination. In our opinion, all mammographically directed biopsies should be completely embedded for microscopic examination.

After the pathologist has completed the evaluation of the specimen radiogram, the surgical margins should be inked. If there is a palpable nodule, it should be incised. If the lesion is an invasive carcinoma at least 10 mm in greatest diameter, a portion of the tumor should be snap frozen and reserved in liquid nitrogen for steroid hormone receptor assay. The remaining biopsy material should be processed in the same manner as any clinically detected invasive carcinomas, with special attention paid to the completeness of excision of the tumor.

Fixation. Although many types of fixation are suitable for breast tissue, we have found that a 15% formalin/alcohol fixative has a number of specific advantages over standard neutral buffered formalin. Most mammographically

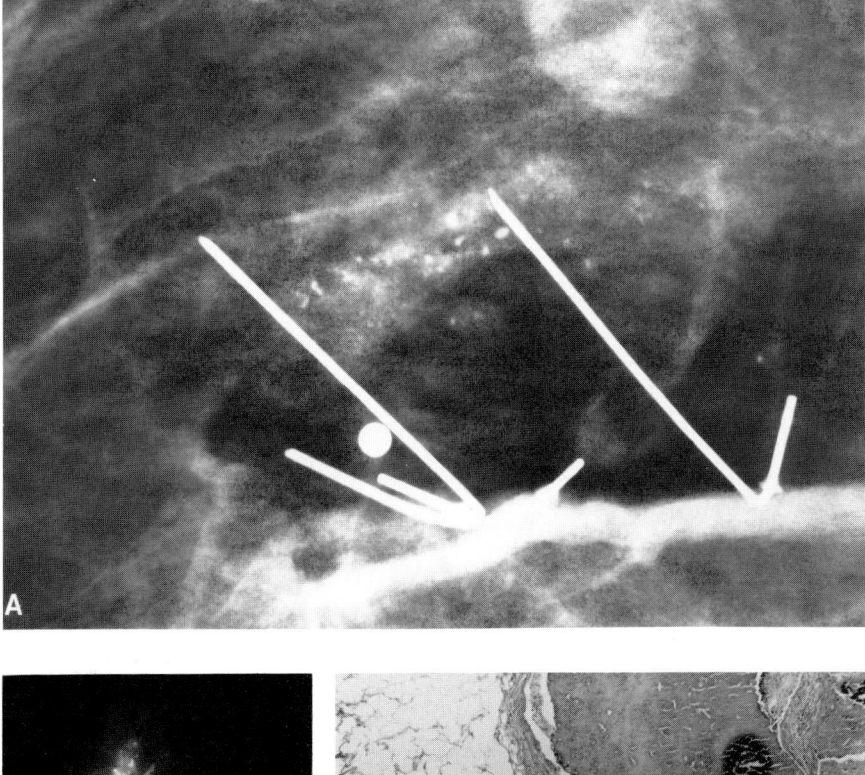

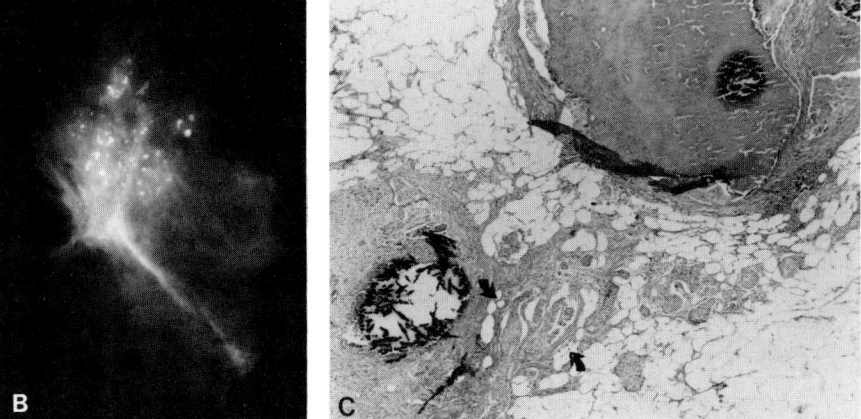

FIGURE 4. *A,* Needle localization film from a 65-year-old woman demonstrating multiple fine and coarse microcalcifications of the breast distributed over an area 12 × 35 mm. *B,* The majority of the microcalcifications seen in the mammogram are demonstrated by the specimen radiogram. *C,* Photomicrograph of duct carcinoma in situ with small focus of invasion (arrows) identified in the mammographically directed biopsy. *D (opposite page),* Radiogram of two segments from the subsequent mastectomy specimen. Residual microcalcifications (arrow) are present at the margin of the biopsy cavity. *E,* Residual invasive duct carcinoma found in the edge of the biopsy cavity in the mastectomy specimen. The lumen of the biopsy cavity is indicated by arrows.

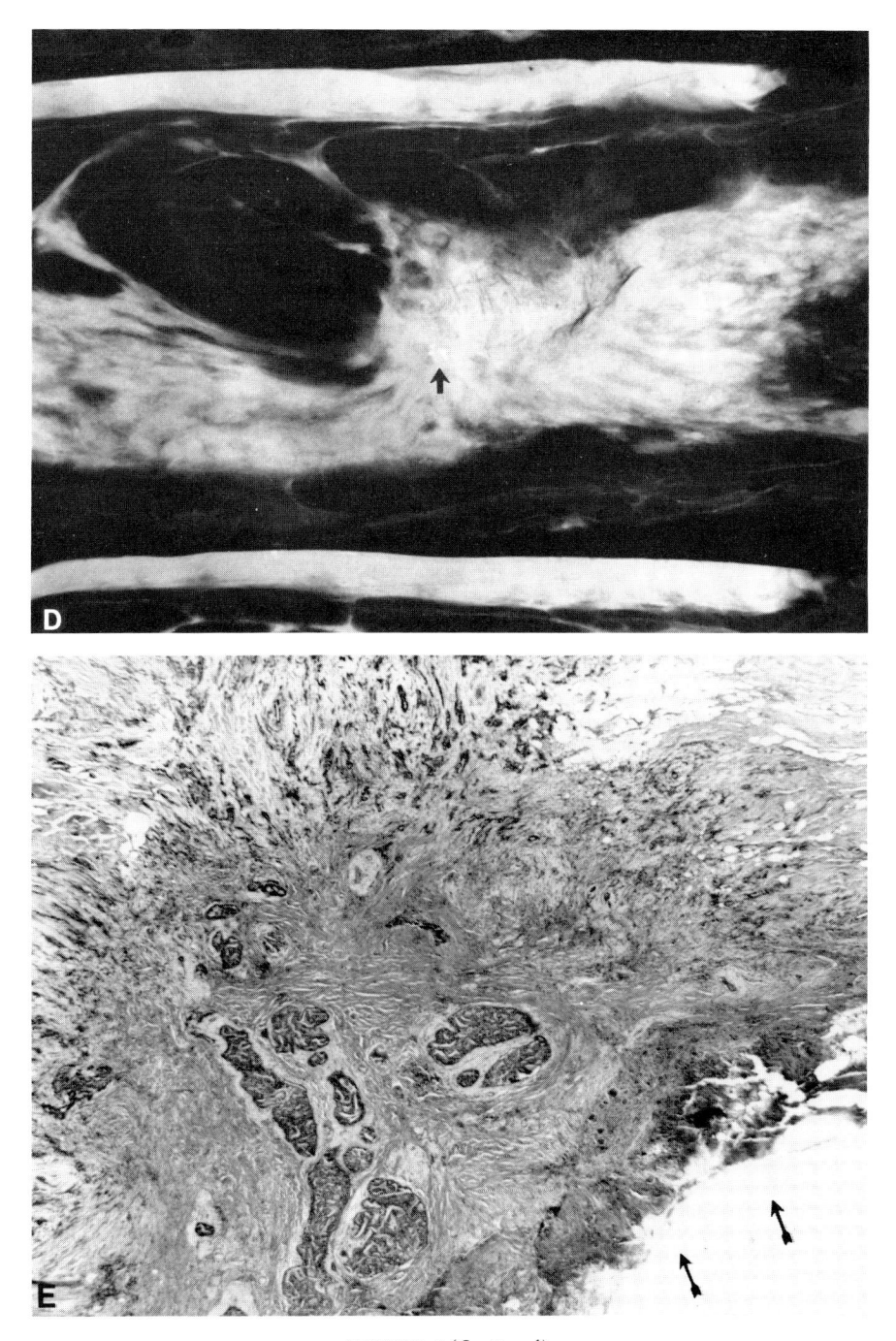

FIGURE 4 *(Continued)*.

FIGURE 5. *A,* Specimen radiogram of a mammographically directed biopsy obtained from a 41-year-old woman. The film demonstrates a small cluster of microcalcifications that extends to one surgical margin (arrow) of the biopsy specimen. *B,* Low-power photomicrograph of the biopsy to show in situ duct carcinoma with microcalcifications seen at one inked surgical margin of the biopsy specimen. *C (opposite page),* Low-power photomicrograph of residual invasive duct carcinoma also present at the inked surgical margin of the biopsy specimen adjacent to the in situ duct carcinoma. *D,* Follow-up mammogram demonstrating fibrosis, but no residual microcalcifications at the site of the mammographically directed biopsy.

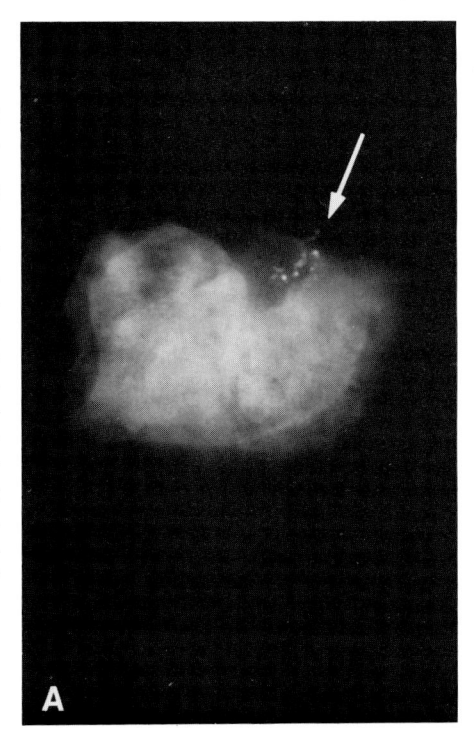

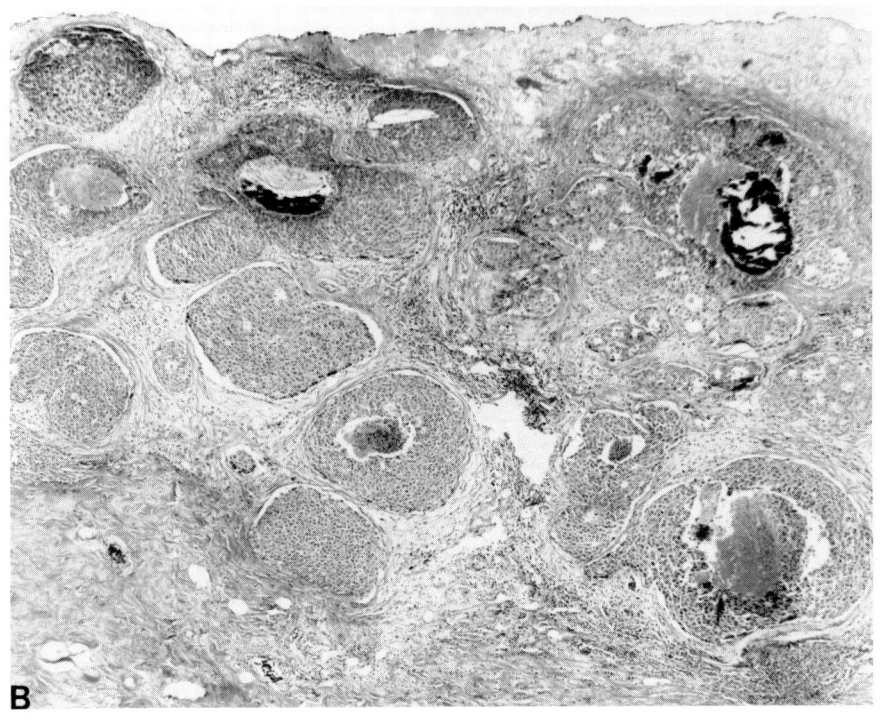

Pathologic Examination of the Mammographically Directed Breast Biopsy 35

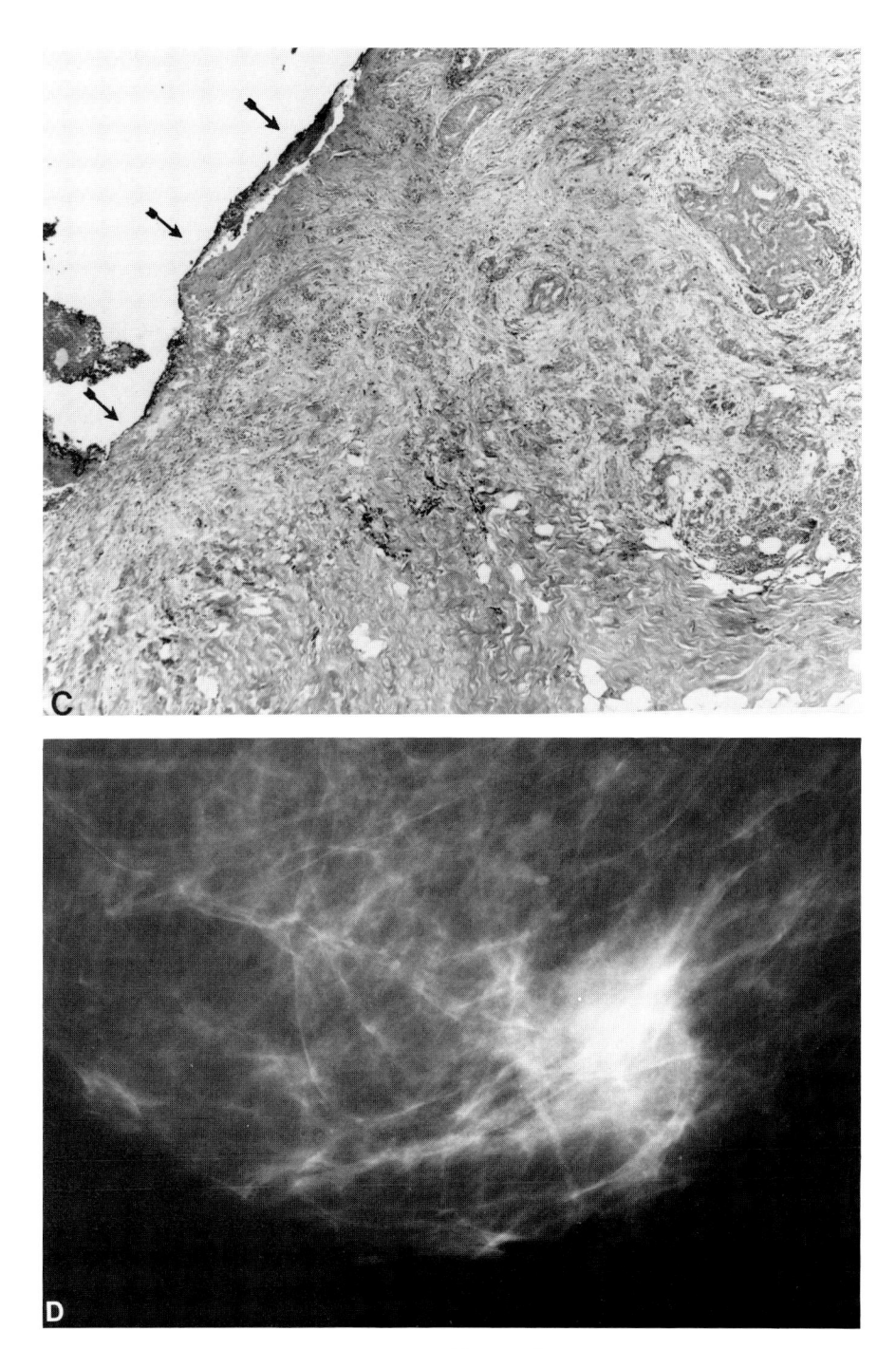

FIGURE 5 *(Continued)*.

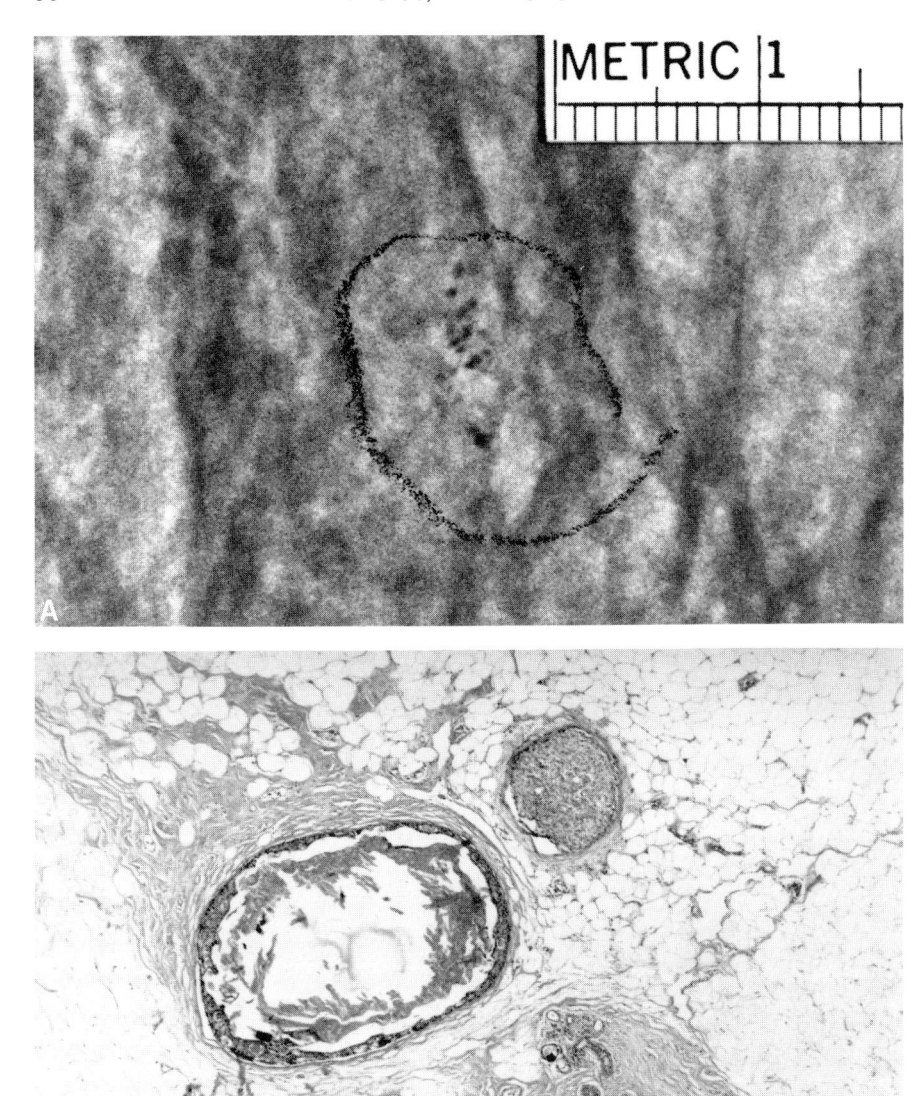

FIGURE 6. *A*, Xeromammogram from a 52-year-old woman found to have a small cluster of suspicious microcalcifications on routine examination. *B*, No lesion, palpable or visible, was demonstrated grossly in the breast biopsy. However, the pathologist took blind samples of the biopsy for estrogen receptor protein analysis, sacrificing the portion of the specimen needed for histologic diagnosis. No microcalcifications could be demonstrated in a specimen radiogram of the remaining biopsy material; a follow-up mammogram documented that the cluster of calcifications had been removed with the biopsy. A solitary focus of duct carcinoma in situ was found in the biopsy specimen, leaving the invasive status of the carcinoma unresolved.

directed breast biopsies are predominantly fatty. Formalin diffuses slowly into fatty tissues and even after complete fixation leaves the fat quite soft. The slow fixation delays processing and the lack of hardening of the fat makes it difficult for the pathologist to adequately section the specimen.

Formalin/alcohol used as a fixative permits processing of biopsies of up to 25 grams in 3 to 4 hours. In this fixative, fatty tissues fix and harden rapidly. This fixative is inexpensive and does not require the special disposal precautions that heavy metal fixatives do.

An additional feature of the formalin/alcohol fixative is that it tends to contract the fatty components of the biopsy such that the fixed specimen is reduced about 10–15% in size. This facilitates specimen sampling by reducing the number of cassettes required for an entire biopsy.

Localization of Microcalcific Lesions. Localization of microcalcifications can be performed in one of two ways: (1) small biopsies, after inking the specimen margins, can be formalin/alcohol fixed and sectioned free hand into 3–4 mm segments; or (2) large biopsies, after inking the specimen margins, can be frozen between blocks of dry ice, and sectioned into 3–4 mm segments using a commercial meat slicer.

With either method, the segments should be laid out in sequence and the segments numbered and radiographed to determine which segments contain the microcalcifications. Microcalcifications may be present in many or all of the segments (Fig. 7); occasionally they are found in only one of many

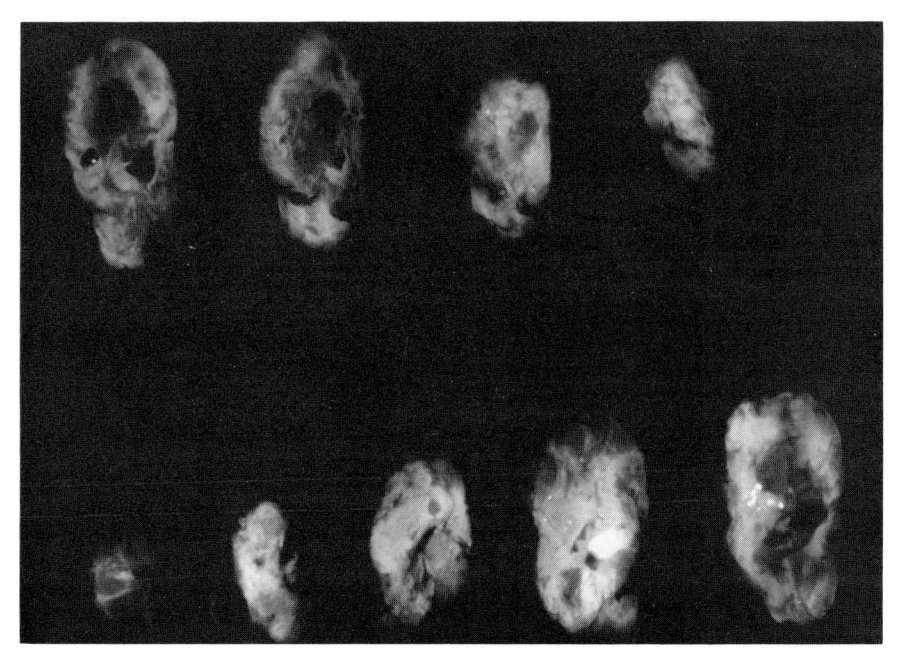

FIGURE 7. Specimen radiogram demonstrating microcalcifications in multiple segments of a mammographically directed breast biopsy (same patient as Fig. 1).

FIGURE 8. *A,* Specimen radiogram of a mammographically directed breast biopsy obtained on a 40-year-old woman demonstrating a small cluster of microcalcifications. *B,* After sectioning, the calcifications were found in only one (arrow) of multiple segments.

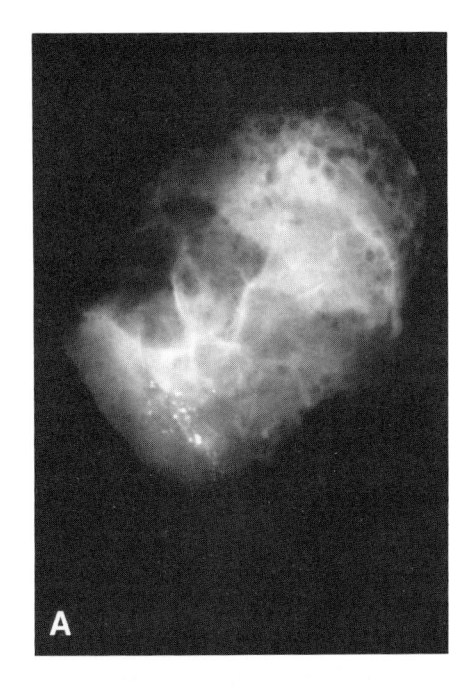

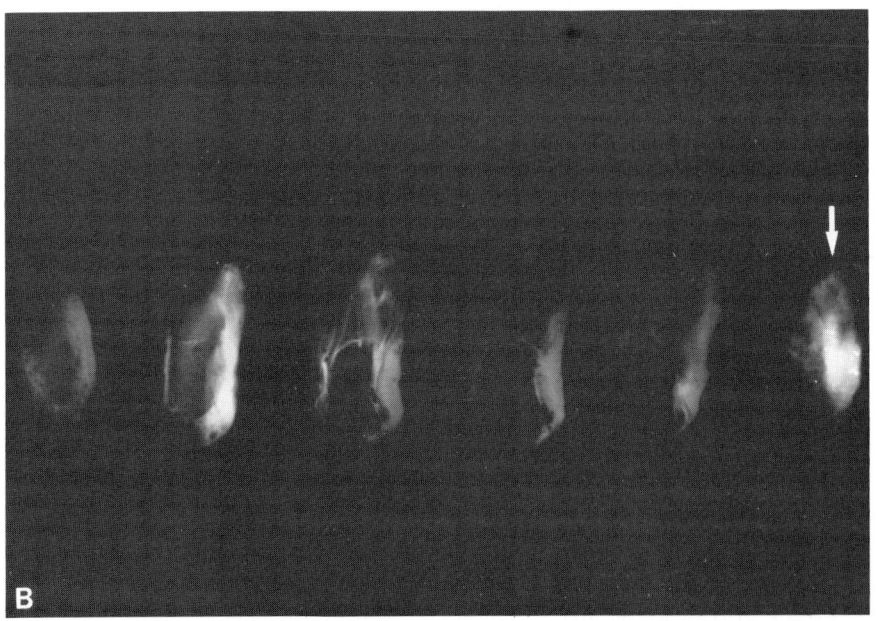

segments (Fig. 8). Blind sampling, particularly of biopsies with microcalcifications limited to a small number of segments, is not adequate to insure that breast neoplasms marked by microcalcifications are detected and completely evaluated. Any segment(s) containing microcalcifications should be embedded individually, identified by unique alpha or numeric characters, and the identifying information recorded in the pathology report.

Trying to short-cut the process by omitting the step of radiographing the sectioned biopsy frequently leaves the pathologist in a quandary as to whether or not the microscopic sections obtained are adequate for interpretation. Without knowing how many and which of the microscopic sections are expected to contain microcalcifications, there is an increased likelihood that significant lesions will not be detected.

If, for whatever reason, specimen radiograms are not obtained at the time the specimen is examined grossly, the paraffin blocks of the biopsy can be radiographed retrospectively to establish which segments contain microcalcifications. However, this approach is less efficient than performing the specimen radiography at the time of gross examination and tends to delay making the diagnosis and completing the pathology report.

SOURCES OF INTERPRETATIVE ERROR IN EVALUATION OF MAMMOGRAPHICALLY DIRECTED BIOPSIES

Biopsies Directed by Microcalcification

Specimen Radiogram Fails to Show the Microcalcifications

Problem. The mammographic lesion has not been adequately localized or the surgeon has not biopsied the area where the lesion was localized.

Solution. Review the localization radiograms and localization procedure. Confirm that the biopsy was taken from the indicated region of localization, not just blindly sampled by the surgeon.

Problem. The region of localization in the mammogram contains no definite microcalcifications.

Solution. Discuss with mammographer.

Problem. Microcalcifications are superficial and are not included in the biopsy.

Solution. The microcalcifications may be located in the dermis of the overlying skin rather than in the breast tissue. Suggest that a small ellipse of skin be obtained to document dermal microcalcifications (Fig. 9).

Problem. Specimen radiogram has been obtained with inadequate (non-dedicated) x-ray equipment, which does not provide a high resolution image of the microcalcifications (Fig. 10).

Solution. Discuss problem with Radiology Department and/or obtain self-contained x-ray unit for the Pathology Department.

Microcalcifications in Specimen Radiogram Do Not Correspond to Those in Mammogram

Problem. Microcalcifications are present in the specimen radiogram but do not appear to correspond to those seen in the preoperative mammogram.

Solution. Carefully compare the specimen radiogram with the preoperative mammogram, looking for distinctive calcifications or other landmarks

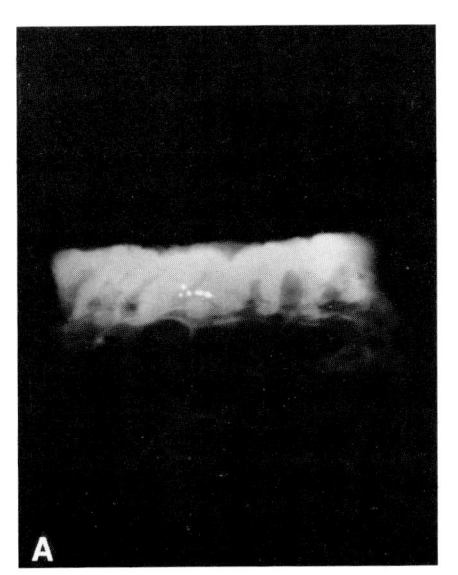

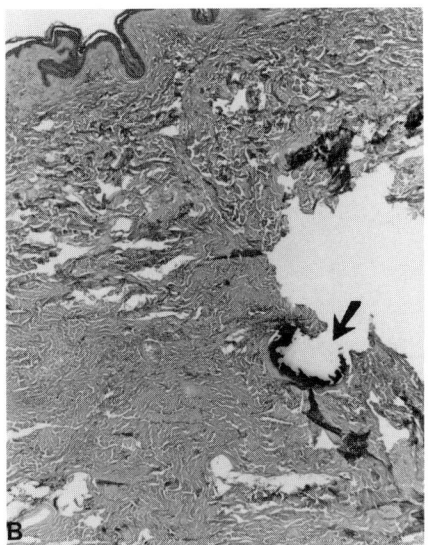

FIGURE 9. Microcalcifications found on a routine screening mammogram of a 68-year-old woman prompted a mammographically directed biopsy. The microcalcifications could not be found in the breast parenchyma. *A,* However, the calcifications were localized in the specimen radiogram to the dermis of the skin included with the breast biopsy. *B,* Low-power photomicrograph demonstrating one of the intradermal microcalcifications (arrow). The calcifications appeared to have formed in branches of cystically dilated sweat gland ducts.

seen in the preoperative mammogram. Specimen radiograms generally provide much better image resolution than do preoperative mammograms. Therefore, additional microcalcifications and other details, not evident in the preoperative mammogram, are frequently seen in the specimen radiogram.

Problem. Microcalcifications are present in the specimen radiogram and correspond to those seen in the preoperative mammogram, but not all of the microcalcifications seen in the preoperative mammogram have been removed with the biopsy.

Solution. Inform the surgeon of the findings and document your estimate of the completeness of the sampling. The pathologist should indicate to the surgeon that additional biopsies of the site are essential for diagnosis.

Problem. Contaminated microcalcifications are seen in the specimen radiogram.

Solution. The specimen or radiographic film has been contaminated with talc or other radio-opaque particulate material. Discard gloves and wash hands before processing film. Rinse off specimen as required before repeating specimen radiography.

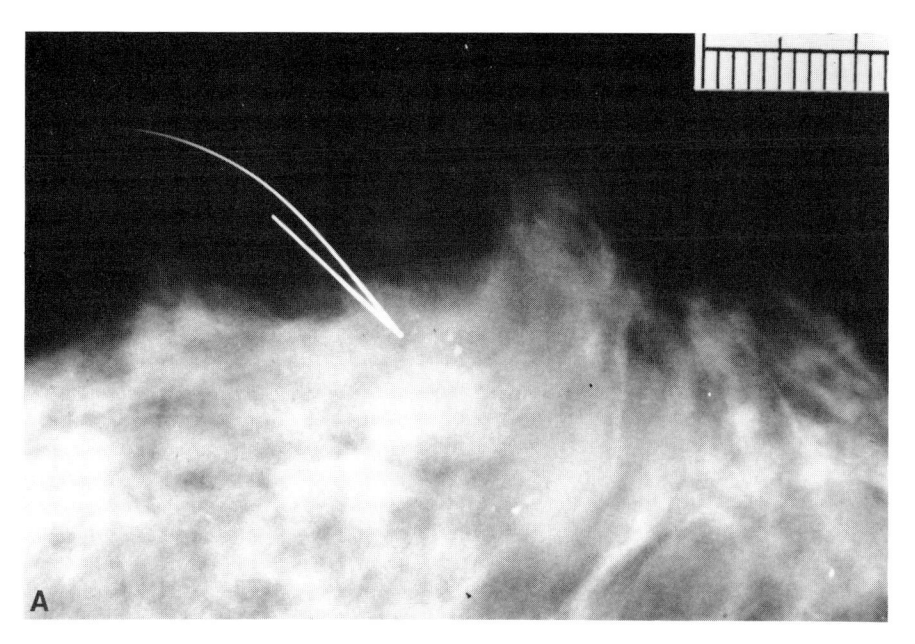

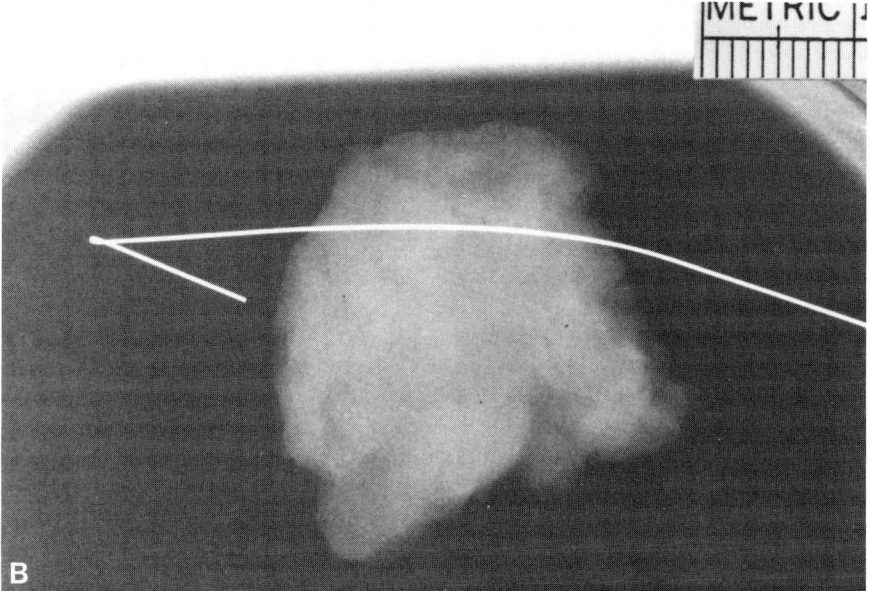

Pathologic Examination of the Mammographically Directed Breast Biopsy   41

FIGURE 10.   *A*, J wire-localization film from the breast of a 55-year-old woman. Numerous fine and coarse microcalcifications are present in the field of interest. *B*, The subsequent specimen radiogram was obtained with inadequate (nondedicated) radiographic equipment. The resulting low-quality image failed to demonstrate the many microcalcifications included in the biopsy.

Specimen Radiogram Demonstrates Adequate Sample of the Lesion, But Microcalcifications Are Not Identified in Microscopic Sections

Problem. Microcalcifications are not seen in the initial microscopic section from a segment recorded as containing microcalcifications.

Solution. The microcalcifications lie deeper in the paraffin block. Make additional sections at deeper levels. Re-radiograph all paraffin blocks, as needed, to establish the identity of the paraffin block(s) containing microcalcifications.

Problem. Microcalcifications seen in the specimen radiogram (Fig. 11A) are not seen in histologic sections even after making multiple deeper sections (Fig. 11B).

Solution. The calcifications may represent oxalate crystals that are transparent with conventional microscopy and easily overlooked.[12] Review tissue sections under plane-polarized light. Oxalate crystals are strongly birefringent when polarized (Fig. 11C).

Problem. Microcalcifications are not seen in deeper sections of the biopsy even after examination of microscopic sections under plane-polarized light.

Solution. Microcalcifications may have been leeched out by acidic fixative or torn out of tissue sections during sectioning in the microtome. Check the pH of the fixative. Carefully examine sections for remnants of calcified material in areas of knife chatter or tissue tearing.

Problem. Microcalcifications do not appear in microscopic slides because of inadequate sampling of the biopsy by the pathologist. Segments containing microcalcifications radiographically are not documented.

Solution. Radiograph all the paraffin blocks and any remaining wet tissue. Process all wet tissue and obtain deeper sections on all paraffin blocks containing microcalcifications.

Biopsies Directed by Soft Tissue Asymmetries and/or Densities Without Microcalcifications

Soft tissue densities can only be identified with certainty by specimen radiography when there is an excision biopsy, and the biopsy includes contrasting fatty breast parenchyma. Then only those soft tissue densities with a characteristic appearance, i.e., a circumscribed or sharply stellate configuration, can be recognized with certainty.

When a biopsy is removed as multiple small fragments of breast tissue of variable density, it is frequently impossible to determine radiologically whether or not the soft tissue density seen in the preoperative radiogram has been removed. However, if the fragments consist entirely of fatty tissue without a radiodense stroma, the surgeon should be informed that it is unlikely that the lesion has been removed and further biopsy of the site is indicated.

THE PATHOLOGY REPORT

Gross Description

The gross description should include the size of the biopsy specimen(s) in three dimensions, aggregate weight, appearance, and presence or absence of

Pathologic Examination of the Mammographically Directed Breast Biopsy   43

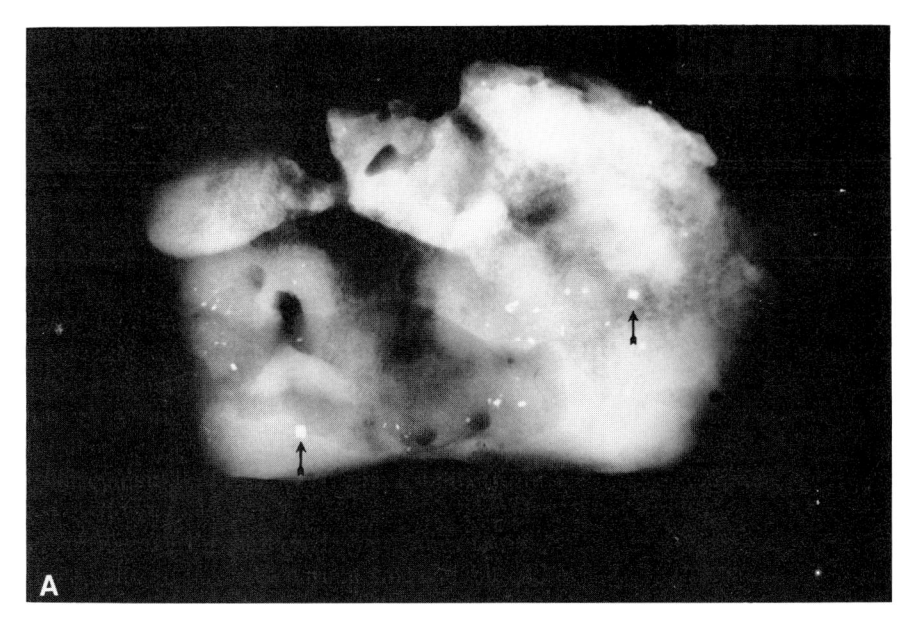

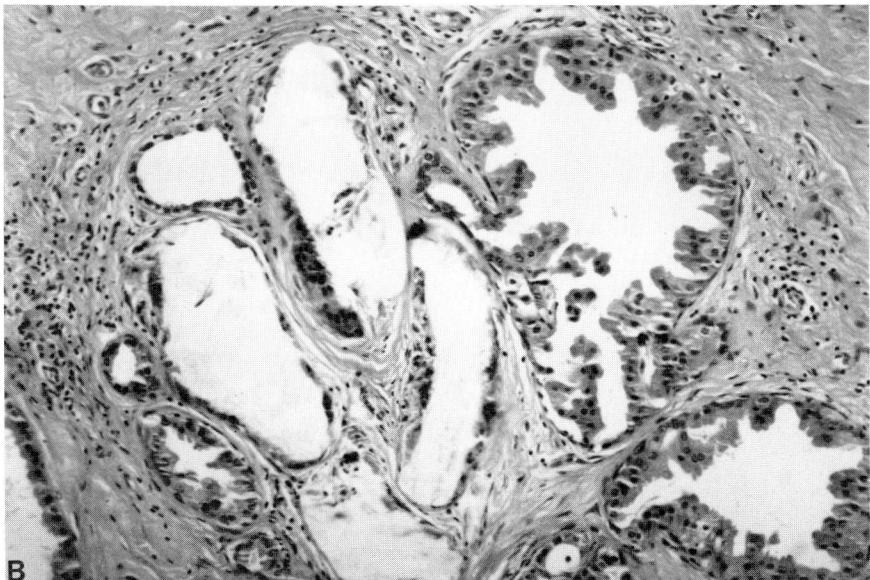

FIGURE 11. *A*, Specimen radiogram demonstrating both fine and coarse microcalcifications in a mammographically directed biopsy performed on a 47-year-old woman. Note that the larger calcifications (arrows) tend to be rectangular, a distinctive feature of oxalate crystals. *B*, Photomicrograph of the breast biopsy taken with a conventional light source, which fails to demonstrate any mineralized crystalline material.

(Figure continued on following page.)

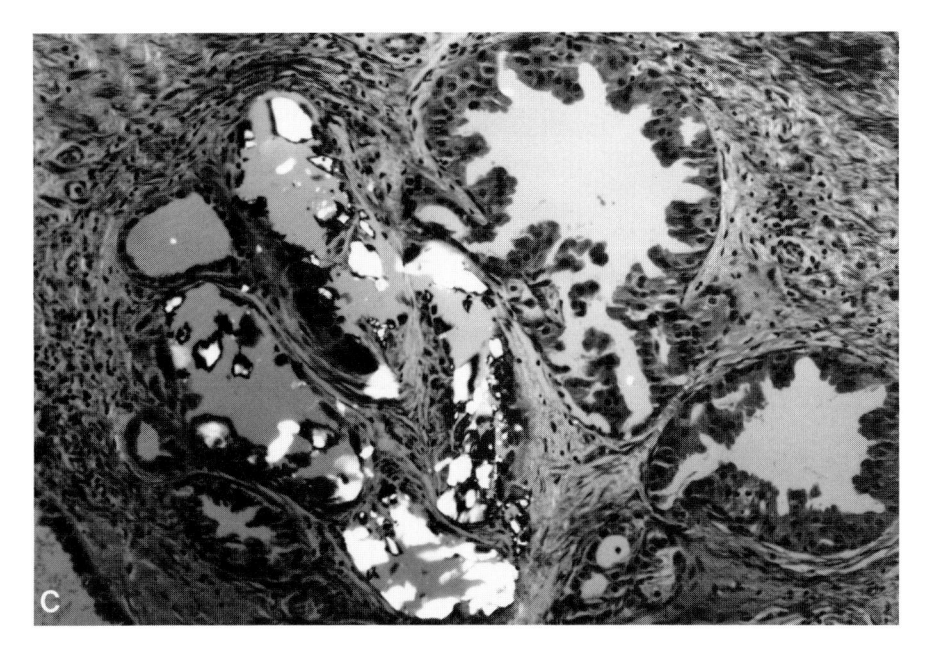

FIGURE 11 *(Continued).* C, The same field as shown in the preceding figure, but photographed with plane-polarized light to reveal the numerous birefringent oxalate crystals present in glandular spaces.

methylene blue staining (if methylene blue was used in the localization procedure), as well as an adequate description of any gross abnormality. The numbered segments of the biopsy containing microcalcifications or soft tissue densities should be specifically identified.

Microscopic Description

The pathologist should identify the histology associated with any significant mammographic (radiographic) lesion. Extension of a carcinoma or epithelial atypia to inked resection margins should be noted. The size of any lesion should be recorded. A corresponding statement regarding the apparent extent of the lesion in the preoperative mammogram also should be provided.

Incomplete sampling of a mammographically identified focus of microcalcifications, e.g., where 10 of 35 microcalcifications appear in the specimen film, and/or extension of a neoplastic process to the inked resection margin should be clearly noted in the report. It is often helpful to repeat this information in a summary comment following the diagnosis. Such a comment should include the clinical significance of incomplete excision and recommendation for appropriate postoperative follow-up mammographic evaluation.

Occasionally the mammographic abnormality represents some benign proliferative process with calcifications, and incidental to this there are foci of in situ duct or in situ lobular carcinoma or some other significant finding. The diagnosis should record the nature of the mammographic lesion and separately record the nature of other incidentally identified lesions.

Diagnosis

The diagnosis should indicate the side and quadrant of the breast biopsied, the nature of the mammographic abnormality that directed the biopsy, the pathologic character of the process(es) noted histologically, and the size of any carcinoma detected. Example: *Right breast, superolateral quadrant, mammographically directed biopsy for microcalcifications—duct carcinoma in situ, 8 mm.*

This approach provides a pathology report that the treating physician can understand. It includes the type of biopsy procedure used, the degree to which the biopsy findings correlate with the mammographic interpretation, the nature, extent and adequacy of excision of the lesion that directed the biopsy, and whether or not even more significant incidental neoplastic change is present. This procedure protects the patient by clearly indicating whether or not an adequate excisional biopsy has been performed, and if it has not, documents the methods used to establish that no lesion was found in the biopsy specimen.

References

1. Shapiro S, Venet W, Strax P, et al: Ten to fourteen-year effect of screening on breast cancer mortality. J Natl Cancer Inst 69:349–355, 1982.
2. Margolin FR, Lagios MD: Mammographic detection of early breast cancer. Ten year experience in a community hospital. West J Med 144:46–48, 1986.
3. UK Trial of Early Detection of Breast Cancer Group: First results on mortality reduction in the UK trial of early detection of breast cancer. Lancet ii:411–416, 1988.
4. Tabar L, Gad A, Holmberg LH, et al: Reduction in mortality from breast cancer after mass screening with mammography. Randomized trial from the British Cancer Screening Working Group of the Swedish National Board of Health and Welfare. Lancet i:829–832, 1985.
5. Anderson I, Aspergren R, Janzon L, et al: Mammographic screening and mortality from breast cancer: The Malmo mammographic screening trial. Br Med J 297:943–948, 1988.
6. Lagios MD: Multicentricity of breast carcinoma demonstrated by routine correlated serial subgross and radiographic examination. Cancer 40:1726–1734, 1977.
7. Lagios MD, Gates EA, Westdahl PR, et al: A guide to the frequency of nipple involvement in breast cancer based on a study of 149 consecutive mastectomies studied in serial subgross and correlated radiographic technique. Am J Surg 138:135–142, 1979.
8. Lagios MD, Rose MR, Margolin FR: Tubular carcinoma of the breast. Association with multicentricity, bilaterality and family history of breast carcinoma. Am J Clin Pathol 73:25–30, 1980.
9. Lagios MD, Westdahl PR, Margolin FR, Rose MR: Duct carcinoma in situ. Relationship of extent of noninvasive disease to the frequency of occult invasion, multicentricity, lymph node metastases, and short term treatment failures. Cancer 50:1309–1314, 1982.
10. Lagios MD: Human breast precancer: Current status. Cancer Surveys 2:383–401, 1983.
11. Lagios MD, Margolin FR, Westdahl PR, Rose MR: Mammographically detected duct carcinoma in situ. Frequency of local recurrence following tylectomy and prognostic effect of nuclear grade on local recurrence. Cancer 63:618–624, 1989.
12. Tornos C, Silva E, El-Naggar A, Pritzker KH: Calcium oxalate crystal in breast biopsies: The missing microcalcifications. Am J Surg Pathol 14:961–968, 1990.

Handling the Mammographically Directed Biopsy: Another Approach

MAHENDRA RANCHOD, M.B.Ch.B., M.Med.

From the Department of
 Pathology
Good Samaritan Hospital
San Jose, California

Reprint requests to:
Mahendra Ranchod, M.D.
Department of Pathology
Good Samaritan Hospital
2425 Samaritan Drive
San Jose, CA 95124

The approach to handling the mammographically directed biopsy described by Dr. Lagios in his article, *"Protocol for the pathologic examination and tissue processing of the mammographically directed biopsy"* in this issue is commendable for its thoroughness. However, because of cost and manpower considerations, we handle our biopsies a little differently. Our approach is described below.

Specimen mammography at our hospital is performed in the Department of Diagnostic Imaging. After the mammographically localized lesion has been removed by the surgeon, the breast biopsy along with the original preoperative mammographs are delivered to the Department of Diagnostic Imaging by an operating room orderly. A specimen radiogram is prepared in the Department of Diagnostic Imaging, and the radiologist communicates with the surgeon directly about the adequacy of the biopsy. The operating room orderly, who has remained in the Department of Diagnostic Imaging during this time, then delivers the breast biopsy specimen to the Pathology Department. The specimen (secured between two sheets of blank radiographic film to maintain orientation), the specimen radiogram, the patient's preoperative mammographs, and the pathology requisition form, are then delivered to the Surgical Pathology gross examination room and handed directly only to a pathologist or to a pathology assistant.

The biopsy and the specimen mammograph are examined immediately by a pathologist. The intact specimen is measured and a note is made about the presence of the J-wire inserted by the radiologist, its location, and any other relevant points. Abnormalities in the specimen radiogram are noted. Where the findings are of a dubious nature, the specimen mammograph is compared with the patient's original mammograms, and, if necessary, the opinion of the radiologist involved in the case is sought.

The J-wire is removed by the pathologist from the biopsy specimen as gently as possible, with either a forceps or pliers. If the specimen was submitted in one piece, it is inked with Davidson's blue dye (Bradley Products, Inc., Bloomington, MN) or India ink, allowed to stand for about a minute, and then dabbed dry with paper towels. We no longer employ Bouin's solution as a mordant, because we are able to achieve good staining with the dye alone. The specimen is cut at 3 to 4 mm intervals and examined grossly.

We only perform frozen sections (or a cytologic preparation from a scraping of the cut surface of the biopsy) in the uncommon situation where there is a lesion resembling an invasive carcinoma and where the lesion is large enough (7–8 mm in maximum dimension) to secure adequate fresh material for steroid hormone receptor assays and ploidy studies. If the frozen section or cytologic preparations are equivocal, all the material is submitted for histologic examination. **We do not perform frozen sections on mammographically directed biopsies in any other situation,** no matter what the persuasion of the surgeon.

Fresh slices of the specimen are then placed on 3 × 5 cards to ensure that the sections remain flat. They are left on the card for a minute or so, to allow the tissue to adhere to the card, and then placed in fixative (formalin, if the tissue is mainly fibrous, or formalin and alcohol, sequentially, if it is predominantly fatty). If the biopsy is received late in the day, we do not hesitate to fix the specimen overnight before submitting sections for tissue processing.

Because we lack facilities for performing specimen radiographs in our department, we do not routinely perform specimen radiography on the sliced specimen. Small specimens are processed for microscopic examination in their entirety. Specimens that are large and that cannot be accommodated in ten or fewer cassettes are handled in one of two ways. If the mammographic lesion of concern can be isolated easily with the help of the specimen radiogram, then that area is generously separated from the rest of the specimen and embedded in its entirety. If, on the other hand, the orientation of the specimen is questionable, or if the area of concern is multifocal, the sliced specimen is subjected to further specimen radiography to ensure proper sampling. In the latter situation, all the slices containing calcium or soft tissue densities of concern (as well as a variable amount of additional fibrous breast tissue) are submitted for microscopic examination. Gross findings are reported to the surgeon verbally whenever there is a significant finding.

We do not submit all the tissue routinely for microscopic examination, because the variation in the amount of nonlesional tissue is related to the surgeon's ability to conservatively excise the areas of concern—more than any other factor. We adopted this protocol for the handling of mammographically directed biopsies some years ago, using common sense as our guide, but without good data to support less than total microscopic evaluation of the mammographically directed breast biopsy. A recent study by Owings et al.[1] provides reassurance of the validity of our approach. Our reporting of the pathologic findings on the mammographically directed biopsy is similar to that of Dr. Lagios, with the exception that, because we do not routinely retain the order of the serial slices of the specimen, we are not able to obtain an accurate three-dimensional measurement of in situ duct carcinomas. This procedure may have to be modified if tylectomy without radiation becomes a popular way to treat small in situ duct carcinomas.

In addition to the above, I believe that the pathology report should include the following: a statement as to whether or not the biopsy was mammographically directed, a note about the presence or absence of calcification, correlation of the location of calcifications in relation to the most significant lesion found in the biopsy, a statement about concordance between histologic and mammographic findings (if appropriate), and pertinent comments about any lesions encountered, as would be done with any breast biopsy.

Reference

1. Owings DV, Hann L, Schnitt SJ: How thoroughly should needle localization breast biopsies be sampled for microscopic examination? Am J Surg Pathol 14:578–583, 1990.

Processing the Small Invasive Carcinoma Detected in the Mammographically Directed Breast Biopsy

JAMES L. BENNINGTON, M.D.

From the Department of
 Anatomic Pathology
 and Clinical Laboratories
California Pacific Medical
 Center, California Campus
San Francisco, California

Reprint requests to:
James L. Bennington, MD
Chairman, Department of
 Anatomic Pathology
 and Clinical Laboratories
California Pacific Medical
 Center, California Campus
P.O. Box 3805
San Francisco, CA 94119

IMPACT OF MAMMOGRAPHY ON THE SIZE OF BREAST CANCERS FOUND AT SURGERY

In recent years, high-resolution mammography has made possible the routine detection of clinically silent, small, nonpalpable invasive breast cancers. Its use, combined with prompt biopsy of mammographically detected suspicious lesions, has resulted in a substantial increase in the numbers of relatively small invasive breast cancers removed surgically (see Bennington J, *"Impact of mammographic screening on the size and relative frequency of invasion in breast cancers seen in a community hospital from 1975 to 1988,"* pp 11–22, this issue).

Prior to the introduction of screening mammography, pathologists rarely encountered invasive breast cancers 10 mm in diameter or less (≤ 10 mm). Tumors of this size were sufficiently uncommon that for almost all published studies from the premammographic era the smallest category of tumor size reported was ≤ 20 mm. The few published studies of clinically detected invasive breast cancers we have located where small invasive breast cancers were recorded reported a range of 2.3–8.5% of all invasive breast cancers ≤ 10 mm,[1-4] and 0.9–1.4% ≤ 5 mm in diameter.[2-4]

These figures may substantially overestimate the numbers of invasive breast cancers ≤ 10 mm that can be detected without the aid of mammography. Kern and Mikkelson[5] in a retrospective slide review of 919 breast cancers treated between the years 1961 and 1970 in one major hospital rejected 38 of the 57 (67%) invasive cancers originally recorded as ≤ 10 mm. Thirty-four of the 38 rejected were found to be larger than originally reported, and the remaining 4 of the 38 were not invasive.

OUTCOME OF PATIENTS WITH INVASIVE BREAST CANCERS < 10 mm IN DIAMETER

In spite of the small number of invasive breast cancers ≤ 10 mm available for study, the concept emerged that tumors of this size rarely metastasize. As a result, invasive breast cancers ≤ 10 mm came to be lumped with a number of histologic tumor types characterized by nonaggressive behavior under the name "minimal breast cancer."[6] Subsequently it was shown that the impression that small invasive breast cancers do not metastasize was incorrect. Axillary lymph node metastases have been reported in as many as 20–24% of patients with invasive breast cancers 5–10 mm,[2-4] and 14–28% of patients with invasive breast cancers ≤ 5 mm.[3-5]

Carter et al.[3] found that the 5-year relative survival rates for patients with invasive breast cancers ≤ 10 mm in relation to lymph node status were: negative lymph nodes, 98.6%; 1–3 positive lymph nodes, 94.8%; and 4 or more positive lymph nodes, 54.8%. These figures would appear to indicate that lymph node status could be used with a high degree of reliability for patients with invasive breast cancers ≤ 10 mm to distinguish those patients likely to remain disease-free from those patients likely to relapse. Unfortunately 5-year survival rates do not give a true picture of clinical course for patients with early breast cancer. Distant micrometastases at the time of surgery may take considerably longer than 5 years to become clinically manifest.

Lymph node-negative patients with invasive breast cancer were reported by Carter[3] to have an 88.4% relative 5-year survival, but only 75% of the patients remained free of distant metastases on long term follow-up. Followed long enough, a substantial number of patients with invasive breast cancers ≤ 10 mm, even those with negative lymph nodes, will develop distant metastases.[4] Metastases from low-grade breast cancers to distant sites frequently become manifest only many years after the initial surgery.[7] Because tumor size, lymph node status, and tumor grade fail to identify a significant number of patients who will develop disseminated metastases, these prognostic variables considered individually are felt to be inadequate for chemotherapy decision making.

RATIONALE FOR SELECTING CHEMOTHERAPY FOR PATIENTS WITH INVASIVE BREAST CANCER

Adjuvant chemotherapy was initially introduced for the treatment of patients with breast cancer in recognition of the fact that lymph node-positive patients without other evidence of disease frequently harbor clinically silent metastases.[8] Subsequently, this approach has become standard practice.[9]

The benefits of adjuvant chemotherapy for lymph node-negative patients with invasive breast cancer also have been demonstrated.[10-12] In the absence of established criteria for selecting which lymph node-negative patients are most likely to relapse, the National Cancer Institute, in a recent clinical alert,[13] has recommended that all patients with invasive breast cancer, irrespective of axillary lymph node status, be considered candidates for adjuvant chemotherapy.

By subjecting all patients with invasive breast cancer to chemotherapy, those with occult metastases are provided whatever benefit is to be derived from this form of treatment; however, this is done at the expense of unnecessary costs and inconvenience for those patients who do not have occult metastases. Ideally, the decision to put a patient on chemotherapy for invasive breast cancer should be based on information about the patient's tumor that can be used to predict with a high degree of accuracy whether or not the patient will develop metastases.

PROGNOSTIC INDICATORS AS THE BASIS FOR SELECTING CHEMOTHERAPY FOR PATIENTS WITH INVASIVE BREAST CANCER

Inasmuch as the most powerful morphologic prognostic indicators, i.e. tumor size and lymph node status, do not adequately discriminate between those patients with invasive breast cancer who will and those who will not develop distant metastases, a number of cell cycle, biochemical, and genetic features of breast cancers are being investigated for this purpose. These features include: (1) tumor nuclear DNA content (ploidy),* (2) rates of tumor cell proliferation (percent of tumor cells in S-phase),* (3) levels of tumor estrogen receptor (ER) and progesterone receptor (PR) protein content,† (4) amplification of tumor oncogenes (HER-2/*neu*),[14] (5) loss of tumor oncogenes (c-Ha-*ras*),[15] (6) tumor epidermal growth factor (EGF) binding,[16] (7) tumor cathepsin D content,[17] and (8) tumor haptoglobin-related protein (Hpr) level.[18]

Preliminary studies suggest that one or more of these eight features, possibly in combination with established morphologically based prognostic indicators, will meet the needs of oncologists for the planning of adjuvant chemotherapy. The implication for pathologists is that all breast biopsies containing invasive breast cancers will need to be processed so as to insure that all essential prognostic information is obtained.

The morphologically based tumor features—i.e., (1) size of the invasive component included in the biopsy, (2) adequacy of biopsy surgical margins, (3) tumor histologic type, (4) tumor grade, and (5) extent of tumor necrosis—

---

*See Bennington J, *"Significance of DNA content and proliferative rate in the invasive carcinoma found in the mammographically directed breast biopsy,"* pp 137–160, this issue.
†See Ross J, et al, *"An update on steroid hormone receptors in surgical pathology,"* pp 103–134, this issue.

can be obtained routinely from formalin-fixed biopsy specimens. However, the most generally used methods for tumor ER, PR, nuclear DNA content, and S-phase analyses require unfixed tumor.

Cytosol assay for quantitative ER and PR, and the various immunochemical methods used for the determination of the percent of tumor cells in S-phase require the use of unfixed fresh or frozen tumor. Collecting such information requires planning ahead to make necessary sample preparations before the specimen is placed in formalin.

However, the pathologist presented with a relatively small breast biopsy (which may or may not contain a palpable mass), a preoperative mammogram showing a small soft tissue density or a suspicious cluster of calcifications, and an anxious surgeon is generally more concerned with the need to establish the correct diagnosis than with processing the specimen in a way that makes it possible to subsequently perform various ancillary studies, which may or may not prove to be needed. Fortunately, special processing of the breast biopsy to insure the availability of all prognostically important morphologic features, in the event that the specimen turns out to contain an invasive cancer, does not need to compromise the timeliness or the accuracy of the diagnosis, nor does it require much incremental effort on the part of the pathologist. Suggested processing procedures to determine accurately the size of an invasive carcinoma found in a mammographically directed biopsy and for assessing the adequacy of biopsy surgical margins are outlined by Lagios in *"Protocol for the pathologic examination and tissue processing of the mammographically directed biopsy,"* pp 22–45, in this issue. The criteria for correctly diagnosing the histologic type of invasive breast cancers identified and for objectively establishing the tumor grade are reviewed by Kamel in *"Breast biopsies: The content of the surgical pathology report,"* pp 161–180, this issue.

The following section describes our approach for routinely obtaining essential prognostically important features of invasive breast cancer that would be lost or compromised by formalin fixation of the tumor.

HANDLING THE MAMMOGRAPHICALLY DIRECTED BREAST BIOPSY SPECIMEN SUSPECTED OF CONTAINING AN INVASIVE CARCINOMA

Rationale

To insure the effective handling of the mammographically directed biopsy that turns out to contain an invasive cancer, the pathologist must assume that **all mammographically directed biopsy specimens removed from women over the age of 30 years that contain a palpable mass or radiographically demonstrated soft tissue density represent an invasive carcinoma until proven otherwise.** Our approach described below for dealing with biopsy specimens meeting these criteria was developed to reduce loss of important prognostic data from breast biopsies containing small invasive carcinomas. Important advantages of this approach are: (1) it does not substantially increase the cost of processing breast biopsy specimens in which no invasive cancer is found, (2) tumor needed for establishing a diagnosis is not lost, and (3) minimal additional effort on the part of the pathologist is required.

Some surgeons are content to submit mammographically directed biopsy specimens for routine pathologic examination without intraoperative documentation that the lesion prompting the biopsy has been removed. However, in our experience most surgeons wish to have the pathologist examine the biopsy in the operating room, and to have the specimen radiograms compared with the preoperative mammograms to be sure that the biopsy is adequate before allowing the patient to leave surgery.

We prefer not to cut into the mammographically directed biopsy specimen until the surgical margins have been marked. Generally, there is no good reason to do so. An exception is the biopsy specimen from the relatively young patient that contains a mass that the pathologist feels is most likely a fibroadenoma. In this situation, especially when the patient is unusually anxious about the diagnosis, the pathologist is justified in immediately sectioning the specimen, because there is little risk of losing important information.

Frozen section examination of the mammographically directed biopsy specimen to establish the diagnosis of invasive cancer should not be performed on mammographically directed biopsies unless all of the following conditions are met: (1) There is a palpable mass large enough to provide adequate material for all essential ancillary studies, (2) the results of the frozen section diagnosis will be used to make an immediate therapeutic decision, and (3) the pathologist is convinced that frozen section examination will not compromise the permanent section diagnosis or evaluation of the adequacy of surgical margins.

Specimen Radiography of the Mammographically Directed Biopsy

After initial gross examination of the mammographically directed biopsy by the pathologist, a specimen radiogram should be obtained. In our hospital, this procedure is performed intraoperatively by the pathologist on call for operating room consultations. The pathologist personally prepares the specimen radiogram using a self-contained, industrial x-ray unit (Faxitron manufactured by Hewlett Packard) and develops the film in an automated film processor located in the surgical suite. The pathologist then compares the specimen radiogram with the preoperative mammogram to determine the extent to which any soft tissue density and/or foci of calcifications that directed the biopsy are included in the biopsy specimen. Correspondence between the findings in the preoperative mammogram and the specimen radiogram are made part of the pathologist's written intraoperative consultation report.

Marking the Margins of the Unfixed Biopsy Specimen

Before cutting into the biopsy, the entire outer surface of the specimen is marked with India ink and blotted dry. The specimen is then cross-sectioned and carefully handled to avoid transferring ink to cut surfaces. If the biopsy contains a lesion suspicious for cancer, touch preparations are made for nuclear DNA analysis and a thin section of tumor is reserved for the determination of the percent of proliferating cells by immunochemical staining. The specimen then is dipped in Bouin's solution to mordant the ink on the surgical margins of the biopsy. Placing the specimen in Bouin's solution immediately to mordant the India ink may make it impossible to obtain adequate touch preparations for nuclear DNA analysis and also may alter immunochemical staining for the percentage of proliferating cells.

Gross Examination of the Biopsy Specimen

After marking the biopsy surgical margins with India ink, the specimen is examined grossly. A magnifying glass may be helpful in identifying small cancers and for examining the specimen radiogram. At the time of the gross examination, any tumor identified should be measured and the maximum length and width recorded in the pathology report.

TOUCH PREPARATION OF SUSPECTED CANCER IN THE BIOPSY FOR TUMOR NUCLEAR DNA ANALYSIS

When a biopsy specimen contains a discrete mass suspicious for cancer, touch preparations are made on specially prepared glass microscope slides of the freshly cut surface of the lesion. We use special slides supplied by Cell Analysis Systems, Inc., 909 South Rt. 83, Elhurst IL, which include normal rat liver control cells. If the breast lesion is small, retracted, and surrounded by fat, it may be necessary to gently scrape the lesion with a scalpel and use the small droplet of material obtained to make the smear. If tumor is readily accessible, it is sufficient to gently touch the slide to the freshly cut surface of the tumor several times. This will routinely provide an adequate specimen, but as an insurance policy, we generally prepare two touch preparation slides. Smears should be air-dried for 10 minutes, fixed in 10% buffered formalin for 10 minutes, and then allowed to air dry until stained by the Feulgen method.

In the event that facilities are not available for determination of nuclear DNA values from touch preparations of the tumor using static (image) cytometry, paraffin-embedded tumor, if it can be spared, can be processed using the Hedley technique[19] to provide cell suspensions for analysis by either flow or static cytometry.

PREPARATION OF SUSPECTED CANCER IN THE BIOPSY FOR S-PHASE ANALYSIS

We have evaluated the specimen-processing procedures involved with immunochemical staining for BrdUrd, Ki-67 and PCNA/cyclin as alternatives for estimating the proliferating fraction of tumor cells. We currently use the Ki-67 or PCNA/cyclin technique, which does not require the in vitro incubation step used for the estimation of BrdUrd uptake.

For Ki-67 staining, fresh frozen tissue is required. For PCNA/cyclin staining a thin slice of tumor is placed in Carnoy's fixative. Histologic sections of the tumor prepared from Carnoy's-fixed material are stained immunochemically for PCNA/cyclin (found only in cell nuclei during the late GI and S-phases of the cell cycle.[20] The percentage of tumor-cell nuclei staining positively provides an indication of the size of the proliferative compartment of the tumor.

Only alcohol-based fixatives work reliably for PCNA/cyclin staining.[20] The advantage of alcohol-based fixatives for the demonstration of antigens masked by formalin fixation has been demonstrated with a number of antibodies.[21] Carnoy's fixation also provides excellent hematoxylin and eosin stained sections for routine histologic examination, if it turns out that the portion of tumor reserved for anti-PCNA/cyclin staining needs to be examined to help establish the diagnosis or the adequacy of the surgical margins.

PREPARATION FOR SUSPECTED CANCER IN THE BIOPSY FOR HORMONE RECEPTOR PROTEIN ANALYSIS

When all of the tumor is not needed for histologic examination, a portion can be reserved for cytosol assay of estrogen and progesterone receptor proteins. If sufficient tumor is not available for cytosol assay, hormone receptor analysis can be performed by immunochemical staining of formalin-fixed, paraffin-embedded tumor sections for both estrogen[22,23] and progesterone receptor protein levels.[24] The stained slides then can be evaluated qualitatively by a pathologist observer, or analyzed quantitatively using an image cytometer with appropriate software.

CASE STUDY OF A MAMMOGRAPHICALLY DIRECTED BIOPSY SPECIMEN CONTAINING A SMALL INVASIVE CARCINOMA

The following case demonstrates the extent to which the pathologist can extract essential prognostic information from a breast biopsy containing an invasive cancer, even when the invasive cancer is relatively small.

Clinical History

The patient, a 62-year-old white woman in general good health, had no increased risk factors for breast carcinoma revealed by her clinical history. On routine mammography, a suspicious, nodular soft density was demonstrated in the 12 o'clock position of the left breast (Fig. 1). A mammographically directed biopsy was performed under local anesthesia. Intraoperative radiography of the specimen confirmed that the soft tissue density had been removed by the biopsy.

Pathologic Findings

The breast biopsy was a 4.1-gram mass of fibrofatty breast tissue that measured 15 × 16 × 30 mm. A suspicious appearing soft tissue density similar in size and shape to that originally identified in the preoperative mammogram was seen on the specimen radiogram (Fig. 2).

After inking the surgical margins, the biopsy specimen was cross-sectioned, revealing a light grey, translucent, sclerotic central tumor measuring

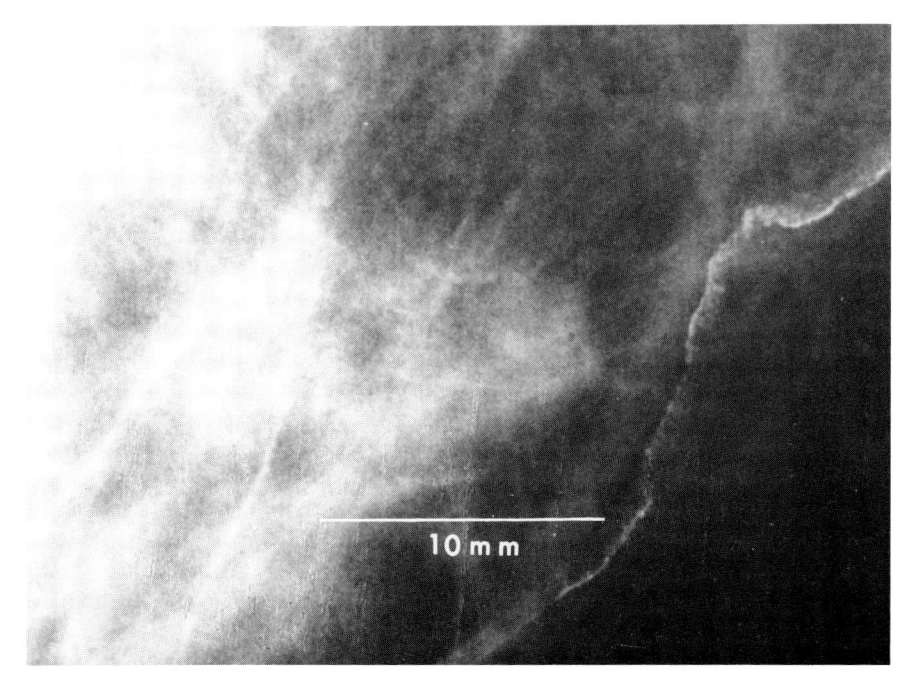

FIGURE 1. Mammogram of the left breast at the level of the nipple demonstrating an 8-mm nodular density with a stellate margin. No calcifications were identified in the lesion.

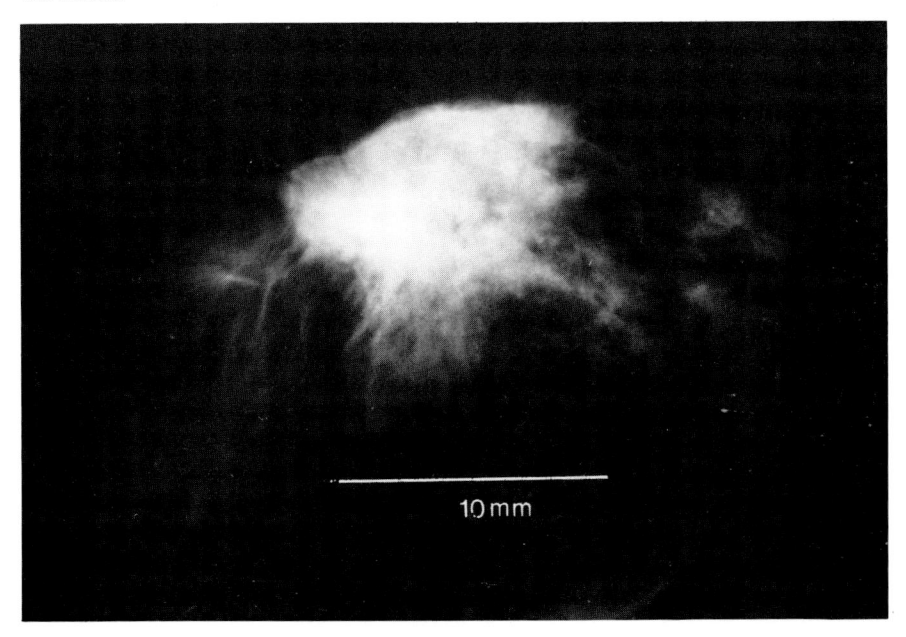

FIGURE 2. Intraoperative radiogram of the mammographically directed biopsy specimen contained a well defined, soft tissue density corresponding in size and shape to the lesion identified in the preoperative mammogram.

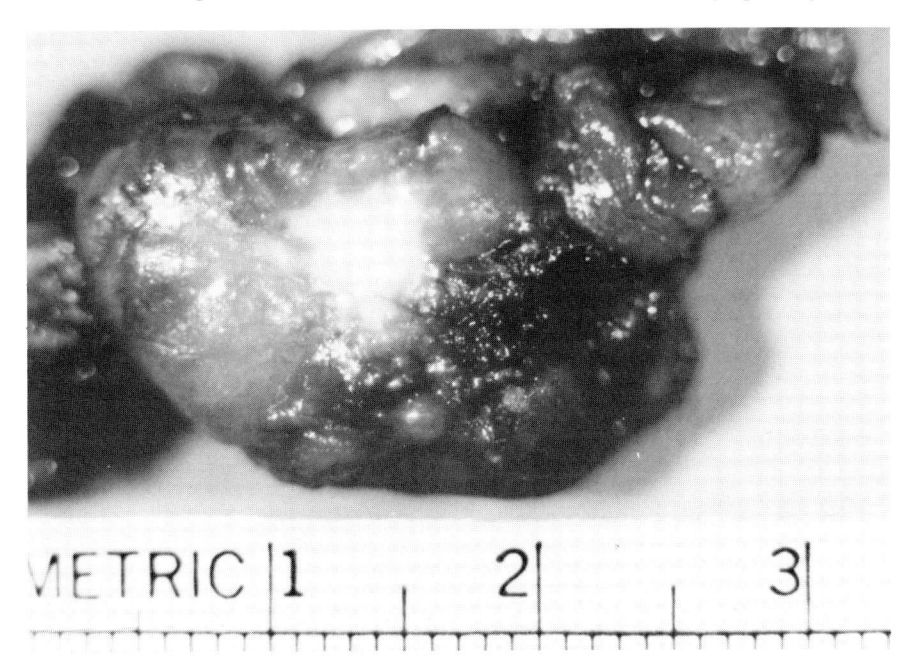

FIGURE 3. The biopsy specimen measured 15 × 16 × 30 mm and contained a firm, grey, well-circumscribed 5 × 8 mm mass consistent with an invasive carcinoma.

6 × 8 mm. The lesion corresponded to the soft tissue density seen in both the preoperative mammogram and specimen radiogram (Fig. 3). The tumor was a well circumscribed invasive duct carcinoma that had a 5 × 8 mm invasive component measured from the microscopic slide (Fig. 4). (We routinely measure the maximum length and width of invasive carcinomas from the specimen radiogram, the gross specimen, and histologic sections on the microscopic slides.) Measurements from these three sources cannot be used interchangeably but do provide a degree of cross-correlation. The invasive carcinoma was well differentiated (Grade I) with good tubular differentiation, no significant nuclear atypia, and a low mitotic count (Fig. 5).

A histogram of the relative nuclear DNA content of the breast cancer revealed a single diploid nuclear DNA peak with a DNA Index of 0.94. Only 3% of the cells had DNA values falling beyond the diploid peak; none had DNA index values > 2 (Fig. 6). Immunochemical staining of the representative section of the Carnoy's-fixed cancer for PCNA/cyclin revealed that 3.5% of the 1000 tumor cell nuclei counted stained positively (Fig. 7). This result corresponded closely to the extimate of cells in S-phase obtained from the nuclear DNA histogram.

The invasive component of the breast cancer was too small to permit conventional cytosol assay for estrogen and progesterone receptor protein levels. Therefore, immunocytochemical staining of formalin-fixed, paraffin-embedded tumor tissue sections was performed with monoclonal antibodies for estrogen and progesterone receptor proteins (Abbott). Positive ER (Fig. 8)

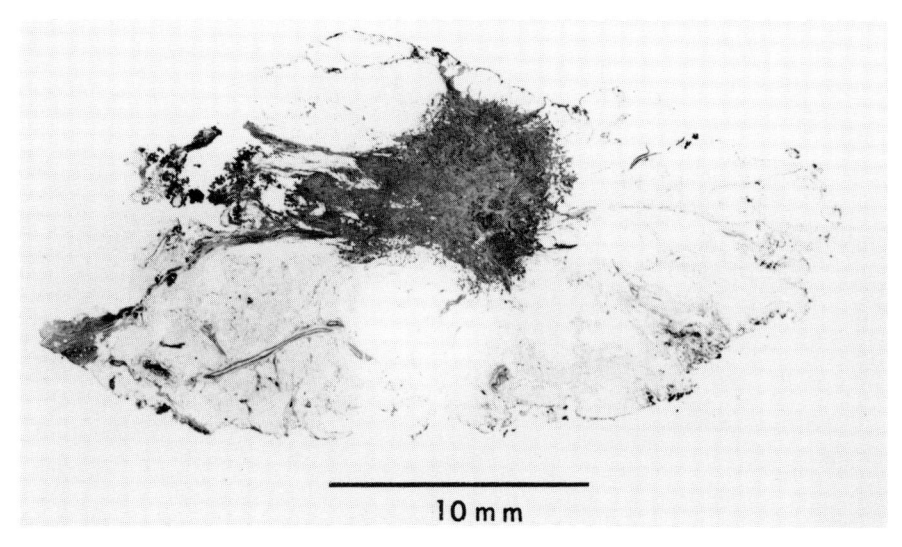

FIGURE 4. Low-power photomicrograph of a cross-section of the biopsy specimen. In this section the invasive carcinoma had a margin of uninvolved tissue, but in deeper sections it extended to the surgical margin.

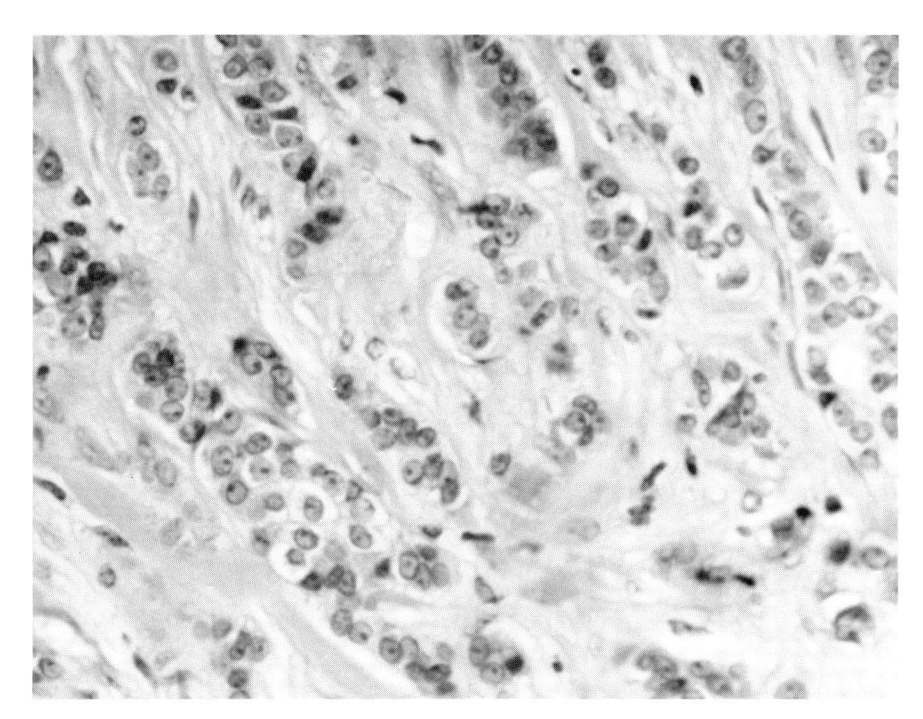

FIGURE 5. Higher power photomicrograph of the invasive duct carcinoma shown in Figure 4. This low-grade carcinoma exhibited good tubular differentiation, minimal nuclear atypia, and only infrequent mitoses in the invasive component. (H & E, negative magnification × 125).

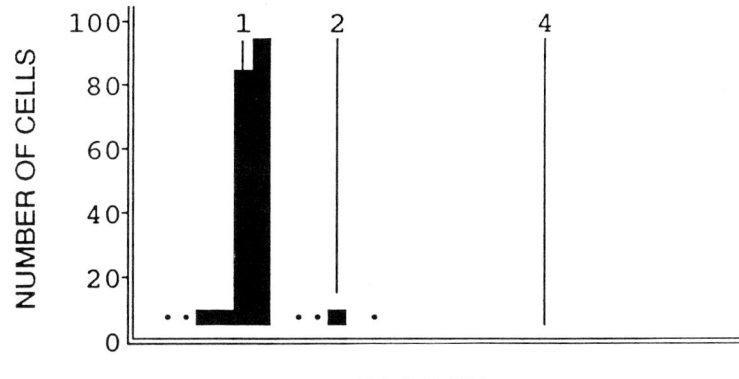

Processing the Small Invasive Carcinoma Detected Mammographically   61

FIGURE 6. Static cytometric nuclear DNA histogram on cells obtained by a touch preparation from the invasive duct carcinoma. The pattern was nuclear DNA diploid (DNA index = 0.94). Fewer than 4% of the tumor cells had nuclear DNA values falling in the range of proliferating diploid cells (S + G_2/M).

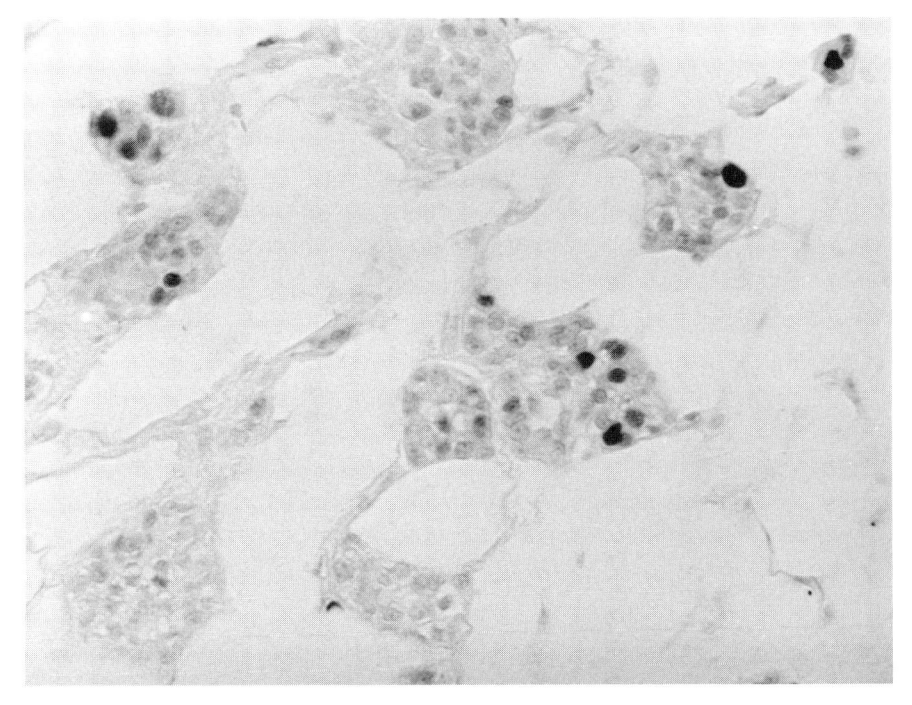

FIGURE 7. The invasive duct carcinoma had a relatively small proliferative component as measured by immunocytochemical staining with a monoclonal antibody to PCNA/cyclin using the peroxidase, anti-peroxidase reaction. The percentage of positive cells (those cells with intense, dark nuclear staining) was less than 4%. This value agrees with the estimate of the percentage of proliferating cells obtained from the nuclear DNA histogram (Negative magnification × 125).

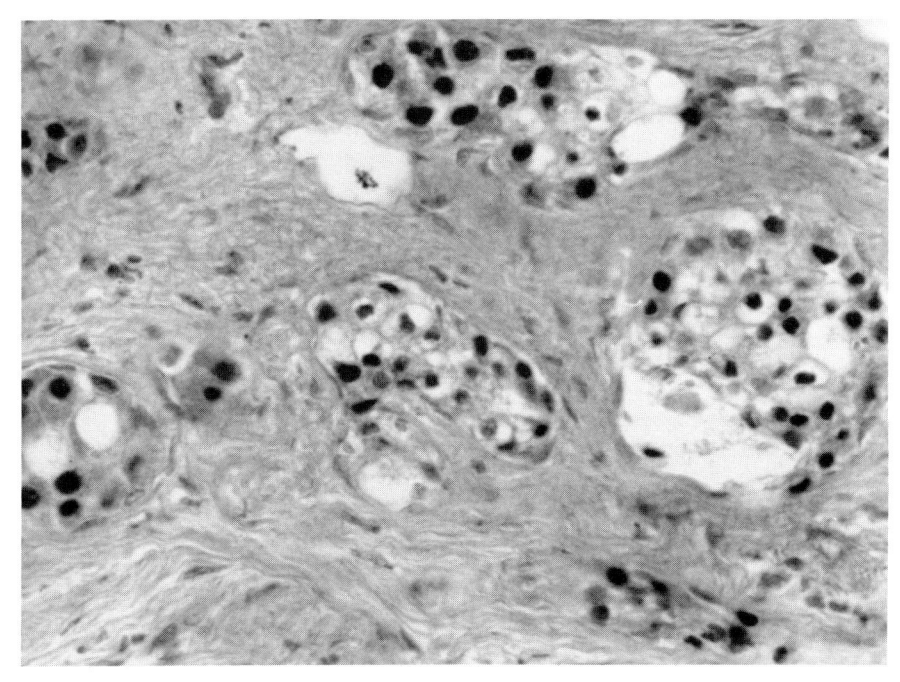

FIGURE 8. The invasive carcinoma was strongly positive for estrogen receptor protein as determined by immunocytochemical staining with a monoclonal antibody to estrogen receptor protein antigen using the alkaline phosphatase, anti-alkaline phosphatase reaction. More than 50% of the invasive cancer cells showed a positive reaction (those cells with intense, dark nuclear staining). (Negative magnification × 125.)

and PR levels were indicated by a strong staining reaction in more than 50% of tumor nuclei.

DISCUSSION AND SUMMARY

In recent years, the use of screening mammography combined with prompt biopsy of mammographically detected suspicious lesions has contributed to a substantial reduction in the size of invasive breast cancers in hospitals with active mammography services. During the same period, a number of new, morphologically based prognostic variables have been identified. Oncologists are coming to rely on these prognostic features for assessing patient prognosis and for helping decide whether or not to use chemotherapy for patients with invasive breast cancer. In this article we have outlined an approach for the handling of mammographically directed breast biopsy specimens that provides for extracting this needed prognostic information from the breast biopsy containing a small invasive carcinoma.

The biopsy chosen to illustrate this approach contained a relatively small invasive duct carcinoma (5 × 8 mm), discovered by mammography. The tumor exhibited a number of favorable prognostic features. It was well differentiated, had a diploid nuclear DNA content, a relative small percentage of proliferating cancer cells, and was positive for estrogen and progesterone receptor protein.

The patient's tumor presented in this case study is fairly typical of well differentiated invasive breast cancers in that all the results of the ancillary prognostic studies were favorable. However, even apparently well differentiated, small invasive breast cancers may exhibit one or more of the following unfavorable prognostic features: (1) aneuploidy, (2) an increased rate of cell proliferation, and (3) negative steroid hormone receptor protein levels (see *"Significance of DNA content and proliferative rate in the invasive carcinoma found in the mammographically directed breast biopsy,"* pp 137–160, this issue).

The classification of an invasive breast cancer as well differentiated, and when the nuclear DNA content is aneuploid, the rate of cell proliferation is high, or the ER and PR levels are negative, should alert the pathologist and oncologist to the possibility of a clinically aggressive tumor. It is most likely that the 20+% of small, low-grade breast cancers that metastasize to axillary lymph nodes and/or distant sites are those that are aneuploid, have unusually high rates of cell proliferation, or are negative for ER and PR in spite of their apparently favorable differentiation.

During the next few years pathologists can expect to be called upon with increasing frequency to extract data on a number of cell cycle, biochemical, and genetic features of breast cancers as a routine part of the specimen examination. Obtaining this information without compromising the histologic diagnosis or losing morphologic-based prognostic information is challenging, particularly with small invasive breast cancers, but is a service pathologists should be able to provide.

References

1. Smart CR, Myers MH, Gloeckler LA: Implications from SEER data on breast cancer management. Cancer 41:787–789, 1978.
2. Fisher B, Slack NH, Bloss JD: Cancer of the breast: Size of neoplasm and prognosis. Cancer 24:1071–1080, 1969.
3. Carter CL, Allen C, Henson DE: Relation of tumor size, lymph node status, and survival in 24.740 breast cancer cases. Cancer 63:181–187, 1989.
4. Nemoto T, Vana J, Bedwanni RN, et al: Management and survival of female breast cancer: Results of a national survey by the American College of Surgeons. Cancer 45:2917–2924, 1980.
5. Kern WH, Mikkelsen WP: Small carcinomas of the breast. Cancer 28:948–955, 1971.
6. Bedwani R, Vana J, Rosner D, et al: Management and survival of female patients with "minimal" breast cancer: As observed in the long-term and short-term surveys of the American College of Surgeons. Cancer 47:2769–2778, 1981.
7. Bloom HJG, Richardson WW: Histological grading and prognosis in breast cancer. A study of 1409 cases of which 359 have been followed for 15 years. Br J Cancer 11:359–377, 1957.
8. Bonadonna G, Brusamolino E, Valagussa P, et al: Combination chemotherapy as an adjuvant treatment in operable cancer. N Engl J Med 292:117–122, 1976.
9. Office of Medical Applications and Research, National Institutes of Health: Consensus Conference: Adjuvant chemotherapy for breast cancer. JAMA 254:3461–3463, 1985.
10. Bonadonna G, Valagussa P, Tancini G, et al: Current status of Milan adjuvant chemotherapy trials for node-positive and node-negative breast cancer. Cancer Res 44:397–400, 1984.
11. Fisher B, Redmond C, Dimitrov A, et al: A randomized clinical trial evaluating sequential methotrexate and fluoracil in the treatment of patients with node-negative breast cancer who have estrogen receptor-negative tumors. N Engl J Med 320:473–478, 1989.

12. Mansour EG, Gray R, Shatila AH: Efficacy of adjuvant chemotherapy in high-risk node-negative breast cancer: An intergorup study. N Engl J Med 320:484–490, 1989.
13. Clinical Alert from the National Cancer Institute, May 18, 1988. Breast Cancer Res Treat 12:305, 1988.
14. Slamon DJ, Clark GM, Wong SG, et al: Human breast cancer: Correlation of relapse and survival with amplification of the HER-2/*neu* oncogene. Science 235:177–182, 1987.
15. Theillet C, Lidereau R, Escott C, et al: Loss of a c-H-*ras*-1 allel and aggressive human primary breast carcinomas. Cancer Res 46:4776–4781, 1986.
16. Fitzpatric SL, Brightwell J, Wittliff JL, et al: Epidermal growth factor binding by breast tumor biopsies and relationship to estrogen receptor and progesterone receptor levels. Cancer Res 44:3448–3453, 1984.
17. Tandon AK, Clark GM, Chamness GC, et al: Cathepsin D and prognosis in breast cancer. N Engl J Med 322:297–302, 1990.
18. Kuhajda FP, Piantadosi S, Pasternack GR: Haptoglobin-related protein (Hpr) epitopes in breast cancer as a predictor of recurrence of the disease. N Engl J Med 321:636–641, 1989.
19. Hedley DW, Friedlander ML, Taylor IW: Application of DNA flow cytometry to paraffin-embedded archival material for the study of aneuploidy and its clinical significance. Cytometry 6:327–333, 1985.
20. Garcia RL, Coltera MD, Gown AM: Analysis of proliferative grade anti-PCNA/Cyclin monoclonal antibodies in fixed, embedded tissues: Comparison with flow cytometric analysis. Am J Pathol 134:733–736, 1989.
21. Mitchell D, Ibrahim S, Gusterson BA: Improved immunohistochemical localization of tissue antigens using modified methacarn fixation. J Histochem Cytochem 33:491–495, 1985.
22. Shintaku P, Said JW: Detection of estrogen receptors with monoclonal antibodies in routinely processed formalin-fixed paraffin sections of breast carcinoma: Use of DNAase pretreatment to enhance sensitivity of the reaction. J Clin Pathol 87:161–167, 1987.
23. Cheng L, Binder SW, Fu YS, Lenin KJ: Demonstration of estrogen receptor by monoclonal antibody in formalin-fixed breast tumors. Lab Invest 58:346–383, 1988.
24. Brastein S, Fruchter R, Greene GL, Pertschuk CP: Immunochemical assay of progesterone receptors in paraffin-embedded specimens of endometrial carcinoma and hyperplasia: A preliminary evaluation. Modern Pathol 2:449–455, 1989.

In Situ Proliferative Epithelial Lesions of the Breast

ONSI W. KAMEL, M.D.
RICHARD L. KEMPSON, M.D.
MICHAEL R. HENDRICKSON, M.D.

From Department of Pathology
Stanford University Medical Center
Stanford, California

Reprint requests to:
Richard L. Kempson, M.D.
Department of Pathology
Stanford University Medical Center
300 Pasteur Drive
Stanford, CA 94305

Considerable progress has been made over the last several years toward understanding the significance of noninvasive epithelial changes in the breast. This progress, in essence, is the result of categorizing in situ alterations according to their clinical significance, or more specifically, according to the risk that such lesions carry to the patient for the development of a subsequent invasive carcinoma. Morphologic definitions, based on this risk, have been provided for the now commonly used diagnostic categories of nonproliferative fibrocystic change, proliferative fibrocystic change, atypical hyperplasia (both ductal and lobular), and carcinoma in situ (including subtypes). We should apply these morphologic definitions when formulating our day-to-day interpretations of breast specimens.

This article summarizes the histopathological criteria that are currently used to define the above-named morphologic categories and, perhaps more importantly, it reviews the clinical implications of the diagnoses that result from this categorization. Moreover, an effort has been made to address diagnostic problem areas that are frequently encountered by practicing surgical pathologists based on our own experience and based on problems that we are frequently asked to address in our consultation practice. The introduction summarizes certain general concepts that pertain to this area of breast pathology, and this introduction is followed by a discussion of each morphologic category, with an emphasis on the definitional histologic features, differential diagnosis, and the clinical implications of each diagnosis.

GENERAL CONCEPTS

The Morphologic Continuum of In Situ Proliferative Epithelial Lesions

The problem of neatly separating the histologic patterns of in situ breast changes into the categories of nonproliferative fibrocystic change, proliferative fibrocystic change, atypical hyperplasia, and in situ carcinoma using morphologic criteria is complicated by the gradual histologic continuum that exists between nonproliferative fibrocystic change on the one extreme and in situ carcinoma on the other. There are no sharp discontinuities in appearance to provide natural divisions along this continuum. As a consequence, the boundaries between diagnostic categories that lie next to one another along the continuum must be considered somewhat arbitrary. Lesions that have all the characteristic morphologic features to place them in the center of the named category will be designated as such by most pathologists familiar with the definitional criteria used to subdivide the continuum. As might be expected, borderline changes (lesions that lie near or on the border between two categories) may be interpreted differently, even by pathologists who routinely examine difficult in situ lesions. A difference of opinion about borderline changes along the morphologic continuum should lead only to an adjustment in the risk status, not significant differences in therapy, because patients with borderline lesions generally are managed conservatively. An effort also should be made to provide standardization and reproducibility in order to avoid the situation in which two observers place the same case in widely separated portions of the continuum, i.e., one interprets it as proliferative fibrocystic change and the other as carcinoma in situ. To this end, familiarity with definitional histologic criteria for these processes cannot be overemphasized. The result of not adhering to the same criteria can be found in the recent report of Rosai, in which considerable variation in interpretation of in situ proliferative lesions was found among experienced surgical pathologists.[31a]

Relative Risk and Absolute Risk

The clinical significance of the in situ epithelial changes that occur in the breast is derived from studies that have demonstrated an increased risk for the subsequent development of invasive carcinoma when certain morphologic patterns are present in a breast specimen. The magnitude of increased risk is conveyed by the term relative risk. The relative risk (RR) is defined as the incidence of a particular observation (invasive breast cancer) in a certain study population (for example, women with biopsies showing florid [significant] epithelial hyperplasia) divided by the incidence of the observation in a certain reference population. Thus, if the incidence of invasive breast cancer in the

TABLE 1. Relative Risk for Invasive Breast Carcinoma Based on Pathologic Examination of Breast Tissue Without Carcinoma*

No increased risk	
Mild sclerosing adenosis	Mild epithelial hyperplasia
Apocrine metaplasia	Fibroadenoma
Apocrine hyperplasia	Solitary papilloma
Cysts, macro and/or micro	Mastitis
Duct dilatation	Periductal mastitis
Fibrosis	Squamous metaplasia
Slightly increased risk (1.5 to 2 times)	
Moderate or florid ductal hyperplasia	
Florid sclerosing adenosis	
Moderately increased risk (4 to 5 times)	
Atypical hyperplasia, ductal or lobular	
High risk (8 to 10 times)	
Lobular carcinoma in situ	
Ductal carcinoma in situ (noncomedo)	

* Modified from Page DL: Risk factors for breast cancer in women with proliferative breast disease. Hum Pathol 17:871–874, 1986.

study population is 20 per 1000 per year and the incidence in the reference population is 10 per 1000 per year, then the study population has a relative risk of 2 for developing invasive cancer. Table 1 presents a summary of the relative risk for a patient to develop invasive breast carcinoma based on morphologic changes in a breast biopsy.

It is important to realize that the RR figure, in and of itself, provides little specific information for individual patient management. If a particular lesion is associated with a RR of 2 for developing invasive carcinoma, that information is not clinically useful without knowing the incidence of invasive carcinoma in the reference population. For example, if the incidence of invasive carcinoma in the reference population is 1 in one million, a RR of 2 has negligible clinical consequences for the individual patient. Because the incidence of breast cancer in the general population varies significantly among various age groups, the clinical significance of a certain RR is strongly dependent on the patient's age at the time of diagnosis. Moreover, because the studies that have reported RRs for various breast lesions have included patients clustered around certain age groups (usually 30 to 60 years), and because they have followed patients for a defined period of time (approximately 15 years), RR figures ideally should be applied within these confines.[27b]

The statistic that most clearly defines the clinical significance of a particular lesion to the individual patient is the absolute risk. This complex statistic is dependent on the RR, the age-specific risk for invasive cancer in the baseline population, the patient's current age, and the patient's competing mortal risk from all other causes.[9] While the determination of absolute risk requires sophisticated mathematics and is not readily applicable to the management of the individual patient, the concept of absolute risk stresses the importance of considering factors other than histologic features when determining the clinical implications of a diagnosis for the patient. Indeed, it must be kept foremost in one's mind that, in this area of breast pathology, a certain histologic diagnosis does not, and should not, always lead to a particular therapeutic intervention.

Precursor Lesions Versus Histologic Markers of Increased Risk

There is an important (and often not well understood) difference between a precursor lesion and a lesion that represents a marker of increased risk for the development of invasive carcinoma. If a lesion is considered to be a precursor, the implication is that, over a specified period of time and in a certain percentage of cases, the lesion will develop into an invasive carcinoma. This has certain important implications regarding treatment. Precursor lesions that give rise to invasive cancer with sufficiently high frequency should be completely excised (to prevent the development of invasive cancer); on the other hand, if a lesion is considered to represent only a marker of increased risk for developing invasive cancer, such a lesion is more akin to a positive family history for breast cancer. Completely excising such a lesion will not erase the risk that such a lesion carries for the subsequent development of breast cancer in the remaining breast tissue. The only two sensible therapeutic options for patients with markers for increased risk for the development of invasive cancer are careful follow-up or removal of all breast tissue.

The group of lesions considered by most investigators to represent a precursor to invasive carcinoma is ductal carcinoma in situ (DCIS). This conclusion has been made more from "guilt by association" than from direct evidence and is primarily based on studies that have shown that a certain percentage of patients with a biopsy showing DCIS will develop invasive carcinoma in the same area of the breast at a later time. The implication is that a part of the in situ lesion was not excised and acted as the precursor for the invasive cancer. However, DCIS, at least of the cribriform or micropapillary types, is not an obligate precursor lesion, because only 25% of women with this lesion develop invasive carcinoma if treatment is no more than simple biopsy.[29] Another way of expressing this is that 75% of patients with cribriform or micropapillary DCIS will not develop invasive carcinoma after biopsy.

Lesions that are currently considered only markers of increased risk rather than precursor lesions include atypical ductal hyperplasia, atypical lobular hyperplasia, and lobular carcinoma in situ (LCIS). Although the presence of these lesions in a breast biopsy places a woman at increased risk for developing invasive carcinoma, both breasts are equally at risk. This fact suggests these changes do not give rise to invasive cancer but rather are morphologic expressions of a state of increased risk. As mentioned above, attempting to completely excise such a lesion does not erase its clinical implications for the patient's remaining breast tissue.

Histologic Appearance Versus Histogenesis

Although considerable time and energy have been invested into dividing in situ and invasive lesions into ductal and lobular types, these designations are based on morphologic appearance and do not necessarily imply histogenesis.

In fact, the morphologic evidence of Wellings and co-workers[46a] has demonstrated that these two morphologic classes of proliferations both appear to have as their site of origin the terminal ductular-lobular unit. Such information should console practicing pathologists who encounter in situ or invasive lesions that seem to demonstrate features of both the lobular and ductal types of lesions. However, one must also keep in mind that the designation of a particular lesion as ductal or lobular based on its morphologic appearance carries certain clinical implications with regard to unilaterality versus bilaterality and "precursor versus marker," regardless of whether or not such lesions share a similar histogenesis.

NONPROLIFERATIVE AND PROLIFERATIVE FIBROCYSTIC CHANGE

The term fibrocystic change encompasses a number of morphologic patterns that can be seen in their most florid state in women who present with nodular or "lumpy" breasts, or, less frequently, in patients who present with a dominant breast mass. However, lesser degrees of these morphologic changes occur in almost all breasts during the reproductive years. Consequently, fibrocystic *change* has replaced the term fibrocystic disease,[18] because the histopathological features of the fibrocystic complex are so common as to be considered normal. The designations of **nonproliferative** fibrocystic change and **proliferative** fibrocystic change have become well accepted in the last several years and are quite useful from a pathologic and clinical standpoint. These two designations allow the pathologist to communicate a set of pathologic findings to the patient's physician and at the same time to indicate whether or not the patient is at a slightly increased risk for developing invasive carcinoma (proliferative fibrocystic change) or not at any risk (nonproliferative fibrocystic change). The distinction between the two entities is based on the presence and extent of epithelial hyperplasia and, more recently, on the presence of extensive sclerosing adenosis.

As has been recommended by the Cancer Committee of the College of American Pathologists,[18] the surgical pathology report should specify the component features whenever the diagnosis of fibrocystic change is made. The histologic features of nonproliferative fibrocystic change (lesions that do not indicate an increased risk for the patient to develop carcinoma) are well known and include fibrosis, duct dilatation, cysts, apocrine change, microglandular adenosis, and mild epithelial hyperplasia. Sclerosing adenosis has historically been included as part of the nonproliferative fibrocystic change complex and, if present in a mild form, should be so included. A recent report by Jensen et al.,[19] however, indicates that when sclerosing adenosis is florid, it carries the risk implications of proliferative fibrocystic change (see below). Moderate and florid ductal epithelial hyperplasia are definitional for proliferative fibrocystic change and imply a slightly increased risk for developing a subsequent invasive carcinoma (see section on ductal hyperplasia). The features of fibrocystic change are well presented in standard texts[2a,27a] and so the following comments will be limited to conceptual, histologic, and clinical aspects of each of the components of the fibrocystic complex that have changed in recent years.

Sclerosing Adenosis

Sclerosing adenosis denotes an increased number of terminal ductules, resulting in enlargement of the lobules, and is associated with fibrosis (sclerosis), which causes varying degrees of distortion of the enlarged lobules. The process can vary from a trivial microscopic focus to one that involves large areas of the breast. Features that help identify sclerosing adenosis are the sharply marginated lobular configuration of the process, the cord-like ducts, the double row of cells often lining the terminal ducts, and the bland nuclear features of the cells (Fig. 1).

There are conflicting reports in the literature as to whether sclerosing adenosis is a risk factor for invasive carcinoma or not. A recent study by Jensen et al.[19] examined this problem. The authors accepted only "well-developed" examples of sclerosing adenosis, which they defined as lesions with "increased numbers of deformed, sclerotic glandular elements in a lobulocentric array approximately double the size of adjacent 'normal' lobular units." In addition the individual lobular units must have at least 50% of their acini involved by the sclerosing process. When sclerosing adenosis was so defined, they found it carried a relative risk of approximately 2 for subsequent invasive carcinoma, even in the absence of any significant epithelial hyperplasia. Based on these findings the authors included sclerosing adenosis among the lesions of proliferative fibrocystic change. In our practice the breast biopsy that contains well-developed sclerosing adenosis is reported as florid sclerosing adenosis, and we indicate that this lesion may place the patient at a slightly increased risk for the development of carcinoma, referencing the above study.

Distinguishing sclerosing adenosis from carcinoma, particularly tubular carcinoma, is the main differential diagnostic consideration. The sharply circumscribed margins and the maintenance of the lobular architecture, as well as the cord-like ducts with closed lumens, are very useful in this regard. In situ carcinoma, both lobular[13] and ductal, as well as atypical hyperplasia can involve sclerosing adenosis, and the presence of abnormal cells in sclerosing adenosis often brings up the problem of invasive carcinoma (Fig. 1). Careful examination of the biopsy, looking for features of carcinoma in situ or atypical hyperplasia elsewhere, is helpful, as is the architecture of sclerosing adenosis that includes the absence of raggedly infiltrating carcinoma cells.

Microglandular Adenosis

This rare type of adenosis features increased numbers of dilated terminal ductules resembling acini or glands randomly arranged without a lobular pattern.[8,32,39,44] The involved glandular elements often contain luminal eosinophilic material. The lining cells are cuboidal, bland, and may occasionally have

---

FIGURE 1 *(opposite page).* An example of "well-developed" sclerosing adenosis featuring a lobular configuration (top) with deformed, sclerotic glandular elements forming cord-like ducts, double row of cells and bland nuclear features (middle). Involvement of sclerosing adenosis by ductal carcinoma in situ (bottom) may mimic infiltrating ductal carcinoma.

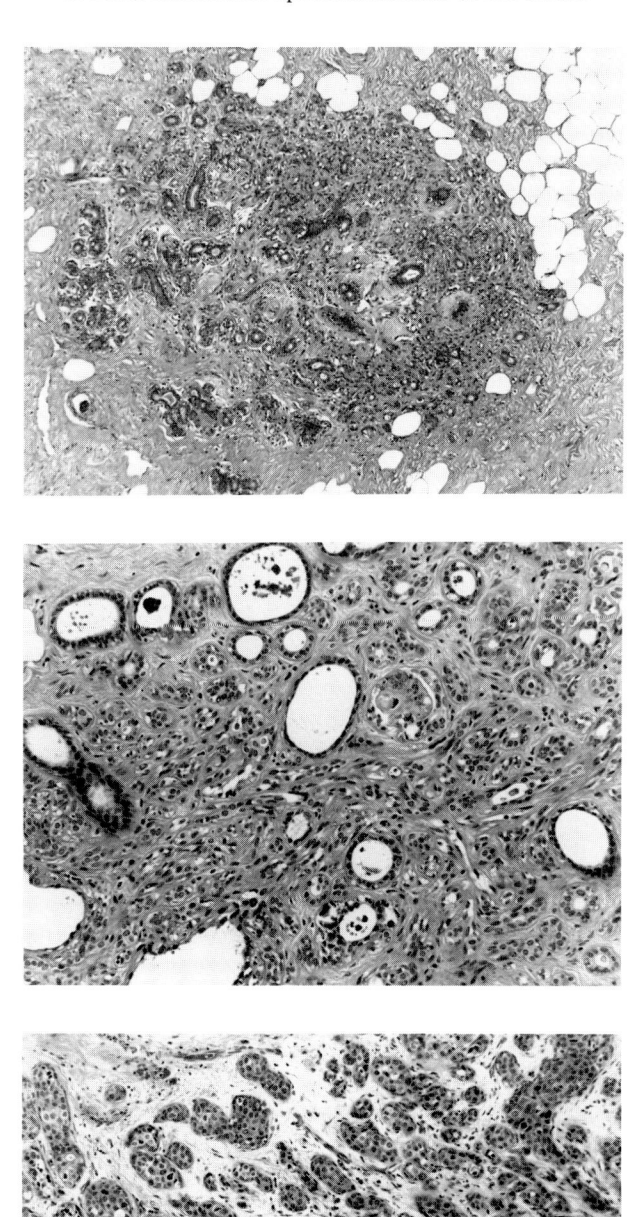

In Situ Proliferative Epithelial Lesions of the Breast

clear cytoplasm. They do not demonstrate significant nuclear pleomorphism. It is this cytologic blandness that helps identify the lesion and distinguishes it from ductal carcinoma. The main differential diagnostic consideration is tubular carcinoma, which is characterized by a low-power stellate architecture with the often pointed neoplastic tubules with gaping lumens set in a dense fibrous stroma. **Blunt duct adenosis** is a phrase sometimes used to describe adenosis in which the terminal ducts are dilated but retain their lobular architecture.

Apocrine Metaplasia and Apocrine Hyperplasia

Apocrine metaplasia is a well recognized component of fibrocystic change in which the cells in some of the ducts display abundant eosinophilic cytoplasm, and they may have apical "snouts." The nuclei of these cells may be small and bland or may be slightly enlarged with prominent nucleoli. In apocrine hyperplasia, these same apocrine cells pile up to the extent that they form two or more cell layers around the duct periphery or form small tufts that may occasionally bridge the duct lumen. Apocrine hyperplasia may also have a papillary architecture in which the apocrine cells line small, thin fibrovascular stalks. Apocrine proliferations, with or without a papillary architecture, may feature cells with enlarged nuclei, nuclear pleomorphism, and prominent nucleoli, and they frequently cause the observer concern. It is important to establish that such lesions are indeed apocrine, a feature that is usually evident once the cells in question are compared with other nonapocrine ductal cells in the same breast-biopsy specimen.

The finding of apocrine metaplasia in a breast biopsy does not place a woman at an increased risk for developing subsequent invasive carcinoma.[31] A recent study of atypical ductal hyperplasia by Tavassoli and Norris[45] also investigated the significance of apocrine lesions and found that neither apocrine metaplasia nor apocrine hyperplasia place women at increased risk for the development of breast cancer. The clinical significance of atypical in situ apocrine lesions has not been well studied, and there are, to our knowledge, no data about the RR that results from their presence in a breast biopsy.

Mild Ductal Hyperplasia and Lobular Hyperplasia

Mild hyperplasia is defined by a proliferation of cells in dilated ducts, to the extent that they are at least 3 cells high but less than 8 to 10 cells high (the latter is the minimal definition for moderate hyperplasia). Since mild hyperplasia has no significance to the patient, it is often called **insignificant hyperplasia** in comparison to moderate or florid (significant) hyperplasia.

It should be noted that the term **epithelial hyperplasia,** as is commonly used, usually refers to a ductal process. A category of lobular hyperplasia, in which the cells found in atypical lobular hyperplasia and lobular carcinoma in situ are present in increased numbers but without filling or expansion of lobular units, may be used. However, the RR associated with such changes is largely unknown.

Moderate and Florid Ductal Hyperplasia

The minimal criteria for moderate hyperplasia is stratification of ductal cells greater than 8 to 10 layers high. The ducts are dilated and the proliferating cells often cross the lumen (Fig. 2). We require stratification of more than 10 cells high and crossing of the lumen before making a diagnosis of florid hyperplasia. Moderate and florid hyperplasia define proliferative fibrocystic change and distinguishing between them is of no clinical importance.

The cells in ductal hyperplasia (whether mild or florid) typically display small, bland, oval-to-elongate nuclei with delicate nuclear chromatin and indistinct cell margins. The cells tend to flow and stream in the same direction, and they often appear to overlap one another. These features may be contrasted with the criteria for atypical hyperplasia and carcinoma in situ, discussed below.

Clinical Implications

Until the study of Page et al.,[31] the risk associated with a benign breast biopsy that did not contain proliferative lesions remained poorly defined in most studies, because the individual morphologic features making up fibrocystic change were not separately analyzed. The results of these authors' 1978 study showed that cysts, fibrosis, and other nonhyperplastic lesions did not put a patient at increased risk for breast cancer if these lesions alone were found in a breast biopsy.[31] Mild hyperplasia is a feature of nonproliferative fibrocystic change, because its presence does not result in an increased risk for the development of invasive breast carcinoma. Moderate-to-florid ductal hyperplasia defines proliferative fibrocystic change, and this change is associated with a 1.5 to 2 times increased risk to the patient for developing a subsequent carcinoma, a risk too low to warrant any clinical action except careful follow-up. There is no difference in cancer risk between moderate and more florid examples of hyperplasia, and, if diagnostic pathologists prefer, both can be incorporated into the term "significant hyperplasia." We prefer moderate and florid hyperplasia, because "significant hyperplasia" may not be generally understood.

Although there are current data supporting the inclusion of florid sclerosing adenosis among the proliferative fibrocystic change lesions,[19] we prefer to reserve the designation of proliferative fibrocystic change for lesions with moderate-to-florid epithelial hyperplasia, and we still report florid sclerosing adenosis as such.

There are no clinical data to justify separating lobular hyperplasia into florid, moderate, and mild types.

ATYPICAL DUCTAL AND ATYPICAL LOBULAR HYPERPLASIA

Page et al. have defined atypical hyperplasia as having "some but not all" of the features of carcinoma in situ.[30] This definition is used for both atypical lobular and atypical ductal hyperplasia. Because we use the outcome information derived from their studies to determine risk, we use their definition. It appears that these authors apply the term "atypical hyperplasia" to lesions that most of us would classify as severely atypical, i.e., lesions that just fall short of cribriform carcinoma in situ. There is little or no information about the relative risk of "minimal atypia" or "moderate atypia" versus atypical hyperplasia, as Page has defined it. It is our impression that the diagnosis of atypical hyperplasia is used more liberally in practice than it has been in the published studies of clinical follow-up of proliferative breast lesions. Specifically, Page and co-workers classified only 3.6% of over 10,000 benign breast biopsies as containing atypical ductal or atypical lobular hyperplasia. If we are too liberal in identifying atypia, our personal categories of atypical hyperplasia will lack comparability with the published data on such lesions. Another reason to explain excess use of the label atypical may relate to the Black-Chabon scale,[4,5] which grades atypia from 1 to 5 (on a scale in which grade 5 equals carinoma in situ) and thus includes mild, moderate, and severe forms. If one wishes to identify those lesions with the level of increased risk equal to the risk Page et al. reported for atypical hyperplasia, then only the high grade Black-Chabon lesions that share some, but not all, of the features of carcinoma in situ should be included in the atypical category.

As noted, atypical ductal hyperplasia is set apart from florid epithelial hyperplasia by the presence of at least some of the features of cribriform or micropapillary DCIS. In our practice we require the cytologic changes of cribriform/micropapillary DCIS to be present (in duct spaces that lack the full architectural features of DCIS) before diagnosing atypical hyperplasia, because it is the cytologic features that set atypical ductal hyperplasia apart from hyperplasia of the usual type. The diagnosis of atypical ductal hyperplasia rather than DCIS is made when there is: (1) involvement of less than the entire duct spaces by the characteristic architectural and cytologic changes of DCIS, or (2) involvement of less than two duct spaces by the characteristic cytologic and architectural changes of cribriform/micropapillary DCIS.

Recently Tavassoli and Norris[45] reported a study of ductal hyperplasia and atypical ductal hyperplasia in which they slightly modified the criteria of Page et al. in an effort to provide a more "precise" definition of atypical hyperplasia. In their study, the diagnosis of atypical ductal hyperplasia was made when: (1) the proliferating cells displayed the cytologic features but lacked the full architectural features of cribriform/micropapillary DCIS, or (2) all the features of cribriform/micropapillary DCIS were present, but the involved ducts/ductules measured less than 2 mm in aggregate dimension. They used the latter requirement because they concluded that the phrase "some but not all" was too vague and that the two-duct minimum criterion used by Page et al. was too restrictive (i.e., if DCIS involves only a single duct

---

FIGURE 2 *(opposite page).* Florid ductal hyperplasia features dilated ducts with stratification of epithelial cells greater than 10 cells high and crossing of the duct lumen (top). The cells of ductal hyperplasia display small, bland, oval nuclei with indistinct cell margins; the cells tend to flow in the same direction or overlap one another (bottom).

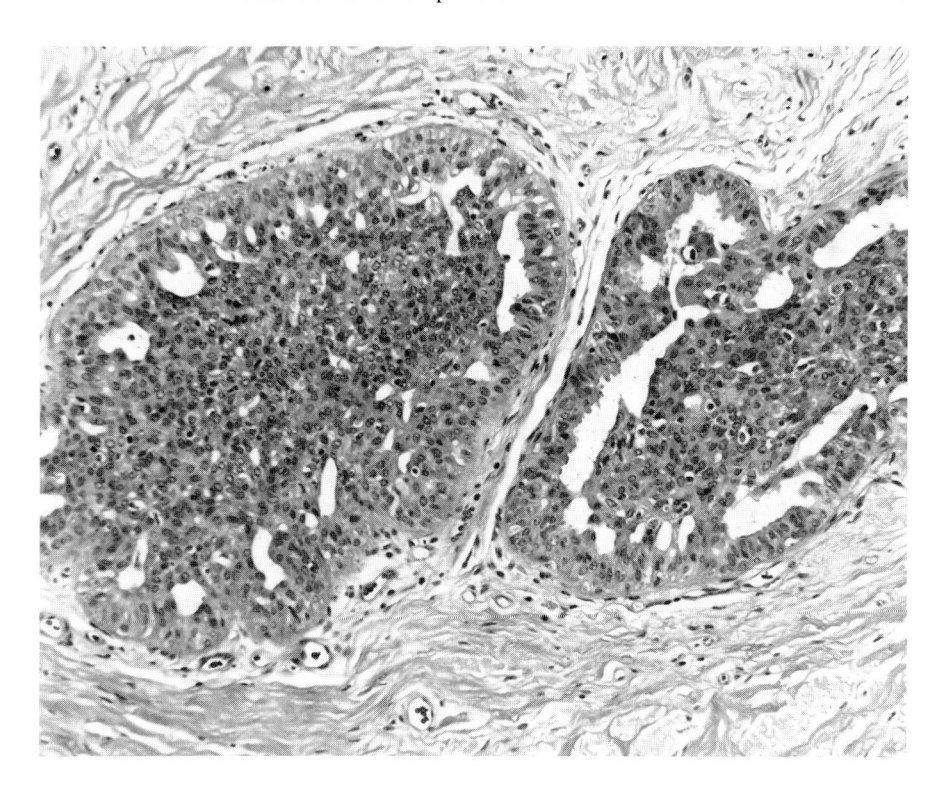

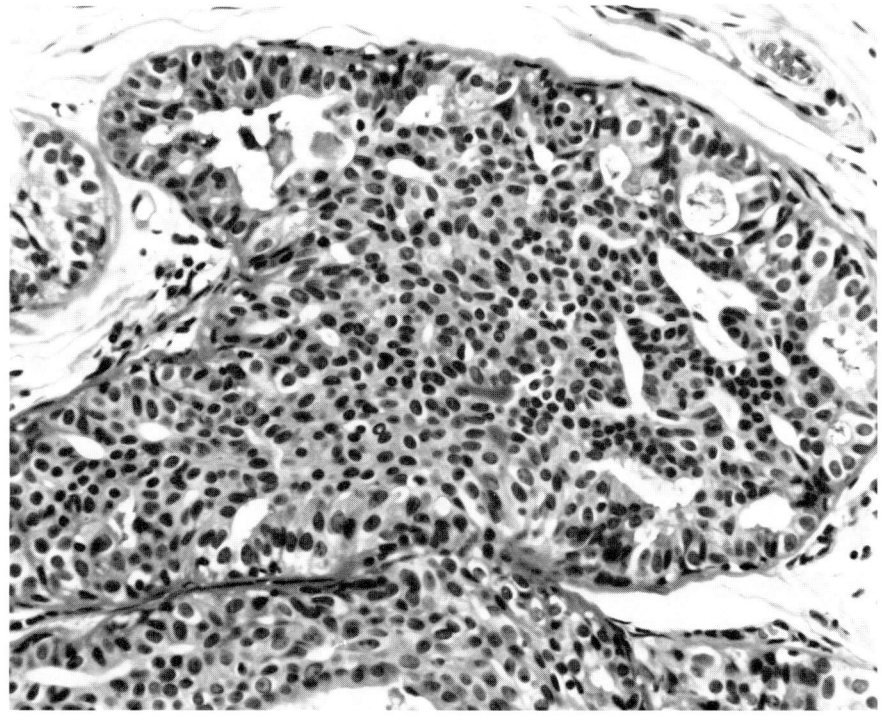

In Situ Proliferative Epithelial Lesions of the Breast

but that duct expands to more than 2 mm in diameter, such a lesion would be designated DCIS by their definition). Unfortunately, instructions about how to measure the area of involvement are not provided. In spite of this, we think the data support using a volume requirement in addition to the cytologic and architectural requirements to diagnose cribriform in situ carcinoma. Tavassoli and Norris emphasized that the cytologic features of atypical ductal hyperplasia are those seen in cribriform/micropapillary DCIS, and as noted we agree this diagnosis should not be made unless at least some of the cells within the ducts show cytologic features of cribriform/micropapillary DCIS.

Atypical lobular hyperplasia is diagnosed instead of lobular hyperplasia when uniform cells characteristic of lobular carcinoma in situ fill some but not all of terminal ductules (acini) in a lobule, or they fill all the lobular units but do not expand at least half of them.

Clinical Implications

An increased risk for invasive breast carcinoma with atypical in situ proliferative lesions was reported by Black et al.[4] in 1972 for patients with benign breast biopsies with grade 3 or 4 atypia. Kodlin et al.[21] also using the Black-Chabon grading system, found that women with grade 4 atypia in benign breast biopsies had an RR of six times that of an age-matched population. Hutchinson et al.[17] also reported that atypical epithelial proliferative lesions in benign breast biopsies place the patient at increased risk to develop a subsequent invasive carcinoma.

The most elaborate follow-up study to date of benign breast disease is the 1985 study of Dupont and Page.[10] This study documented that patients with significant atypical hyperplasia of either the ducts or lobules, as defined above, had a risk 4.4 times as great for developing subsequent invasive carcinoma as the general population for women their age, and 5.3 times as great as that for women whose breast biopsies showed only nonproliferative fibrocystic change. Women with a biopsy displaying atypical hyperplasia and a family history of an immediate relative with breast carcinoma had a risk elevated to 8.9 times that of the general population and 11 times that of women who had neither of these two features. Tavassoli and Norris,[45] using the somewhat different definition of atypical hyperplasia described above, essentially confirm Dupont and Page's risk estimates.

It is important to realize that atypical hyperplasia, whether ductal or lobular, results in an increased risk to both breasts[30] and that the risk from these lesions decreases with time from diagnosis.[11] When the cells of atypical lobular hyperplasia extend from the terminal ductules to involve the larger ducts, Page et al. found the risk for subsequent carcinoma to be intermediate between that for atypical lobular hyperplasia and that for LCIS.[28]

DUCTAL CARCINOMA IN SITU

Ductal carcinoma in situ does not represent a single, uniform morphologic entity, but a spectrum of lesions that ranges from the single microscopic focus of cribriform/micropapillary DCIS in the setting of proliferative fibrocystic change to widespread ductal involvement and cancerization of lobules by comedo-type DCIS that may be visible as a mass lesion.[15] We divide the DCIS spectrum into four major histologic types: (1) cribriform/micropapillary DCIS, (2) intraductal (intracystic) papillary carcinoma, (3) solid-type DCIS, and (4) comedo DCIS. The features that define the histologic types of DCIS are: architecture, cytology, and the presence or absence of necrosis. However, as is almost always the case for morphologic entities, there is overlap between these. The intraductal (intracystic) papillary carcinoma is discussed after the other types of in situ carcinoma, because information about its RR has not been as fully evaluated as the other types of in situ carcinoma.

It is becoming increasingly clear that the histopathologic characteristics of DCIS and the extent of involvement of the breast by the process are important features that define the biologic potential of DCIS lesions.[23,24,24a,42] Thus, it is perhaps more clinically relevant to consider the DCIS spectrum as consisting of low, intermediate, and high-grade lesions. DCIS grade is assessed predominantly on the basis of cytologic features and, to a lesser extent, on the presence or absence of necrosis. Low-grade DCIS lesions are those without cytologically malignant cells and with little or no necrosis and include the following histologic categories: cribriform, micropapillary, papillary, and some solid DCIS lesions. High-grade DCIS is defined by cytologically malignant cells and necrosis, i.e., comedo-type DCIS. Intermediate-grade DCIS is composed of cells with cytologic features intermediate between those of cribriform DCIS and comedo DCIS. While these are often solid lesions, they may have papillary or microacinar architecture with variable amounts of necrosis. The concept of "grade of DCIS" is evolving from clinicopathologic studies that indicate a difference in the biologic behavior of various types of DCIS lesions; these studies are helping to clarify some of the confusion associated with the carcinoma in situ diagnosis.[20] The pathologist should therefore be familiar with the spectrum of DCIS, the histologic categories within this spectrum, the biologic potential of the lesions (based on the grade and extent of the process), and the clinical implications of the diagnosis.

Ductal Carcinoma In Situ of the Cribriform/Micropapillary Type

The cribriform and micropapillary patterns of DCIS are considered together because they are commonly present in the same biopsy, sometimes in the same duct, and because the constituent cells may be identical. Because the constituent cells are not cytologically malignant, we think it important that both the architectural and cytologic features described should be present before making a diagnosis of this type of intraductal carcinoma.

Cribriform DCIS is histologically defined as dilated ducts filled with or lined by a stratified population of monotonous cells arranged around cleanly punched out spaces. These spaces have also been described as supported by rigid bars of cells giving rise to a "crisp" punched out or "Roman bridges" appearance. The cells (particularly the nuclei) distinctly stand apart from each other. Cytologically, the cells may be one of two types. One type is characterized by rather enlarged nuclei with fairly abundant, eosinophilic cytoplasm and distinct borders. The nuclei are round and often contain a small but conspicuous nucleolus. The other type of cells are smaller and their nuclei have dense, often clumped chromatin and inconspicuous nucleoli. Cell margins may not be distinct in the latter cells (Fig. 3). These two cell types are in sharp contrast to the elongate or oval, streaming and overlapping cells with evenly distributed chromatin that are typically found in ductal hyperplasia.

Micropapillary DCIS (clinging carcinoma of Azzopardi) features dilated ducts lined by a few layers of uniform cells that focally stratify to form finger-like or club-shaped protuberances with bulbous ends, which extend into the dilated lumen. The cells may form arches against the duct wall. The protruding structures do not contain fibrovascular cores and are composed of the same cell type that lines the rest of the duct. The constituent cells of this lesion typically are the smaller cells with less cytoplasm containing basophilic, dense nuclei with inconspicuous nucleoli (Fig. 4).

In both cribriform and micropapillary lesions, necrosis is usually not present, and if it is present it is inconspicuous. Mitotic figures are usually sparse. Table 2 contrasts epithelial hyperplasia with DCIS of the cribriform type.

The minimal criteria for the diagnosis of cribriform DCIS are at least two, and preferably more, dilated duct spaces lined completely by a uniform population of one or the other abnormal cell types described above arranged in the required architectural patterns. Lesions that have the cytologic features of cribriform DCIS but not the architectural features required for the diagnosis are placed in the category of atypical ductal hyperplasia. We think the *quantity* requirements of Page et al. and Tavassoli and Norris are very important and should be observed (because only those lesions that fulfill the quantity requirements result in the risk associated with ductal carcinoma in situ; see section on atypical hyperplasia.) Cribriform micropapillary lesions that otherwise qualify for in situ cribriform carcinoma but are less than 2 mm in aggregate dimension (and which nearly always involve less than two duct spaces) are designated **atypical ductal hyperplasia.** Cribriform/micropapillary lesions with cytologic and architectural features of in situ cribriform carcinoma greater than 2 mm in aggregate dimension (and which nearly always involve greater than two duct spaces) are designated **DCIS of the cribriform/micropapillary type.**

Ductal Carcinoma In Situ of the Comedo Type

Comedo-type DCIS represents the high-grade extreme of the in situ proliferative epithelial process, and, as is more fully discussed below, manifests qualities associated with cancer. It likely represents an in situ process that

---

FIGURE 3 *(opposite page).* Cribriform ductal carcinoma in situ with "crisp" punched out spaces or spaces supported by "rigid bars of cells." The constituent cells may display small nuclei with dense, often clumped chromatin and inconspicuous nucleoli (top) or may display fairly abundant cytoplasm with rather enlarged nuclei and small but conspicuous nucleoli (bottom).

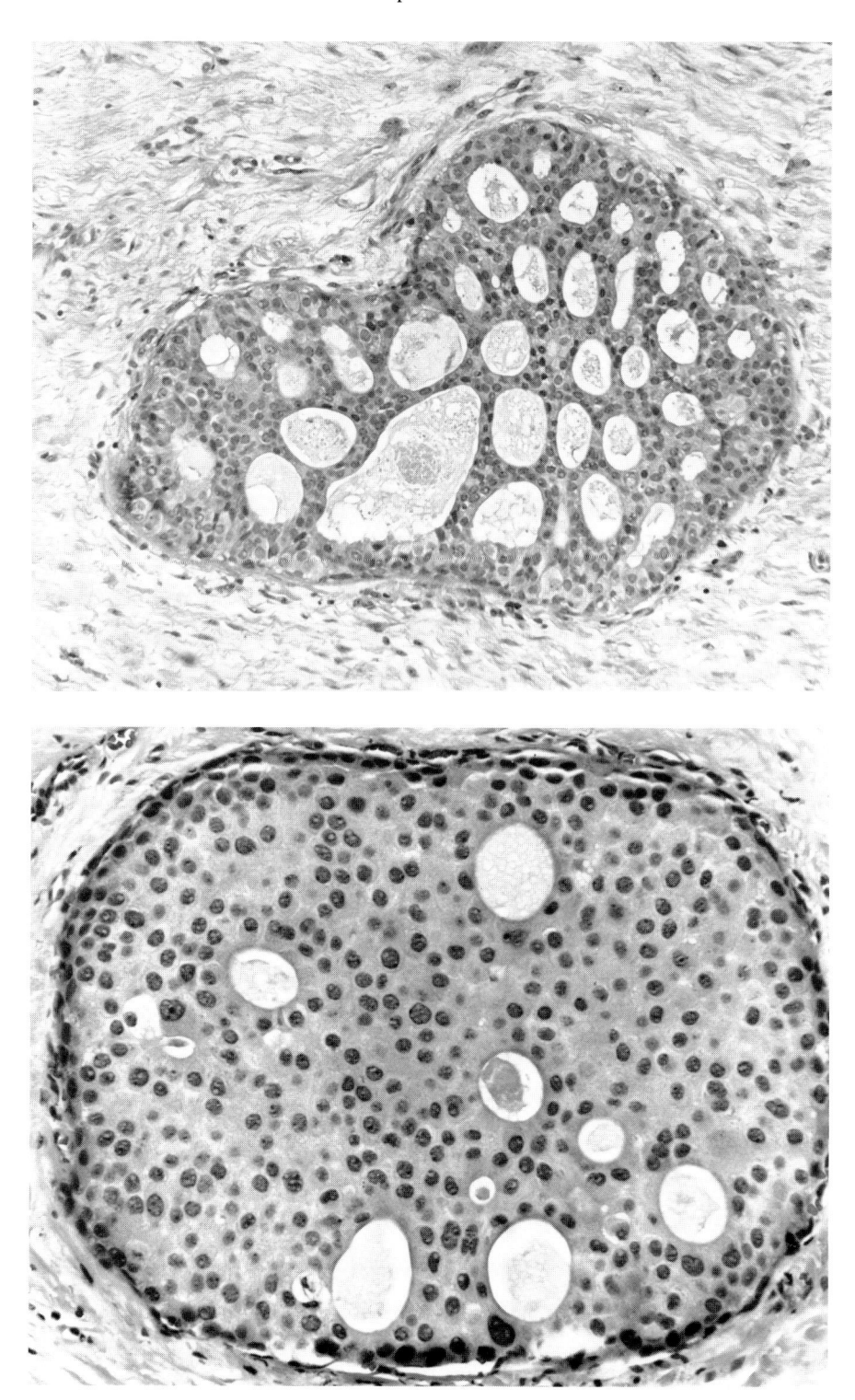

In Situ Proliferative Epithelial Lesions of the Breast

TABLE 2. Histologic Features Useful in Distinguishing Ductal Epithelial Hyperplasia from Cribriform DCIS

Ductal Hyperplasia	Cribriform DCIS
1. Spaces collapsed, slit-like, trabeculae not rigid	Spaces sharply punched out, curved and round; trebeculae rigid
2. Necrosis rare	Necrosis may be present
3. Streaming or flip-flopping of cells	Streaming or flip-flopping absent
4. Cells ovoid or elongate with overlapping nuclei, nuclear membranes collapsed, nucleoli inconspicuous	Cells are round to columnar; may show prominent nucleoli; nuclei stand apart; rigid nuclear membranes *or* nuclei are small and dense but still uniform and round with rigid nuclear membranes
5. Syncytial pattern of cells	Cell margins often distinct
6. Apocrine metaplasia may be present	Cells can be large and eosinophilic; but characteristic apocrine metaplasia unusual
7. Calcifications infrequent	Calcifications frequent

DCIS = ductal carcinoma in situ.

gives rise to invasive carcinoma rather frequently; however, there is little evidence that it is an obligate preinvasive lesion.

Histologically, comedo DCIS is defined as dilated ducts lined by stratified, cytologically malignant cells with central necrosis of tumor cells. The architectural pattern may be a solid lining of stratified cells or a cribriform pattern of cells around the duct periphery. The cells demonstrate striking nuclear enlargement, nuclear pleomorphism, prominent nucleoli, and frequent mitotic figures, some of which may be abnormal (Fig. 5). Cytologically, malignant cells are the essential feature of comedo DCIS, a point that requires emphasis, because necrosis may be associated with a number of other intraductal lesions, including florid papillomatosis of the nipple, atypical hyperplasia, and cribriform/micropapillary DCIS.

Because the constituent cells are cytologically malignant and because necrosis is usually extensive, there is seldom difficulty in diagnosing this type of intraductal carcinoma. The most frequent type of diagnostic problem is determining whether early stromal invasion is present or not. This problem arises because comedo DCIS often extends as an in situ process into ramifying small ducts and lobular acini, and this growth pattern may be associated with a stromal, granulation tissue-like reaction of the type often seen in invasive carcinoma. We insist on finding jagged infiltration of tumor nests extending beyond the lobular units before interpreting suspicious areas as definite evidence of stromal invasion. Sometimes one cannot be certain whether invasion is present or not; in such cases, this uncertainty should be expressed

FIGURE 4 *(opposite page).* Micropapillary ductal carcinoma in situ characterized by dilated ducts lined by a few layers of uniform cells which focally stratify to form finger-like or club-shaped protuberances that occasionally bridge the duct lumen (top). The club-shaped protuberances often have bulbous ends and are composed of the same cell type which lines the rest of the duct (bottom).

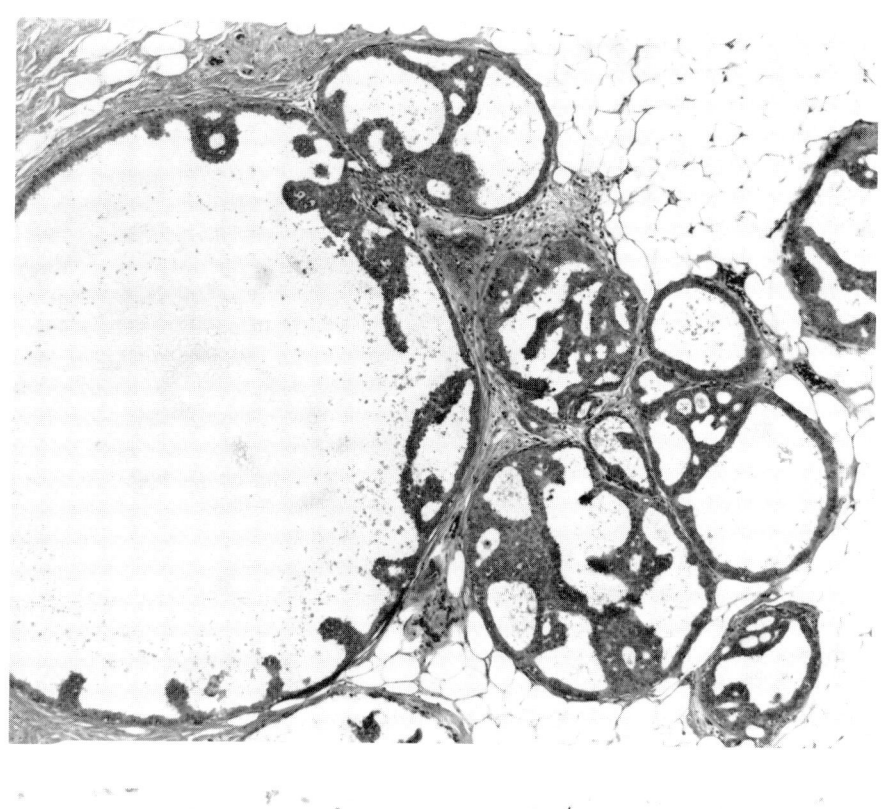

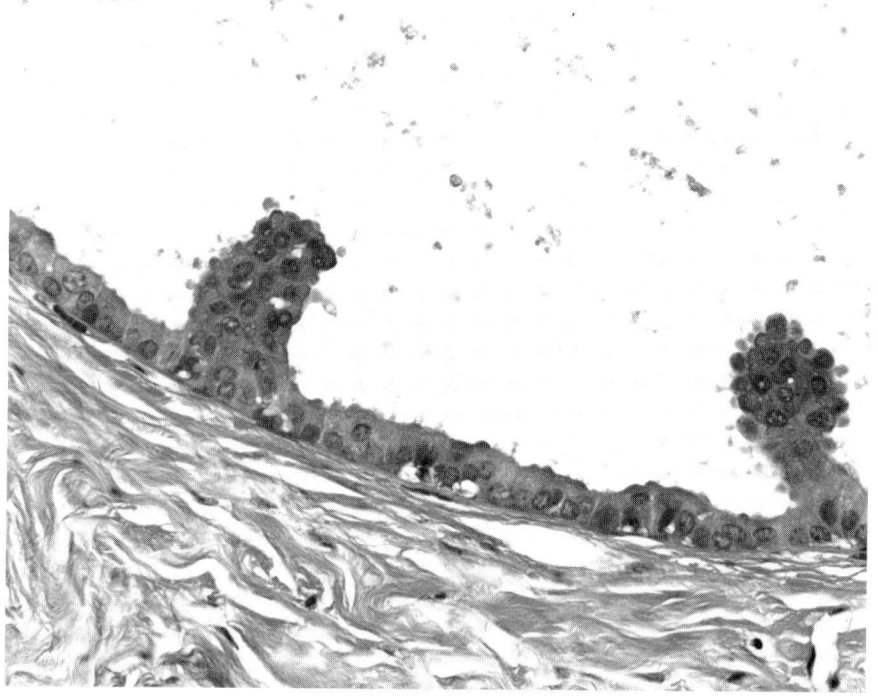

In Situ Proliferative Epithelial Lesions of the Breast 81

in the surgical pathology report using such terms as "suspicious for invasion" or "early microinvasion cannot be excluded" (Fig. 6).

Investigators have reported on various biologic and clinical characteristics of comedo DCIS in contrast to other DCIS types. Comedo DCIS has been found to be composed of cells with an aneuploid DNA content.[24,24a] a not unexpected finding given the cytologic appearance of the cells that constitute the lesion. The comedo lesion has a proliferative rate that is significantly higher than other types of in situ carcinoma and which in fact is similar to that observed with invasive carcinoma.[26] The cells in comedo DCIS usually express the Neu oncogene,[46] a feature that has been associated with aggressive breast carcinomas. Unlike other types of DCIS, the comedo lesion is by far the one most frequently associated with foci of microinvasion in which jagged nests of malignant epithelial cells extend from the duct or ductule into the surrounding stroma.

Ductal Carcinoma In Situ of the Solid Type: An Intermediate Lesion

Occasionally, the uniform, relatively bland cells of the type found in cribriform/micropapillary in situ carcinoma grow in a solid pattern. These lesions are most often found in association with areas of cribriform DCIS, and we include such lesions in the cribriform DCIS category (i.e., low-grade DCIS).

The designation of solid-type DCIS is used by us when the cytologic features of a DCIS lesion are significantly worse than are seen in the cribriform lesion. Such lesions usually display a solid pattern of atypical epithelial cells filling dilated ducts, some of which form microacini or small spaces. Necrosis may be present but is not usually as extensive as that found in comedo DCIS. The cells that constitute such lesions show features intermediate between those of cribriform DCIS and comedo DCIS (Fig. 7). Although the solid type of DCIS does not feature cytologically malignant cells, nuclear enlargement, nuclear chromatin abnormalities, and occasional mitotic figures are found in solid-type DCIS (intermediate lesion). When such lesions are encountered, we clearly indicate in the pathology report that the features present are intermediate between those of cribriform and comedo DCIS.

The biologic significance of such lesions has not been extensively evaluated, so it is expected that some pathologists may feel this category is unnecessary. However, we think it is useful because it allows the pathologist to more clearly designate a DCIS lesion that does not fit well into the cribriform/micropapillary or comedo DCIS "boxes." The possible clinical significance of such a designation is discussed below.

Clinical Implications of Noncomedo DCIS

Although it has not been possible to study the "true" natural history of DCIS (because the procedure required for diagnosis can alter the natural

---

FIGURE 5 *(opposite page).* Comedo-type ductal carcinoma in situ defined by stratified cytologically malignant cells with central necrosis of tumor cells (top). The cells demonstrate striking nuclear enlargement, nuclear pleomorphism, prominent nucleoli, and mitotic figures (bottom).

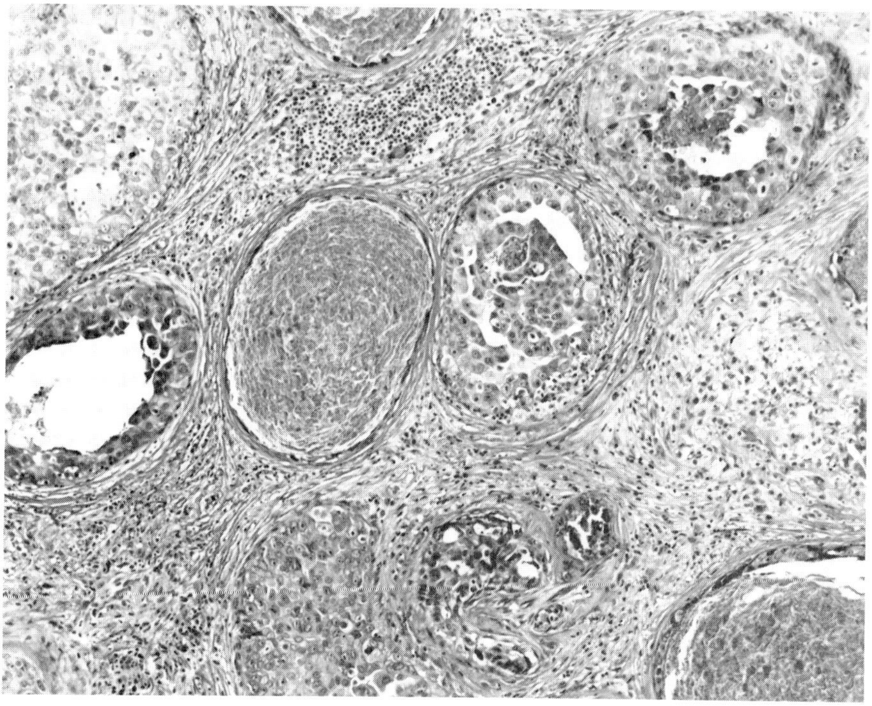

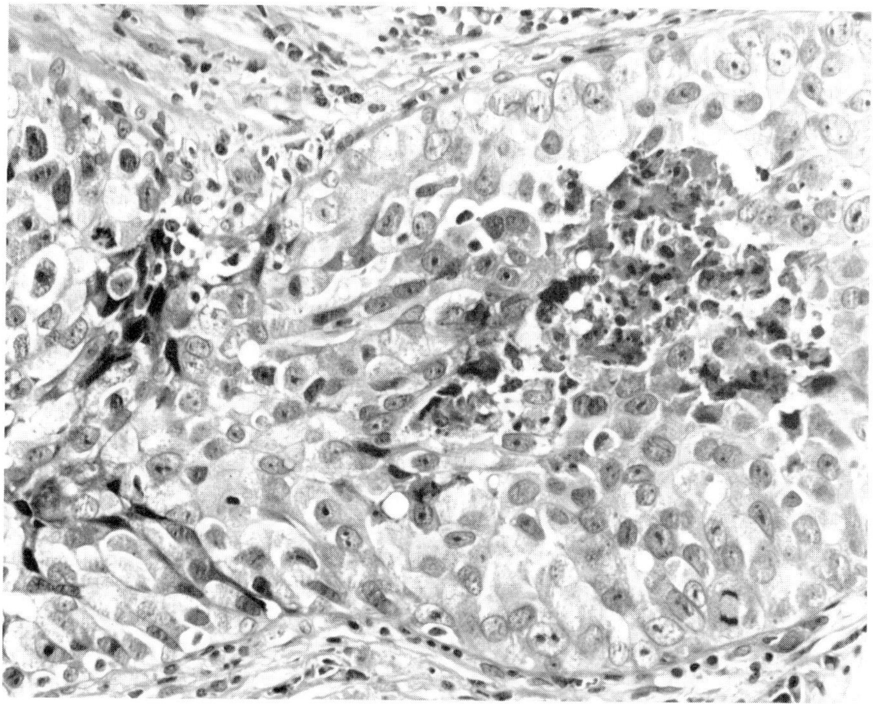

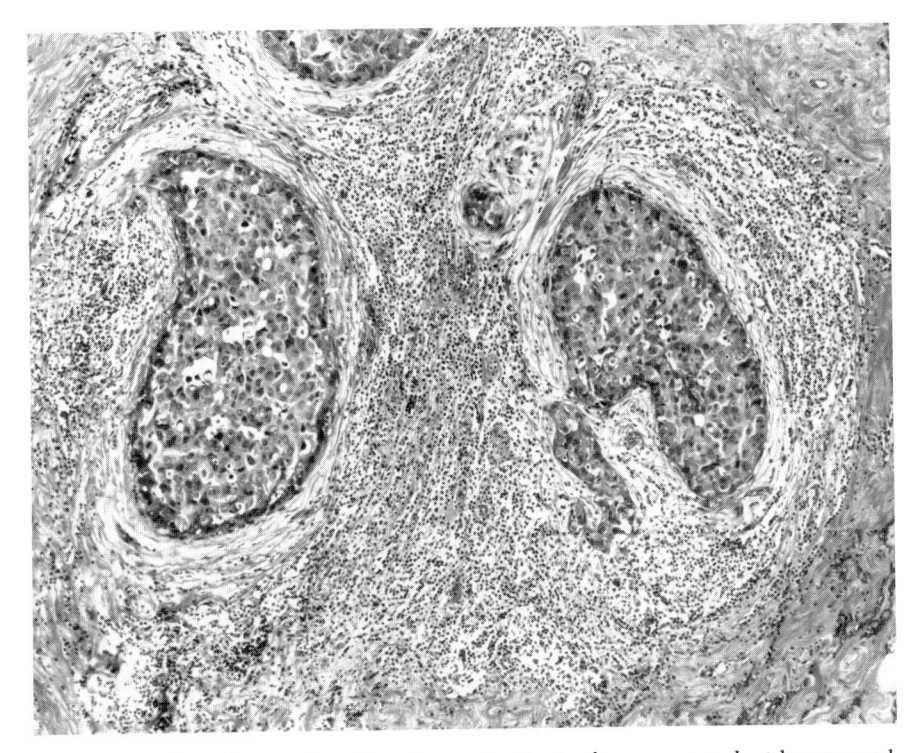

FIGURE 6. Comedo-type ductal carcinoma in situ is often associated with a stromal, granulation tissue-like reaction and extends into small ducts, features that may mimic invasive carcinoma.

history of the disease), there have been at least three published studies[3,12,29] with long-term outcome data that have examined the clinical implications of noncomedo DCIS found in a breast biopsy after which there is no further therapy. Probably, the most widely known study is that by Page et al.[29] who reviewed 11,760 "benign" breast biopsies and identified 28 cases that fulfill the current criteria for cribriform/micropapillary DCIS. The report does not indicate the size (extent) of the lesions or the status of the biopsy margins. Follow-up data (avg. 15 years) was available on 25 women of whom seven (28%) developed subsequent invasive carcinomas between 3 and 10 years after biopsy. All invasive carcinomas occurred in the same quadrant of the same breast as the initial biopsy. These results indicate that a woman with a biopsy showing noncomedo DCIS has a 25% chance of developing invasive

---

FIGURE 7 *(opposite page).* Solid type ductal carcinoma in situ in which the ducts are essentially filled by cells that show features intermediate between those of cribriform DCIS and comedo DCIS (top). Solid type DCIS with microacini and central necrosis (bottom). The cytologic features are more atypical than those seen in cribriform DCIS but do not show the cytologic malignancy required for the diagnosis of comedo type DCIS (bottom).

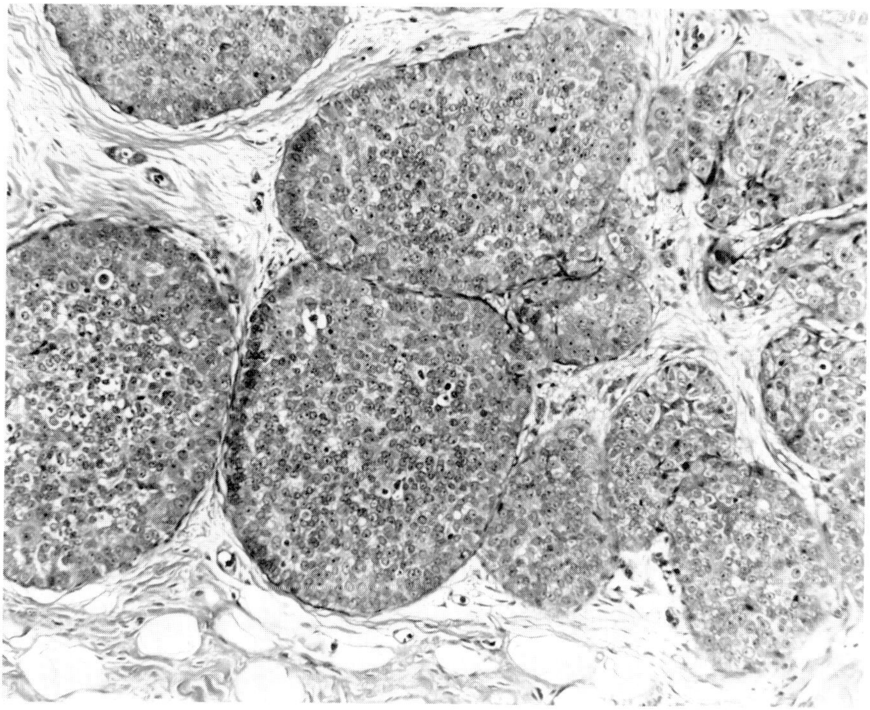

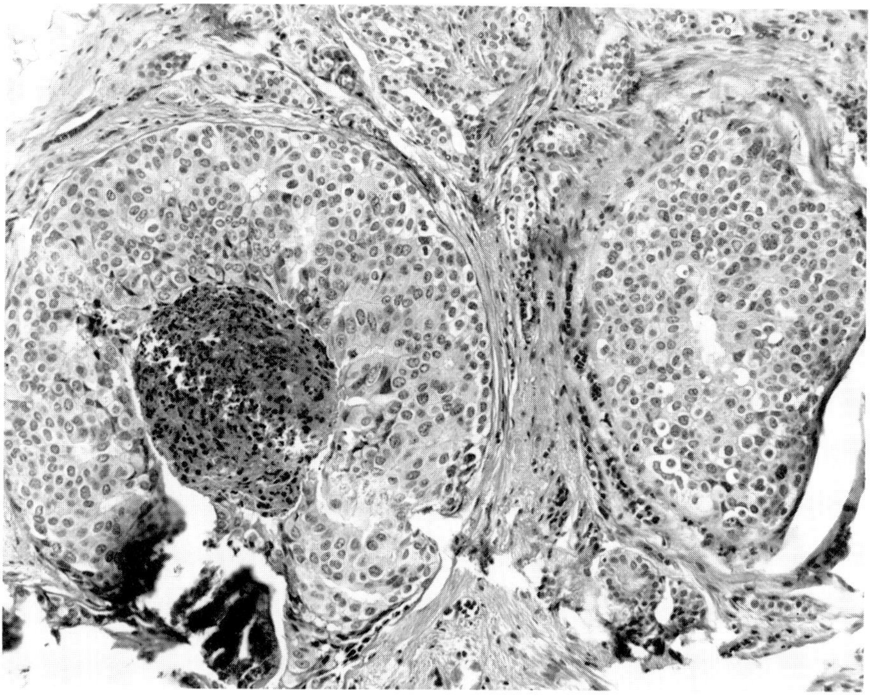

carcinoma over the following 15 years or, looked at another way, she has a relative risk of 11, i.e., such a woman is 11 times more likely to develop invasive carcinoma than an age-matched control. This relative risk is not per year; it is the risk over the entire follow-up period which in the study by Page et al. was 15 years.

Bestill et al.[3] reported a similar study in which 25 cases of noncomedo DCIS (the histologic descriptions indicate cribriform, micropapillary, and papillary types) were identified following review of 8609 "benign" breast biopsies. Follow-up data were available on 10 patients (avg. 21.6 years), six (60%) of whom developed subsequent invasive carcinoma an average of 9.7 years following biopsy. At least four of the recurrent carcinomas were in the area of the original biopsy site.

Eusebi et al.[12] have also reported a similar study in which they reviewed 4,371 biopsies and identified 42 evaluable cases of carcinoma in situ (avg. follow-up, 16.7 years) which they divided as follows: seven cases of DCIS (cribriform and comedo), 21 cases of clinging carcinoma (micropapillary DCIS), and 14 cases of LCIS. These authors also estimated the extent of disease (focal: $< 10\%$ of breast units involved; intermediate: 10–40% of breast units involved; and diffuse: $> 50\%$ of breast units involved by DCIS). In the first group of seven patients, one, who had diffuse comedo DCIS, developed invasive carcinoma 5 years following biopsy and died of widespread disease. In the second group, 2 of the 21 patients with clinging carcinoma (micropapillary DCIS) developed invasive carcinoma and both patients died of disease. The authors combined the data of these first two groups (3 of 28 patients, or 10%, developing invasive carcinoma) and calculated a relative risk of 4.3 for such lesions. Interestingly, none of the patients in the LCIS group developed subsequent invasive carcinoma in the follow-up period.

The results of these three studies are difficult to compare, because the histopathologic groups are not identically defined and none of the studies clearly reports the size of the lesion or the status of margins. Although these studies give variable results regarding the risk that DCIS lesions carry for the development of subsequent invasive carcinoma, all three studies indicate that DCIS is a marker for increased risk for developing invasive carcinoma. The relative risk figures of Page et al. are in-between those of the other two studies and are the most widely quoted.

Clinical Implications of Comedo DCIS

The only well-known study that has examined the clinical significance of comedo DCIS in a biopsy for which no further treatment is performed is a 1938 report by Lewis and Geschickter.[25] In their study of 47 patients, there were eight patients who were initially treated by local excision alone. Six of these eight patients developed local recurrence, five within 18 months and the other after 4 years. In three of the patients, axillary metastases were found at the second operation. It should be noted that the patients in this study clinically presented with a palpable breast mass, and most had, by today's standards, relatively extensive disease (the sizes of the eight lesions were as follows: 0.5 cm, 1 cm, 2 cm, 3 cm, 6 cm (2), 9 cm, "grapefruit"). Although these data may not be applicable to mammographically detected lesions, it is generally accepted that comedo DCIS results in an RR for developing invasive carcinoma equal to or greater than the risk that results from the noncomedo DCIS lesions.

Significance of Size (Extent) and Grade of DCIS

The studies by Lagios et al.[23,24,24a] have provided some very useful information regarding mammographically detected DCIS. The technique that the authors use to examine breast biopsies allows for fairly accurate determination of the size (extent) of the DCIS lesion. Moreover, in a more recent study investigating recurrence following lumpectomy, these authors have documented the type of DCIS as well as the status of the excision margins. Their recent publications have addressed two main questions: (1) What significance does the size (extent) of the DCIS lesion have on the probability of finding multicentric disease and occult invasive disease elsewhere in the breast; and (2) What is the relationship between histologic type of DCIS and recurrence in small ($<$ 2.5 cm), mammographically detected lesions that are treated only by lumpectomy with tumor-free margins?

In addressing the question of occult invasion and multicentricity, the authors examined mastectomy specimens using a serial subgross method following an initial biopsy diagnosis of DCIS. The authors found that the incidence of multicentricity was rare and that occult invasion was absent in women whose initial biopsy showed the DCIS lesion to be less than 2.5 cm in size (extent). In contrast, lesions larger than 4.0 cm had a significant incidence of multicentricity (14 of 17) and occult invasion (10 of 17).[23] Their most recent study of 115 cases showed that approximately 40% of the 31 biopsies with DCIS lesions greater than 4.5 cm were associated with occult invasion when the mastectomy specimens were examined by the serial subgross technique; this finding did not occur in the 84 biopsies with DCIS lesions less than 4.5 cm.[24] These studies document that small DCIS lesions are very rarely associated with invasive carcinoma and that as the size of the lesions increases (particularly nearing 4 or 5 cm) so does the probability of finding associated invasive carcinoma elsewhere in the breast.

Lagios et al. have also reported on the significance of the histologic grade of DCIS on recurrence in small ($<$ 2.5 cm), mammographically detected DCIS lesions, nearly all of which were completely excised. Their study group of 79 cases was divided into DCIS types based on architecture, nuclear morphology, and necrosis, resulting in categories similar to the comedo DCIS (Types I and II), solid DCIS or intermediate lesion (Type III), and cribriform/ micropapillary DCIS (Type IV) categories described above. In that study, 19% (7 of 36) of patients who had high-grade nuclear morphology and comedo-type necrosis developed recurrence; only 1 of 10 patients with intermediate grade histology developed a recurrence; and none of the 33 patients with DCIS of the micropapillary/nonnecrotic cribriform type and low-grade nuclear morphology developed a local recurrence.[24]

Silverstein et al. have confirmed that by far the majority of women who develop a recurrence following a diagnosis of DCIS are those with comedo-type DCIS in the initial biopsy.[42]

DCIS: Content of the Surgical Pathology Report

It is becoming increasingly clear that the current designation of ductal carcinoma in situ (DCIS) represents a spectrum of lesions that vary from a small focus of cribriform/micropapillary DCIS in the setting of proliferative fibrocystic change to widespread comedo DCIS with cancerization of lobules. As might be expected, this has caused some confusion regarding the clinical biology of these lesions.[20] Documentation of certain pathologic features, however, helps to define the expected behavior and may well affect the therapy that is offered to and/or the therapy that is chosen by the patient. Thus, it is important that the surgical pathology report in which the diagnosis of DCIS is made (in the absence of invasive carcinoma) contains certain information that helps to define the particular lesion being diagnosed (Table 3).

Once a diagnosis of DCIS is made, the surgical pathology report should indicate the type of DCIS lesion, the size (extent) of the lesion, and the status of the excision margins whenever possible. The type of DCIS can be determined using the criteria summarized above. The terms cribriform/micropapillary, solid, and comedo are most widely used. We support the use of an intermediate designation (solid DCIS or intermediate lesion) for lesions warranting this designation. Determining the size (extent) of the DCIS lesion may be difficult because DCIS is not usually identified grossly and because most pathologists do not employ the labor and time-intensive subserial sectioning technique Lagios et al. use to study breast biopsies. Adequate methods for reporting an estimate of the size (extent) of a DCIS lesion include: (1) providing an estimate of the percent of breast units involved by DCIS with an indication of the size of the breast biopsy specimen, (2) sectioning the biopsy from one end of the specimen to the other and submitting the sections in sequence, thus allowing for an estimate of the size of the lesion based on the sections in which the lesion is present, or (3) in very small DCIS lesions, a measurement of size of the lesion may be obtained directly from the slide. Status of excision margins should be indicated as involved or uninvolved by focal or extensive disease.

General Guidelines for the Treatment of DCIS

There seems little question that the treatment of DCIS should be individualized to each patient, because the choice of treatment depends on

TABLE 3. DCIS: Content of the Surgical Pathology Report

1. Diagnosis
2. Histologic type
   Cribriform/micropapillary
   Solid (intermediate lesion)
   Comedo
3. Size (extent) of lesion
4. Status of margins

many factors, including the nature and size of the lesion, the size of the breast, mammographic findings, family history, patient age, and the patient's own thoughts and feelings about the risk of developing invasive carcinoma and about the various treatment options. Converting relative risk to absolute risk is a complex task that takes into account various factors of each patient.[9] Even in view of these individual factors, however, it is possible to provide general guidelines or recommendations for treatment based on knowledge of data from clinicopathologic studies that have defined the general behavior of these lesions.

It is generally well accepted that DCIS is cured by mastectomy; however, such surgery is considered excessive for most DCIS lesions under 2-3 cm, particularly as more conservative therapy is being used successfully for local control of invasive carcinoma.[41] It is also generally well accepted that an axillary lymph node dissection is not necessary for DCIS,[45] except perhaps for widespread comedo DCIS or for extensive DCIS in which microinvasion cannot be excluded,[43] because axillary lymph node involvement is present in a very low percentage (1-3%) of patients with DCIS only.[1,6,40]

The studies that have investigated the adequacy of excisional biopsy (lumpectomy) alone for the treatment of DCIS indicate that recurrence occurs between 4% and 23% of the time, usually over a short follow-up period (3 to 5 years).[14,20] While some authors have found radiation therapy to decrease the likelihood of recurrence, others have not found a significant difference. The difficulty with many of these studies is that the diagnosis of DCIS is not further specified with regard to the histologic grade of the lesion, size (extent) of the lesion, or the status of the excisional biopsy margins.

The studies of Lagios et al. indicate that complete excision (lumpectomy) with clear margins is adequate treatment for small (< 2.5 cm), mammographically detected, low-grade (cribriform/micropapillary) DCIS (average follow-up 48 months). Very close follow-up or some sort of therapy in addition to complete excision may be needed for small, completely excised, high-grade (comedo) lesions, because these have an approximately 20% chance of recurrence. Wide excision and radiation therapy or mastectomy is likely required for adequate local control of large (> 5 cm), high-grade (comedo) DCIS lesions, because these lesions appear to show a very high rate of recurrence following biopsy only and are frequently (40-45%) associated with invasive carcinoma elsewhere in the breast. There are no data on which to make recommendations for low-grade DCIS lesions larger than 2.5 cm or for intermediate lesions; however, complete excision with clear margins and close follow-up with or without radiation therapy well may be adequate treatment.

LOBULAR CARCINOMA IN SITU

Risk data for patients with in situ lobular lesions have been determined by dividing the morphologic continuum into atypical lobular hyperplasia and lobular carcinoma in situ (LCIS). As a result "lobular neoplasia,"[16] a term coined to encompass both atypical lobular hyperplasia and LCIS, should no longer be used.

The criteria for the diagnosis of LCIS are derived from studies evaluating the risk of these lesions. The diagnosis requires certain architectural and cytologic features that are considered definitional. All of the terminal ductules (acini) of a lobule must be completely filled by relatively small, round, uniform cells that stand apart from each other and are evenly distributed throughout each acinus; there should not be any intercellular spaces. In addition, at least one-half of the terminal ductules (acini) must be expanded and/or distorted by the process. Other features that may be present but are not considered definitional include mitotic figures (usually rare) and the presence of signet ring cells and/or vacuolated cells that are helpful in identifying a process as lobular. The spectrum of lobular hyperplasia, atypical lobular hyperplasia, and LCIS is depicted in Figures 8 and 9.

Involvement of Ducts by LCIS (Pagetoid Spread)

Not infrequently, the characteristic small, round, uniform cells of LCIS will be found either singly or, more commonly, in groups beneath the epithelium of ducts. The lobular cells are distinct from the epithelial, ductal-lining cells that most often are flattened, although they may occasionally retain their cuboidal or columnar appearance (Fig. 10). This lesion has been previously called "pagetoid spread." In the presence of LCIS, its identification is usually not difficult. However, such lesions may be subtle and, in the absence of LCIS, may be missed altogether. Occasionally, a problem may arise in the distinction of "pagetoid spread" from myoepithelial cell hyperplasia, because this latter process also occurs beneath the ductal epithelium and the myoepithelial cells also have a very uniform appearance. However, the cytoplasm of the majority of the cells in myoepithelial cell hyperplasia is usually clear and the nuclei are small and oval in contrast to the eosinophilic cytoplasm and round nuclei of lobular cells.

At times the only feature of LCIS found in a breast biopsy is the spread of the characteristic cells into ducts, and this feature should not be ignored. However, both atypical lobular hyperplasia and LCIS may grow in this fashion; consequently, identification of ductal involvement by atypical lobular cells necessitates a careful search for atypical lobular hyperplasia or LCIS elsewhere in the biopsy. It is generally agreed that in the absence of identifying the lobular process, a diagnosis of atypical lobular hyperplasia or LCIS should not be made. Rather, a phrase such as "involvement of ducts by atypical lobular cells" should be used with the provision of an explanation that such lesions are usually associated with LCIS or atypical lobular hyperplasia.

FIGURE 8 *(opposite page).* Lobular hyperplasia features increased numbers of the characteristic small, round, uniform cells without complete filling or expansion of the acini (top). Atypical lobular hyperplasia showing filling of most of the acini without significant expansion or distortion of more than half of the acini (bottom).

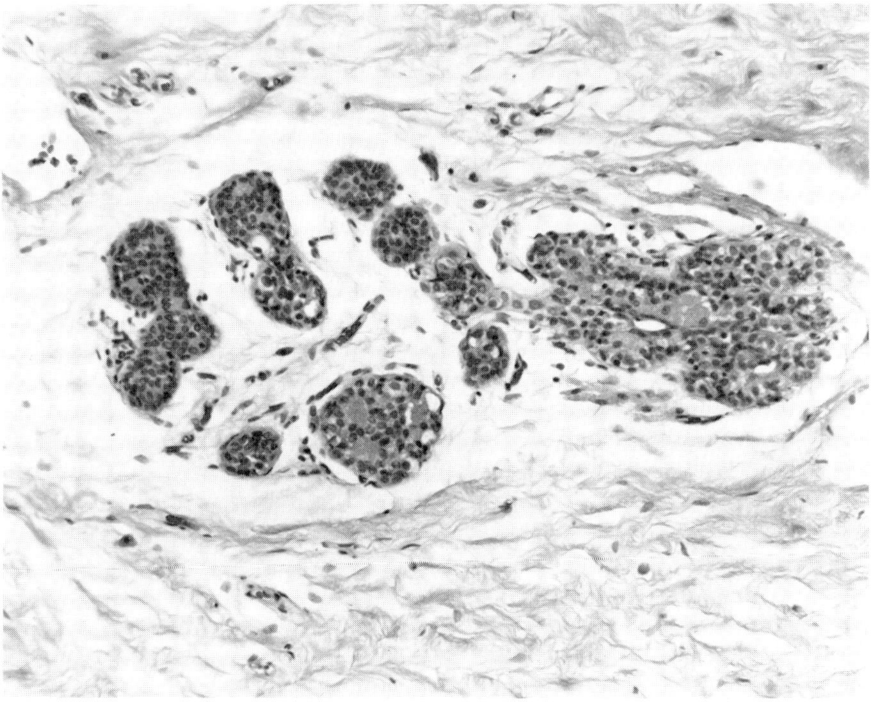

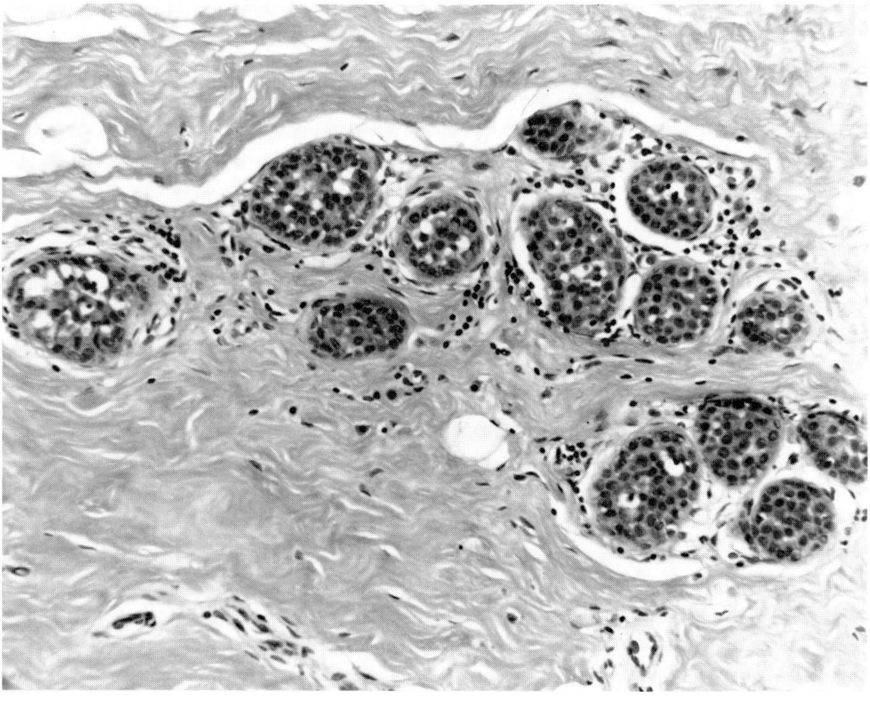

LCIS Versus Involvement of Lobules by DCIS

The distinction between LCIS and involvement of lobules by DCIS (cancerization of lobules) is usually straightforward. However, occasionally the cells of cribriform DCIS may be quite bland when they involve lobules and as a result may closely mimic the cells of LCIS. Examination of several levels of the paraffin block is quite useful in this situation. When DCIS involves lobules, it usually does so in an uneven distribution instead of the uniform filling typically seen in lobular proliferative processes. DCIS cells will occasionally form gland-like spaces within the acini, something lobular cells rarely do. The DCIS cells are relatively large, with appreciably enlarged nuclei and distinct cell borders, and there is usually a noticeable cytologic and nuclear variability between the cells. In contrast, the features that help to set apart LCIS are the uniform, complete, and even filling of the terminal ductules and the small, round cells, which are uniform one to the next. Vacuolated and signet ring cells, when present, are also helpful in identifying a process as lobular (Table 4). It is important to realize that it is the histologic features (architectural and cytologic) that define a process as ductal or lobular and not the location of the process.

Clinical Implications

Numerous studies have demonstrated that lobular carcinoma in situ is a marker for an increased risk for developing subsequent invasive carcinoma and that both breasts are equally at risk.[16,38] The magnitude of this risk varies slightly from series to series, but the average estimate is roughly 10 times that of the normal population. There are a number of treatment options that have been proposed for LCIS. We think that all options should be explained to the patient and that the patient's desires, the status of the remaining breast tissue, patient age, and family history should influence the treatment decision. Almost all patients at our institution choose local excision and careful, regular follow-up.

TABLE 4. Histologic Features Useful in Distinguishing LCIS from Involvement of Lobules by DCIS

LCIS	DCIS in Lobules ("Cancerizaton" of Lobules)
1. Complete filling of acini by uniform, evenly distributed cells	Uneven distribution of cells often with formation of gland-like spaces
2. Small, round cells very uniform one to the next	Noticeable cytologic and nuclear enlargement and variability between cells
3. Vacuolated and signet-ring cells helpful	Vacuolated and signet-ring cells usually not present

LCIS = lobular carcinoma in situ; DCIS = ductal carcinoma in situ.

FIGURE 9 (opposite page). Atypical lobular hyperplasia in which essentially all of the terminal ductules (acini) are filled by small, round, uniform cells with expansion or distortion of less than half of the acini (top). A well-developed example of lobular carcinoma in situ showing filling of all of the acini and expansion of over half of the acini by the characteristic cells (bottom).

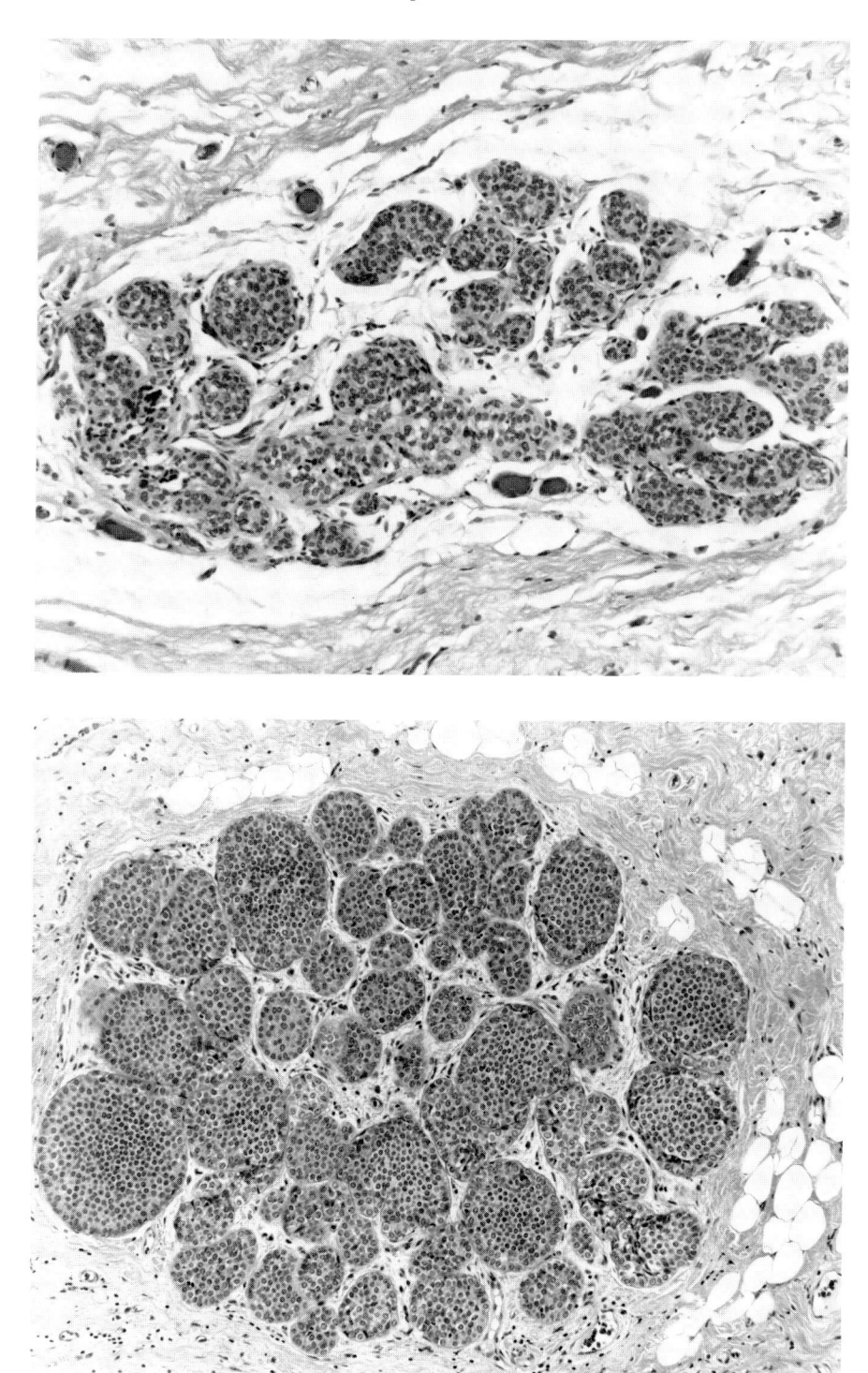

In Situ Proliferative Epithelial Lesions of the Breast

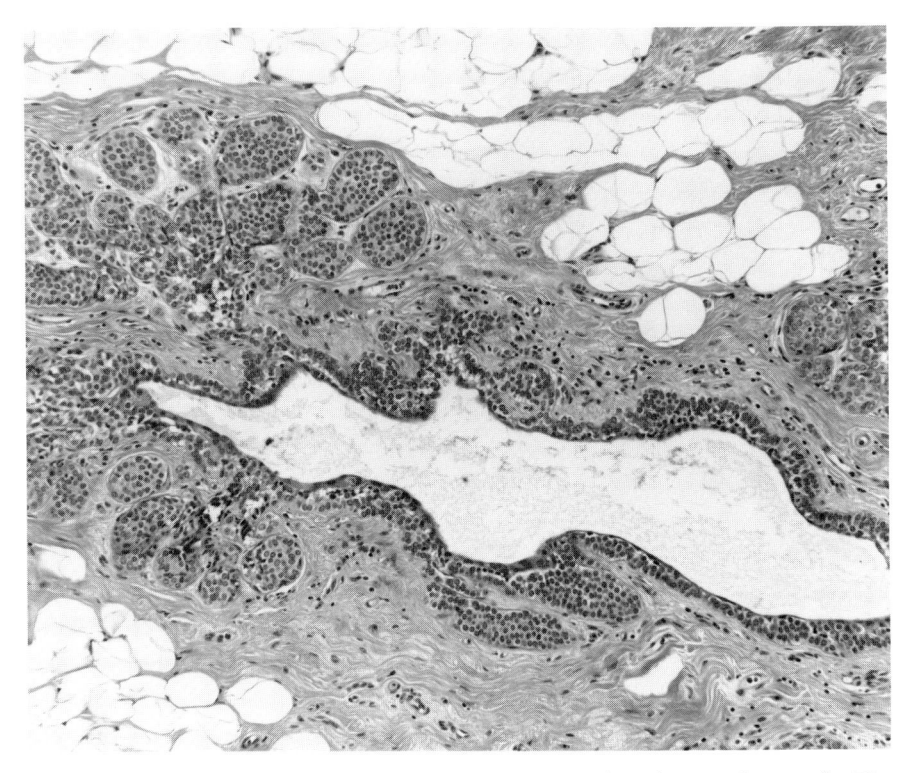

FIGURE 10. Lobular carcinoma in situ involving a duct (pagetoid spread). The characteristic small cells are found either singly or in groups beneath the flattened duct epithelium.

INTRADUCTAL (INTRACYSTIC) PAPILLARY CARCINOMA

Intraductal (intracystic) papillary carcinoma is a noninvasive papillary epithelial proliferation occurring within a large dilated duct, which is designated as carcinoma primarily on the basis of cytologic features. It is considered apart from the other lesions in the DCIS category because of its distinctive histologic appearance and because its significance as a risk lesion has not been fully investigated.

Intraductal papillary carcinoma is usually a solitary lesion. Architecturally, the defining feature is a large dilated duct or cystic space containing a complex arborization of generally thin, delicate fibrovascular stalks on which is found a single population of epithelial cells. Cytologically, three main patterns are recognized. In one, the pattern is that of cribriform/micropapillary DCIS extending from the fibrovascular stalks. Atypical ductal hyperplasia may be associated with the process; however, diagnostic areas of DCIS should be identified (Fig. 11).

FIGURE 11 *(opposite page).* Intraductal (intracystic) papillary carcinoma (top) showing the pattern of cribriform ductal carcinoma in situ extending from thin, delicate fibrovascular stalks (bottom).

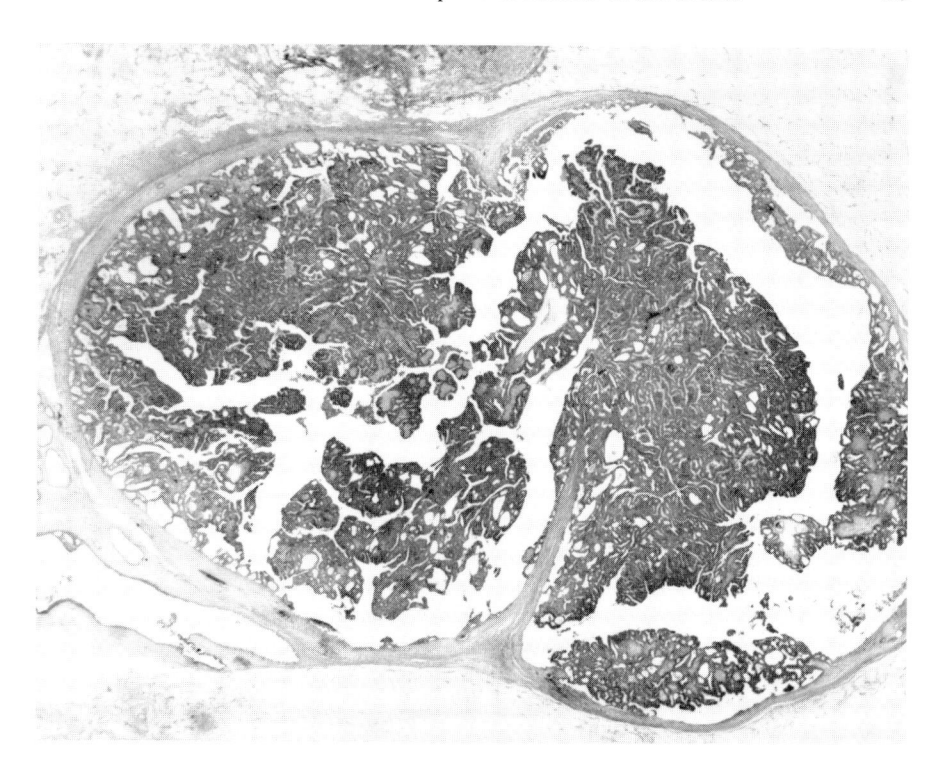

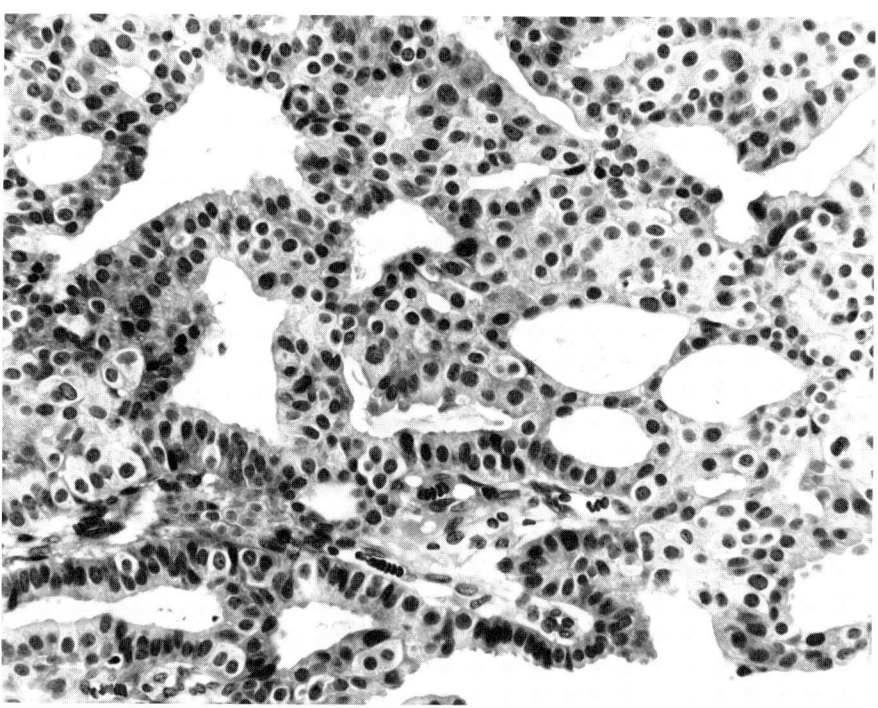

In Situ Proliferative Epithelial Lesions of the Breast

Cribriform/micropapillary DCIS may be present in adjacent smaller duct spaces. In the second type (the "tall-hyperchromatic cell type"), the stalks are lined by a single population of tall cells with elongated, hyperchromatic nuclei that are arranged perpendicular to the stalks. The cells are closely packed together and often display a pseudostratified appearance. The nuclei are enlarged and the chromatin is dense (Fig. 12). A third pattern is sometimes described in which cribriform DCIS and atypical ductal hyperplasia are mixed together with areas of benign papilloma. In all three types, mitotic figures may be present and are a very useful diagnostic feature. In addition, focal necrosis is much more common in carcinoma than in papillomas in women over 40 years of age.

The main differential diagnostic consideration, of course, is intraductal papilloma (Table 5), which is usually characterized by broad, hyalinized stalks, two distinct cell types, and a complex, adenosis-like ductal proliferation within the hyalinized stroma. Necrosis is unusual and mitoses are rare in papillomas. Any proliferative lesion that features necrosis and large numbers of mitotic figures should be interpreted very carefully. However, it is also important to remember that considerable atypia, mitotic activity, and even necrosis are allowed within the definition of papillomas in younger individuals and in subareaolar papillomas (also called papillomas of the nipple).

Clinical Implications

The follow-up study of Carter et al.[7] has stressed the importance of examining the ducts adjacent to the intraductal papillary carcinoma. From the limited data available, patients with intraductal (intracystic) papillary carcinoma are essentially cured by complete excision as long as there is no typical DCIS present in the tissue adjacent to the cystic space and no involvement of the capsule.

TABLE 5.   Features Helpful in Distinguishing Intraductal Papillary Carcinoma from Intraductal Papilloma

Papilloma	Intraductal Papillary Carcinoma
1. Broad fibrovascular stalks often with hyalinized stroma	Thin, delicate stalks with complex, arborizing pattern
2. May show trapping of benign duct elements, apocrine metaplasia, squamous metaplasia, and/or adneosis pattern within stalk	Usually not present
3. Two cell types: epithelial and myo-epithelial	One cell type: either "tall-hyperchromatic" or cribriform DCIS type
4. Mitotic figures and necrosis rare	Mitotic figures and necrosis may be present

DCIS = ductal carcinoma in situ.

FIGURE 12 *(opposite page).* Intraductal papillary carcinoma of the "tall-hyperchromatic cell" type. The single population of tall cells demonstrates elongate, hyperchromatic, dense nuclei arranged perpendicular to the stalks, often showing a pseudostratified appearance (bottom).

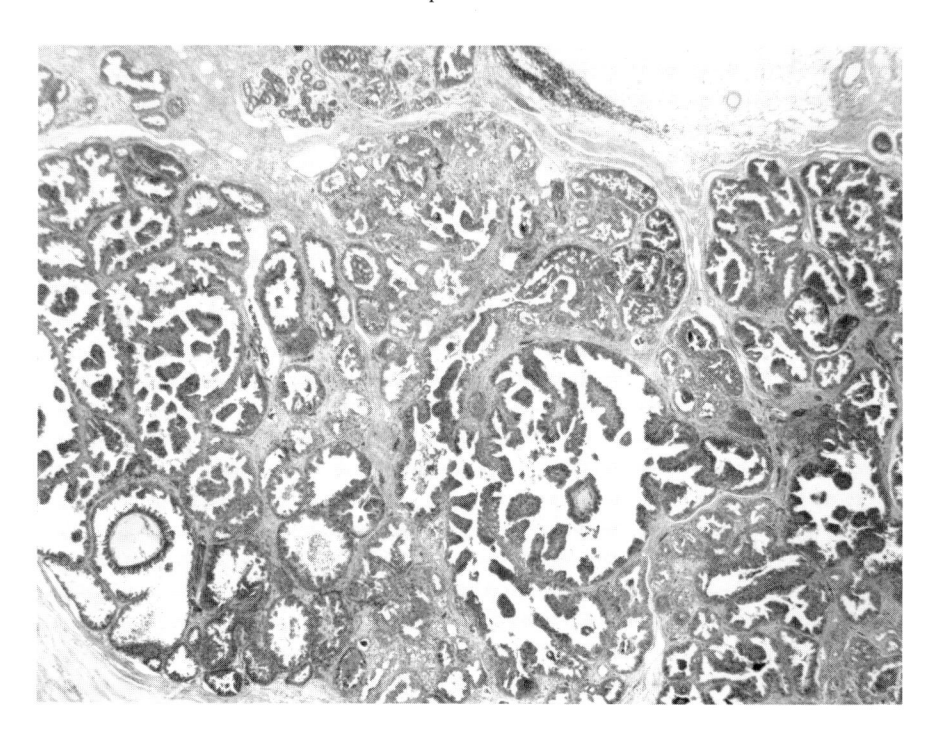

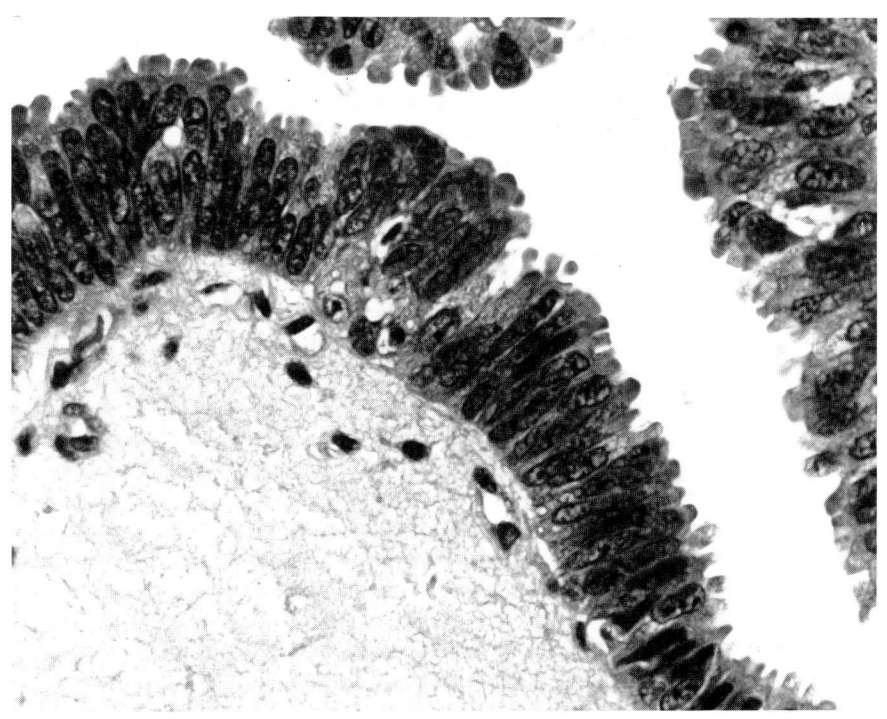

In Situ Proliferative Epithelial Lesions of the Breast

PAPILLARY LESIONS OF VARIABLE OR UNCERTAIN RISK

In our definition, papillomas are proliferative lesions in which the constituent cells cover cores of fibrovascular stroma. The covering epithelium usually consists of two cell types, columnar cells lining the spaces and myoepithelial cells beneath. Characteristically, the fibrous cores are broad and often extensively hyalinized. Extensive hyalin can trap glands, giving a pseudoinfiltrative appearance. Epithelial hyperplasia can occur within papillomas, including atypical hyperplasia, and, at times, carcinoma in situ may be found in a portion of an otherwise benign papilloma. Papillomas occur within both the lactiferous ducts and in the smaller ducts in the periphery of the breast distant from the nipple. Papillomas may extend along ducts for a considerable distance, particularly the larger ones near the nipple. We consider adenoma of the nipple and florid papillomatosis of the nipple[33,34] as forms of papilloma. The former is characterized by areas of hyperplasia as well as adenosis-like change within the fibrous stroma. A considerable degree of nuclear atypia may be present, and this can cause diagnostic problems. As noted, papillomas may be multiple. The main differential diagnostic consideration for papillomas is intraductal papillary carcinoma.[22] The features we use to make this distinction have been discussed above.

Another form of papillomatous proliferation of the breast is **juvenile papillomatosis** or "Swiss cheese disease."[35,36,37] This lesion presents as a discrete mass typically in an adolescent or young adult. The gross specimen is multicystic and the large numbers of varying-size cysts easily can be appreciated by holding the histologic sections up to the light. The cysts are lined by varyingly hyperplastic epithelium as well as papillary structures. The hyperplasia may be quite atypical, and foci of necrosis and large numbers of mitotic figures may be present. Young women may also have extensive papillomatosis and hyperplasia without cysts and without a discrete lesion. Histologic distinction from DCIS and intraductal papillary carcinoma may be difficult because of the atypia, necrosis, and mitotic activity; close attention to the clinical presentation and the age of the patient as well as the numerous cysts can help to make a correct diagnosis.

Clinical Implications

The risk for a patient with a papilloma, or papillomas, to develop a subsequent carcinoma is somewhat controversial. However, there is general agreement that the solitary subareolar papillary lesions do not constitute a significant increased risk. If atypical hyperplasia or carcinoma in situ are mixed within the papilloma, it is assumed that the risk of these lesions will be the same as those lesions without papillary architecture. Haagensen and others have presented evidence to suggest that multiple papillomas do constitute a significant increased risk of developing a subsequent carcinoma, but it is not clear that atypical hyperplasia and/or carcinoma in situ within the papillomas were excluded. Today, most investigators put single papillomas, whether subareolar or in the periphery of the breast, into the "no increased risk/only slightly increased risk" categories.[10,27b]

The studies by Rosen have suggested that women with florid papillomatosis, particularly those that are atypical, may have an increased risk of developing invasive carcinoma, but the magnitude of this risk is largely unknown at the present time. Recent data suggest that juvenile papillomatosis represents an increased risk for carcinoma only for patients with recurrent, bilateral juvenile papillomatosis and a family history of breast carcinoma.[35]

PAGET'S DISEASE OF THE NIPPLE

Paget's disease of the nipple represents ductal carcinoma in situ involving the epidermis of the nipple, although the adjacent breast ducts usually contain DCIS as well.[2,47] Microscopically, carcinoma cells are present in the epidermis either singly or in groups. These cells are characteristically large, with enlarged nuclei, and they have conspicuous nucleoli, abundant eosinophilic-to-clear cytoplasm, and distinct cell borders (Fig. 13).

Lesions that most commonly arise in the differential diagnosis of Paget's disease of the nipple include actinic keratosis, squamous carcinoma in situ, and intraepidermal involvement by malignant melanoma. Although epidermal squamous lesions show atypical cytologic features, the abnormal cells do not stand apart from normal adjacent keratinocytes, as in Paget's disease.

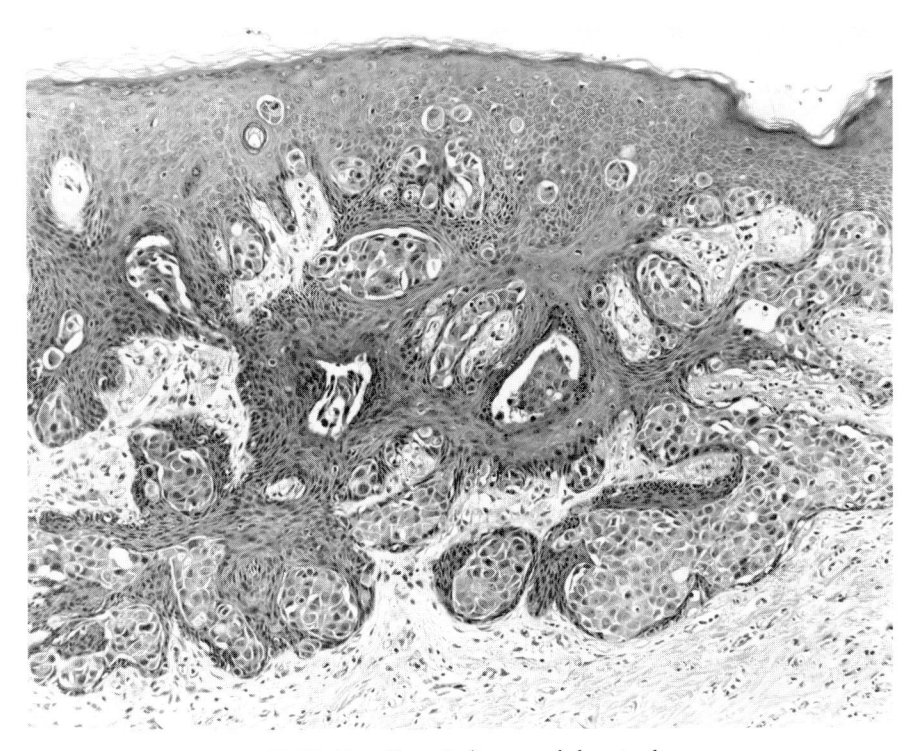

FIGURE 13. Paget's disease of the nipple.

Distinction from melanoma in situ may also present problems. The identification of DCIS in neighboring ducts usually will resolve the issue. In the absence of this finding, however, mucin stains may help to document the DCIS cells. In rare cases, immunohistochemical stains against keratins and S-100 protein may be required to distinguish DCIS involving the nipple from melanoma.

Clinical Implications

The finding of Paget's disease of the nipple indicates DCIS involving at least the epidermis of that part of the breast. In nearly all excisional breast biopsies, the ducts of the adjacent breast tissue will also harbor DCIS; therefore, the clinical implications are considered to be those of the DCIS of the ducts. In a significant percentage of cases, invasive carcinoma will also be present in the underlying breast. It has not been clearly shown that Paget's disease independently affects prognosis beyond that expected for DCIS. If a nipple biopsy demonstrates Paget's disease, mammography and excisional biopsy should be performed to document the type and extent of underlying neoplastic process in the breast.

Acknowledgment

The authors thank Mrs. Kelley Ramey for preparation of the manuscript.

References

1. Ashikari R, Hajdu SI, Robbins GF: Intraductal carcinoma of the breast. Cancer 28:1182–1187, 1971.
2. Ashikari R, Park K, Huvos AG, et al: Paget's disease of the breast. Cancer 26:680–685, 1970.
2a. Azzopardi JG: Problems in Breast Pathology. Philadelphia, W.B. Saunders, 1979.
3. Bestill WL, Rosen PP, Lieberman PH, et al: Intraductal carcinoma: Long-term follow-up after biopsy only. JAMA 239:1863–1867, 1978.
4. Black MM, Barclay THC, Cutler SJ, et al: Association of atypical characteristics of benign breast lesions with subsequent risk of breast cancer. Cancer 29:338–343, 1972.
5. Black MM, Chabon AB: In situ carcinoma of the breast. Pathol Annu 4:185–210, 1969.
6. Carter D, Smith RRL: Carcinoma in situ of the breast. Cancer 40:1189–1193, 1977.
7. Carter D, Orr SL, Merino SJ: Intracystic papillary carcinoma of the breast. After mastectomy, radiotherapy or excisional biopsy alone. Cancer 52:14–19, 1983.
8. Clement PB, Azzopardi JG: Microglandular adenosis of the breast—a lesion simulating tubular carcinoma. Histopathology 7:169–180, 1983.
9. Dupont WD: Converting relative risks to absolute risks: A graphical approach. Stat Med 8:641–651, 1989.
10. Dupont WD, Page DL: Risk factors for breast cancer in women with proliferative breast disease. N Engl J Med 312:146–151, 1985.
11. Dupont WD, Page DL: Relative risk of breast cancer varies with time since diagnosis of atypical hyperplasia. Hum Pathol 20:723–725, 1989.
12. Eusebi V, Foschini MP, Cook MG, et al: Long-term follow-up of in situ carcinoma of the breast with special emphasis on clinging carcinoma. Sem Diag Pathol 6:165–173, 1989.
13. Fechner RE: Lobular carcinoma in situ in sclerosing adenosis. A potential source of confusion with invasive carcinoma. Am J Surg Pathol 5:233–239, 1981.
14. Fisher ER, Sass R, Fisher B, et al: Pathologic findings from the National Surgical Adjuvant Breast Project (Protocol 6). I. Intraductal carcinoma (DCIS). Cancer 57:197–208, 1986.
15. Gump FE, Jicha DL, Ozello L: Ductal carcinoma in situ (DCIS): A revised concept. Surgery 102:790–795, 1987.
16. Haagensen CD, Lane N, Lattes R, et al: Lobular neoplasia (so-called lobular carcinoma in situ) of the breast. Cancer 42:737–769, 1978.

17. Hutchinson WB, Thomas DB, Hamlin WB, et al: Risk of breast cancer in women with benign breast disease. J Natl Cancer Inst 65:13–20, 1980.
18. Is "fibrocystic disease" of the breast precancerous? (Consensus meeting, October 3–5, 1985, New York). Arch Pathol Lab Med 110:171–173, 1986.
19. Jensen RA, Page DL, Dupont WD, et al: Invasive breast cancer risk in women with sclerosing adenosis. Cancer 64:1977–1983, 1989.
20. Ketcham AS, Moffat AL, Vexed surgeons, perplexed patients, and breast cancers which may not be cancer. Cancer 65:387–393, 1990.
21. Kodlin D, Winger EE, Morgenstern LL, et al: Chronic mastopathy and breast cancer: A follow-up study. Cancer 39:2603–2607, 1977.
22. Kraus FT, Neubecker RD: The differential diagnosis of papillary tumors of the breast. Cancer 15:444–455, 1962.
23. Lagios MD, Westdahl PR, Margolin FR, et al: Duct carcinoma in situ. Relationship of extent of noninvasive disease to the frequency of occult invasion, multicentricity, lymph node metastases, and short term treatment failures. Cancer 50:1309–1314, 1982.
24. Lagios MD, Margolin FR, Westdahl PR, et al: Mammographically detected duct carcinoma in situ: Frequency of local recurrence following tylectomy and prognostic effect of nuclear grade on local recurrence. Cancer 63:618–624, 1989.
24a. Lagios MD: Duct carcinoma in situ: Pathology and treatment. Surg Clin North Am 70:853–871, 1990.
25. Lewis D, Geschickter CF: Comedo carcinoma of the breast. Arch Surg 36:225–234, 1938.
26. Meyer JS: Cell kinetics of histologic variants of in situ breast carcinoma. Breast Cancer Res Treat 7:171–180, 1986.
27. Page DL: Cancer risk assessment in benign breast biopsies. Hum Pathol 17:871–874, 1986.
27a. Page DL, Anderson TJ: Diagnostic Histopathology of the Breast. New York, Churchill Livingstone, 1987.
27b. Page DL, Dupont WD: Premalignant conditions and markers of elevated risk in the breast and their management. Surg Clin North Am 70:831–851, 1990.
28. Page DL, Dupont WD, Rogers LW: Ductal involvement by cells of atypical lobular hyperplasia of the breast. A long-term follow-up study of cancer risk. Hum Pathol 19:201–207, 1988.
29. Page DL, Dupont WD, Rogers LW, et al: Intraductal carcinoma of the breast: Follow-up after biopsy only. Cancer 49:751–758, 1982.
30. Page DL, Dupont WD, Rogers LW, et al: Atypical hyperplastic lesions of the female breast. A long-term follow-up study. Cancer 55:2698–2708, 1985.
31. Page DL, Vander Zwaag R, Rogers LW, et al: Relationship between component parts of fibrocystic disease complex and breast cancer. J Natl Cancer Inst 61:1055–1063, 1978.
31a. Rosai J: Borderline epithelial lesions of the breast. Am J Surg Pathol 15:209–221, 1991.
32. Rosen PP: Microglandular adenosis. A benign lesion simulating invasive mammary carcinoma. Am J Surg Pathol 7:137–144, 1983.
33. Rosen PP: Subareolar sclerosing duct hyperplasia of the breast. Cancer 59:1927–1930, 1987.
34. Rosen PP, Caicco JA: Florid papillomatosis of the nipple. A study of 51 patients, including nine with mammary carcinoma. Am J Surg Pathol 10:87–101, 1986.
35. Rosen PP, Kimmel M: Juvenile papillomatosis of the breast: A follow-up study of 41 patients having biopsies before 1979. Am J Clin Pathol 93:599–603, 1990.
36. Rosen PP, Cantrell B, Mullen DL, et al: Juvenile papillomatosis (Swiss cheese disease) of the breast. Am J Surg Pathol 4:3–12, 1980.
37. Rosen PP, Holmes G, Lesser ML, et al: Juvenile papillomatosis and breast carcinoma. Cancer 55:1345–1352, 1985.
38. Rosen PP, Lieberman PH, Braun DW, et al: Lobular carcinoma in situ of the breast. Detailed analysis of 99 patients with average follow-up of 24 years. Am J Surg Pathol 3:225–251, 1978.
39. Rosenblum MK, Purrazzella R, Rosen PP: Is microglandular adenosis a precancerous disease? A study of carcinoma arising therein. Am J Surg Pathol 10:237–245, 1986.
40. Rosner D, Bedwani RN, Vana J, et al: Noninvasive breast carcinoma. Results of a national survey by the American College of Surgeons. Ann Surg 192:139–147, 1980.
41. Schnitt SJ, Silen W, Sadowsky NL, et al: Ductal carcinoma in situ (intraductal carcinoma) of the breast. N Engl J Med 318:898–903, 1988.
42. Silverstein MJ, Waisman JR, Gamagami P, et al: Intraductal carcinoma of the breast (208 cases). Clinical factors influencing treatment of choice. Cancer 66:102–108, 1990.
43. Silverstein MJ, Rosser RJ, Gierson ED, et al: Axillary lymph node dissection for intraductal breast carcinoma—is it indicated? Cancer 59:1819–1824, 1987.

44. Tavassoli FA, Norris HJ: Microglandular adenosis of the breast. Am J Surg Pathol 7:731, 1983.
45. Tavassoli FA, Norris HJ: A comparison of the results of long-term follow-up for atypical intraductal hyperplasia and intraductal hyperplasia of the breast. Cancer 65:518–529, 1990.
46. van de Vijver MJ, Peterse JL, Mooi WJ, et al: Neu-protein overexpression in breast cancer. Association with comedo type ductal carcinoma in situ and limited prognostic value in stage II breast cancer. N Engl J Med 319:1239–1245, 1988.
46a. Wellings RR, Jensen HM, Marcum RG: An atlas of subgross pathology of the human breast with special reference to possible precancerous lesions. J Natl Cancer Inst 55:231–273, 1975.
47. Wood WS, Hedgedus C: Mammary Paget's disease and intraductal carcinoma: Histologic, histochemical and immunocytochemical comparison. Am J Dermatopathol 10:183–188, 1988.

Steroid Receptors in Surgical Pathology
With Special Reference to Small Mammographically Detected Breast Lesions

JON C. ROSS, M.D.
SCOTT BINDER, M.D.
MARK C. ROUNSAVILLE, M.D.
KLAUS LEWIN, M.D.

From Department of Anatomic
   Pathology and Clinical
   Laboratories
California Pacific Medical
   Center, California Campus
San Francisco, California (JCR,
   MCR)

Department of Dermatopathology
Scripps Clinic and Research
   Foundation
La Jolla, California (SB)

and Departments of Pathology
   and Medicine
UCLA School of Medicine
Los Angeles, California (KL)

Reprint requests to:
Jon C. Ross, M.D.
Department of Anatomic
   Pathology
California Pacific Medical
   Center, California Campus
3700 California Street
San Francisco, CA 94118

The cellular receptors for estrogen, progesterone, and other steroid hormones appear in the cytosol fraction of homogenated specimens of hormonal target tissues. These receptors have traditionally been detected and quantitated by biochemical techniques that involve binding tritium-labelled marker steroids to the receptor proteins. An important recent development has been the creation of various monoclonal antibody reagents that specifically recognize antigenic determinants on receptor molecules.[47] These monoclonals are valuable tools for better understanding the biology of steroid receptors. They have been used to show, for example, that the primary cellular locus of estrogen receptor is within the nucleus, not within the cytoplasm as had been previously believed.[45,63,70] Commercially available monoclonal reagents are now the basis of improved clinical laboratory techniques for measuring estrogen and progesterone receptors—both for assays of the cytosol fraction of tumor homogenates and for newer immunohistochemical analyses.

These immunohistochemical methods extend determination of receptor status to even small needle localized breast lesions.

Prior to the availability of monoclonal antibodies directed against human receptor proteins, pathologists often encountered problems in providing both optimal histopathologic evaluation and receptor analysis for small breast tumors. It is very possible in the near future, if the results of many recent immunohistochemical studies are confirmed, that the pathologist will be able to submit the entire quantity of the small tumor specimens obtained by mammographically directed biopsy for permanent section, and thus obtain not only a complete look at the tumor but also, by immunohistochemistry, the most accurate detection of the tumor's hormone receptor status from the same specimen.

This article is not limited to consideration of the mammographically directed breast biopsy, but generally surveys the application of steroid receptor measurement in surgical pathology. Various aspects of this topic have been well reviewed elsewhere.[45,62,63,90,108,113,141] Here the emphasis is on a practical review for pathologists—with special attention to the recent developments in receptor immunohistochemistry and to the proper handling of small mammographically localized biopsy specimens.

THE PATHOLOGIST'S ROLE

The surgical pathologist is directly responsible for obtaining appropriate breast cancer samples for receptor determination by cytosol assay, and it is generally a pathologist who supervises the assay and reports the results. However, in many instances a consulting laboratory performs the assay. This distances many practicing pathologists from knowledge of receptor assay techniques and interpretation. Nevertheless, given his role in obtaining tissue for study, the pathologist will be asked to interpret results. He may be asked to integrate receptor determinations with other variables that determine prognosis of breast cancer. If anything goes wrong, the pathologist will certainly be asked to explain and justify why hormone receptor assay results are unavailable in a particular case. The pathologist may be asked why results appear discordant with a prior study from the same patient. Furthermore, the pathologist must appreciate the *relative* clinical value of knowing the hormone receptor status of a neoplasm, vis-à-vis other prognostic information. He will then be able to divide and allocate small specimens wisely for various competing pathologic examinations.

What is the clinical significance of estrogen receptor (ER) and progesterone receptor (PgR) measurements in the management of breast cancer patients?

Prognosis

The preponderance of evidence suggests that breast carcinoma patients with ER-positive tumors have longer disease-free survival and overall survival than those with ER-negative tumors.[90,134,146] Patients with PgR-positive tumors generally also have shown longer disease-free survival,[1,21,90,146] although not all studies have shown this effect.[142] Of course, the value of such prognostic information depends on its degree of independence from other well-known and generally available prognostic indicators, such as axillary lymph node status, tumor size, and histologic and nuclear grade.

Although nodal status is the dominant prognostic indicator for breast carcinoma, several studies have affirmed that receptor status does have independent prognostic significance for Stage I and Stage II breast cancer patients (i.e., those without and those with axillary lymph node metastases). Skoog and his colleagues found that ER-rich tumors were associated with a lower mortality than ER-poor tumors for both premenopausal and postmenopausal women, irrespective of the number of lymph nodes involved by carcinoma.[134] The relative prognostic importance of various factors in node-negative patients is, however, debated. Fisher and his colleagues found that nuclear grade was a relatively more important prognostic factor than estrogen receptor status for node-negative patients, and that progesterone receptor status was of little or no prognostic value for this group.[38] For Stage I patients, McGuire asserts that ER status and tumor size appear most prognostically important[90] and questions the reproducibility of tumor grading.[91]

For Stage II patients, including the group of Stage II patients with more than 3 positive axillary nodes, both ER positivity and PgR positivity have shown favorable prognostic effect as measured by disease-free survival and overall survival.[37,146] In Stage II, the most important prognostic factors appear to be the number of positive axillary nodes, the size of the primary tumor, and the steroid receptor status.[90] Interestingly, several multivariate studies have shown that the prognostic importance of PgR status, as opposed to ER status, may be greater for Stage II patients, especially as regards disease-free survival.[1,17,37,90]

In a multivariate study of Stage I–III breast cancer patients, which included nuclear DNA analysis of tumors, Kallioniemi et al.[64] found progesterone receptor content to be an independently significant prognostic factor (along with nodal status, tumor size, and DNA ploidy). Klintenberg et al. also found ER status to be an independent prognostic indicator, along with proliferative index, when considered together with nodal status in a multivariate study of breast cancer disease-free survival.[73]

Response to Therapy

Results of endocrine therapy for disseminated breast carcinoma vary greatly in accord with the steroid receptor content of the neoplasms. More than 60% of ER+ lesions respond to endocrine manipulations, whereas less than 10% of ER– lesions respond.[20,146] Approximately 70% of ER+PgR+ lesions respond, and many ER–PgR+ tumors also respond favorably.[1,20,146] Of course, the clinical value of being able to predict response to a therapy varies considerably with the potential toxicity of the treatment being contemplated. When hormone receptor data first became available for clinical management of breast cancer patients, ablative surgery was the common form of endocrine treatment. That is not the case today. Drug therapy with tamoxifen, an antiestrogen, has generally replaced oophorectomy, adrenalectomy, and hypophysectomy in the treatment of these patients. Furthermore, tamoxifen is remarkably nontoxic and is probably one of the best tolerated drugs in the pharmacopeia.

Response of breast cancer to chemotherapy has also been studied as a function of hormone receptor status. Increased, decreased, and unchanged response rates to chemotherapy have been reported for ER+ tumors.[26,67,78,146] Corle et al. reported improved response rates only for tumors with high ER levels, a finding that may account for some of the disparities found elsewhere in the literature.[26] Some investigators have hypothesized that chemotherapy's effect on breast cancer in premenopausal women is mediated partly through chemical castration.[11]

Combined chemoendocrine therapy regimens have been designed to eliminate both hormone-dependent and hormone-independent clones of neoplastic cells.[108] Most such trials have not shown a change in response rate or significant changes in response duration. None has shown a significant effect on overall length of survival.[108,113] New clinical studies of such combined therapy modalities are in progress at this time.[8,41,53]

Treatment Decisions

Adjuvant Therapy. Systemic therapy decisions are often based on the patient's steroid receptor status. The National Institutes of Health adjuvant therapy guidelines for breast carcinoma are summarized in Table 1.[45,101] These guidelines, based on a consensus conference sponsored by the NIH in 1985, are generally accepted by clinical oncologists. An update from the NIH Consensus Development Panel concerned with treatment of early stage breast cancer was adopted in June of 1990.[101a] The 1990 NIH-sponsored panel agreed that the majority of node-negative breast cancer patients are cured by local surgery plus axillary dissection alone, but that the rate of local and distant recurrence can be somewhat decreased by either adjuvant chemotherapy or tamoxifen. They left the issue whether or not to employ such adjuvant therapy

TABLE 1. Summary of National Institutes of Health Guidelines for Breast Carcinoma

Women with negative nodes:
 1. Adjuvant therapy not recommended as a routine.
 2. Consider chemotherapy for high risk patients (large tumor, **ER-** and **PgR-**, high histologic grade, aneuploid, high labelling index or S-phase).

Premenopausal women with positive lymph nodes:
 1. Combination chemotherapy preferred.
 2. No known benefit of adjuvant endocrine therapy and not recommended outside clinical study setting.

Postmenopausal women with positive nodes:
 1. **ER+**: tamoxifen.
 2. **ER-**: weigh toxicity of chemotherapy against minor increases in survival and disease-free survival, especially if 4 or more positive nodes.

in a node-negative woman to be decided on a case-by-case basis, balancing risks and benefits.

Adjunctive systemic therapy is not now considered routine in node-negative patients, although its use, particularly in high-risk lesions (e.g., ER– and PgR–) is becoming more common. A great deal of controversy now surrounds the question of a standard therapy for node-negative patients.[54,129] This was generated in part in mid-1988 by the release, as a National Cancer Institute Clinical Alert, of preliminary results from trials testing the value of systemic adjuvant therapy for node negative patients.[100,120] This media release suggested that chemotherapy or tamoxifen therapy may be advantageous and should be considered for node-negative patients. The early results of several node-negative adjuvant therapy trials have recently been published, indicating a modest improvement in disease-free survival after systemic treatment.[9,35,38,54,80] Patient selection for these studies is commonly based on estrogen receptor status. In general, ER-negative cases are entered on trials testing the role of cytotoxic chemotherapy and ER-positive cases are entered on tamoxifen trials. An exception, is the Novaldex Adjuvant Trial Organization (NATO) study, a randomized European tamoxifen trial that includes pre- and postmenopausal patients, node-negative and node-positive, ER-positive and ER-negative. In this trial, tamoxifen appears to benefit all subgroups of women with breast cancer, including those with ER-negative tumors.[104]

Premenopausal patients with positive axillary lymph nodes generally are treated with chemotherapy in the United States, the steroid receptor status being irrelevant to that treatment decision. However, tamoxifen has recently been advanced as a safe and effective alternative to chemotherapy in node-positive premenopausal women whose neoplasms are ER-positive.[8] For postmenopausal patients with positive nodes, the hormone receptor status is key in deciding the type of adjuvant approach to be followed.[53] The PgR status appears to be of special importance in predicting the results of tamoxifen therapy in this adjuvant setting.[90] If the ER and PgR status were unknown in such a case, employing tamoxifen as an adjuvant would appear to have little toxicity for a postmenopausal woman with positive nodes. But insofar as chemotherapy might prove advantageous for high-risk receptor-negative postmenopausal patients, it is obviously preferable to know the receptor status. Now that immunohistochemical analysis for ER is available, an archived block may be studied to resolve the question of ER-status, even years after the original presentation.

Palliative Therapy. For women with disseminated metastatic breast carcinoma requiring palliative management, ER and PgR status will guide treatment as well. For patients whose tumors do contain ER, tamoxifen is standard treatment. For steroid receptor-negative women, both premenopausal and postmenopausal, and for patients whose pattern of visceral metastases is less likely to be favorably affected by endocrine manipulations, combination chemotherapy is generally employed. Bone, skin, and soft tissue metastases generally respond more favorably to endocrine therapy than do metastases in brain, lung, liver, and other viscera. Tamoxifen may be employed by oncologists at some point in the management of even the steroid receptor-negative cases, in the slim chance (< 10%) of achieving a response.

In Situ Carcinoma

Currently, there is no established clinical utility of steroid receptor determinations for in situ carcinomas of the breast. In fact, as will be further elaborated below, it is a disservice to the patient to homogenize biopsy material for cytosol receptor determinations of in situ neoplasms. With the advent of immunohistochemistry, which allows receptors to be identified while still conserving the tissue for histopathologic examination, analysis of in situ carcinoma for ER and PgR is feasible, although of no current clinical use. Fifty-six cases of in situ breast carcinoma have been studied for steroid receptors by Bur and Chowdhary.[13]

What correlations exist between steroid receptor content and other pathologic characteristics of breast carcinomas?

Histologic Type and Grade

A high frequency of ER positivity has been reported for invasive lobular carcinomas[127] and for all breast carcinomas regarded as well differentiated.[40,84,115] Differentiation can be imputed from a variety of characteristics; Fisher and colleagues have shown that high overall histologic grade, nuclear anaplasia alone, and tumor necrosis are all significantly correlated with negative ER status.[40] Results are mixed as regards a possible association of negative ER status with lymphocytic host response seen in breast carcinomas.[15,40,127] The association of ER positivity with histologically better differentiated neoplasms has earned for the receptor status the reputation as a "biochemical" measure of differentiation. The strong correlation of tumor grade with steroid hormone receptor status has prompted questions about the independence of these variables as prognostic indicators.[25,39]

Ploidy and Growth Fraction

Reinforcing the viewpoint of steroid receptors as biochemical indicators of neoplastic differentiation are correlations between absence of receptors, on the one hand, and both aneuploid nuclear DNA content and high growth fraction of breast carcinomas, on the other. The inverse relationship appears well established between measures of growth fraction (such as thymidine labeling index or flow cytometrically determined S-phase fraction) and ER and PgR content.[32,51,65,89,94,107] Early results are more varied for correlations of receptor status with stem cell ploidy. Those authors who have been able to demonstrate a statistically significant association have shown that tumors which have diploid nuclear DNA pattern (or which have lower DNA indices in the spectrum from diploid to markedly aneuploid) are more likely to have positive receptors.[32,57,94,106] Others have not been able to demonstrate significant associations.[7,31,51,89]

What proportion of breast cancer specimens contain steroid receptor proteins and how are the results reported?

The reported rates of positivity of breast carcinomas for ER and PgR vary significantly from study to study.[141] Those recorded here are representative and are based on biochemical (radioligand) cytosol receptor assays. Detectable ER is found in breast cancers of approximately 60% of premenopausal patients and in 75% or more of postmenopausal patients. Detectable PgR is found in 50–70% of breast carcinomas. In contrast to ER, PgR is somewhat more common in tumors from premenopausal patients.[141]

ER and PgR content are usually correlated, both positive or both negative, in breast carcinomas. ER is thought to have a role in the induction of synthesis of PgR in breast cancer cells.[109] This hypothesis may account for the fact that PgR is relatively infrequently found in ER negative tumors. The exceptions are interesting in that they occur primarily in younger premenopausal or perimenopausal women. On closer study such tumors can sometimes be shown to be false negative for ER (as, for example, when sensitive assays of nuclear fractions are performed).[141] ER+PgR− tumors occur mostly in postmenopausal patients, and the absence of PgR is considered clinically significant because it correlates with a somewhat lower response rate to endocrine therapies.[109]

The amount of hormone receptor is generally reported as the specific activity, i.e., as a ratio of receptor content to the protein content of the cytosol. Because cellularity varies markedly in cancer specimens used to prepare the cytosols, some laboratories have reported the receptor content as a ratio to the weight of the tissue homogenized. This type of reporting should not, however, replace a report of the specific activity. Almost all of the correlative data relating receptor content of breast and other carcinomas to prognosis and response to endocrine therapy are presented in terms of specific activities of receptor. Because receptor is reported in this manner, proper attention must be given to the method of protein assay and its standardization.[51,145] Some studies have employed DNA rather than protein content of cytosols to obtain a specific activity, but again this results in data that are difficult to compare to the rest of the literature.[73]

The range of receptor concentrations in human breast cancers is a wide one. For ER, this range extends from 0 to over 1000 femtomoles per milligram of cytosol protein (fmol/mg prot). Cut off thresholds for reporting "positive" and "negative" results of ER determinations vary from laboratory to laboratory, generally from a low of 3 fmol/mg protein up to 20 fmol/mg protein. In the borderline range of 3–19 fmoles/mg protein an intermediate frequency of response of metastatic breast carcinoma to hormonal therapies has been observed.[145] In this regard, Paridaens has emphasized the significance of the quantitative level of ER, as distinguished from the categorical classification of lesions as receptor positive or negative.[114] On the other hand, the prognostic significance of ER status has been suggested by Thorpe et al.[142] to lie in a simple qualitative distinction between receptor positive and negative patients, and not in the quantitative level of ER per se.

Also generally reported with the molar quantity of receptor protein is the dissociation constant, which characterizes its binding to the hormone ligand in question. This dissociation constant, generally abbreviated as Kd, is inversely correlated with the affinity of the binding being described (the smaller the Kd, the greater the affinity of the binding). Since ER and PgR bind their respective hormone ligands very strongly, one should anticipate appropriately low values for Kd. For ER, the dissociation constant for estradiol is in the range of 1×10^{-10} M. Estrogens and progestins may be bound with lower affinity by other cellular constituents, and this lower affinity binding may be nonspecific. These are important concepts to recall in the interpretation of indirect methods of histochemistry, which attempt to evaluate steroid hormone binding to tissue sections (discussed in more detail below).

How reproducible are the results of hormone receptor assays?

Coefficients of variation for multiple determinations of ER levels from the same cytosol using traditional biochemical techniques are in the range of 5–16%.[108] However, the majority of discordant assays are for ER levels in the equivocal range of 3–10 fmol of receptor per milligram of cytosol protein. The occurrence of major discordance (i.e., clearly negative [< 3 fmol/mg] versus clearly positive [> 10 fmol/mg]) is much less common, about 3%.[42] Small tissue samples lead to higher discordance rates. Also, patients biopsied while on tamoxifen or within a 2-month period after stopping this drug frequently have false negative tumor ER values by conventional biochemical cytosol assays.[59] The latter problem of interference by estrogens or anti-estrogens is not a problem with the newer immunoassays (vide infra). The newer cytosol immunoassays also have a lower coefficient of variation for multiple determinations on the same cytosol, in the range of 5–10%.[76]

How does the receptor status of a breast carcinoma evolve over time and after treatment?

As a general rule the ER status of a breast carcinoma tends to "breed-true" over the course of the patient's disease, unless there has been intervening endocrine therapy between the assays.[2,30,113] More precisely, the rates of discordance of ER content determinations between metachronous (sequential) biopsies on the one hand and between concurrent biopsies on the other are similar (about 12–34%).[2,108] Thus, results of assays at different points in a patient's course may occasionally differ from one another, just as they may at a single point in time, but several careful studies suggest that they do not do so in a systematic way when groups of patients assessed with multiple ER assays are studied. This suggests that heterogeneity of steroid receptor content may be as great within the primary tumor as between samples from spatially separate sites (or that methodological errors obscure variation due to heterogeneity). This seems particularly to be the case when no therapy, or a course of chemotherapy, has intervened between the two assays. Some literature supports the finding of greater discordance rates for ER assays when two biopsies are separated by intervening endocrine therapy,[2] but this may be due to factors other than treatment selection against ER-positive clones of neoplastic cells. These factors have been reviewed by Osborne and include confounding effects produced by the drug tamoxifen (which may block receptor binding sites), decrease in receptor concentrations due to decrease in tumor cellularity after treatment, and false-negative results due to small biopsy size at the second determination.[59,68,108]

Some studies have shown apparent loss of ER in metastatic sites when compared to the primary tumor, but these data must be interpreted in the light of discordance rates for simultaneous assays, as noted above. Nevertheless, these data will be cited. Klinga et al. found that estrogen and progesterone receptor assay results varied from the primary lesion to the axillary nodal metastasis, usually by loss of the receptor from the metastatic deposits.[72] Others have also documented discordance in the results of ER assays from primary and metastatic sites.[128] The essential question regarding ER status and tumor progression is whether the ER-receptor status determined at the time of mastectomy allows one to predict the response to endocrine manipulations after a variable, sometimes prolonged, interval to metastasis. DeSombre and Jensen found that, despite a tendency toward decreased estrophilin content with time in their data from sequential biopsies, prediction of endocrine response could accurately be based on initial mastectomy specimen receptor assays.[30]

The story is different for progesterone receptor, for which a definite trend to loss of the PgR appears to result from endocrine therapy. Gross et al. reported the discordance rate for simultaneous biopsies to be 9%, whereas that for subsequent versus original biopsies was 44% (when the initial PgR assay was positive).[48] Importantly, this was shown to be due to intervening endocrine therapy. Specifically, 56% of patients in the cited study treated with endocrine therapy lost tumor PgR. Survival was much worse for those patients whose tumors converted to PgR negative.[48] This provides a reason for gathering material for progesterone receptor assay from recurrent or metastatic breast carcinoma specimens, even when a prior receptor assay on the primary tumor has already been obtained, and when there has been an intervening course of endocrine therapy.

What are the advantages and disadvantages of the various clinical laboratory methods used to determine ER and PgR content in tumors, and are they all measuring the same things?

Biochemical and Immunochemical Cytosol Techniques

Traditional methods for measuring steroid receptor molecules in tumor specimens have relied upon biochemical means of identifying specific high-affinity binding of radiolabelled estrogens or progestogens in cytosols. Cytosols are prepared by homogenizing a sample of the neoplasm and subjecting the homogenate to ultracentrifugation. Two widely used methods of demonstrating the specific steroid binding in cytosols are: (1) multipoint titration, and (2) sucrose density gradient centrifugation. Both depend on the binding of radioligands to the receptor. Multipoint titration methods often employ the use of dextran-coated charcoal to remove unbound estrogen from the assay mixtures (hence, the common abbreviation for this technique as the "dextran-coated charcoal method"). These biochemical techniques are labor intensive and therefore costly. The recent introduction of monoclonal antibodies directed against steroid receptor molecules has altered the way these tests are being done by many laboratories.

There are several disadvantages of the traditional biochemical (radioligand) cytosol techniques:

1. Conventional biochemical radioligand binding cytosol techniques require relatively large sample size and therefore tend to exclude effusions and needle biopsies (250 mg of tumor tissue per assay).
2. Conventional cytosol techniques do not measure all receptor, namely, that portion of the receptor already bound to steroid molecules in vivo.
3. Measurement of cytosols does not allow direct assessment of tumor cell heterogeneity.
4. Cytosol assay does not allow for convenient assessment of specimen adequacy (i.e., percent necrosis, fibrosis, cellularity) or allow distinction of in situ from invasive components.
5. Conventional cytosol methods are laborious and expensive, and necessitate handling of radioactive substances.

Some of these disadvantages are corrected by the currently available **cytosol monoclonal immunoassay** for steroid receptors (EIA by Abbott Laboratories Diagnostics Division, North Chicago, IL). Specifically, the immunoassay: (1) allows analysis of smaller specimens (only 200 μl of cytosol, as little as 20 mg of tumor tissue, is required; (2) assays all of the receptor (whether bound to steroid in vivo or not); (3) is substantially less laborious than conventional cytosol techniques; and (4) does not employ radiolabelled steroids. The immunoassay is also less expensive, if assays are appropriately batched, but it is still subject to criticisms 3 and 4 in the previous listing of disadvantages.

The cytosol immunoassay (Abbott EIA) is subject to potentiation rather than interference by anti-estrogens (4-hydroxytamoxifen) and diethylstilbesterol. When they bind to the estrogen receptor, these molecules are thought to cause a conformational change in the receptor. This exposes an additional antigenic site to the monoclonal antibody and results in a doubling of the apparent estrophilin content by cytosol immunoassay in the presence of these substances.[82]

Measurement of estrogen and progesterone receptors using the cytosol immunoassay technique has been extensively compared to the standard radioligand binding assay method with good results,[56,102a] and the Abbott EIA method may be used with confidence. Successful application of the cytosol immunoassay technique to specimens obtained by fine needle aspiration has been reported.[79]

Direct Methods of Immunohistochemistry

False negative cytosol assays for steroid hormone receptors may be obtained because the sample of tissue that was reserved for the assay contained little neoplastic tissue. This may happen when the neoplastic tissue is necrotic, extensively fibrotic, or paucicellular for any other reason. One traditional method for dealing with this tissue is to examine histologically a section of tissue immediately adjacent to that reserved for the cytosol assay, to ensure that viable neoplastic tissue has been sampled. An attractive alternative approach, especially for the surgical pathologist, is to depart from measurement of cytosols and instead to demonstrate the steroid receptors immunohistochemically. Several methods have been proposed to accomplish this goal.

Recent development of monoclonal antibodies directed against determinants on the ER molecule (estrophilin) have made possible the direct visualization of receptor protein in its nuclear habitat.[70] A number of reports have shown good correlation of the histochemical technique of determining ER status with both the results of cytosol assays for ER and the results of endocrine therapy.[33,69,71,83a,86,88,117,135a] These studies are summarized in Table 2.

These histochemical preparations for ER tend to have clean backgrounds, with little evidence of nonspecific staining. The monoclonal antibody can be employed with either frozen sections or paraffin-embedded tissues, the latter having crisper morphologic detail as well as offering the convenience of using routinely processed material. The positive stains show a reassuring internal control for specificity, in that the receptor is located in the nucleus and not elsewhere (Figs. 1 and 2).

When first introduced, this histochemical method for identifying ER was only applicable to frozen tissue sections or fresh specimens (Abbott ER-ICA

TABLE 2. Studies of Correlation Between the Histochemical Technique of Determining ER Status and Cytosol Assays for ER and Endocrine Therapy

Study	Specificity	Sensitivity
McClelland et al.[88]	100% (for response to endocrine therapy)	100%
McCarty et al.[86]	93% (for response to endocrine therapy)	89%
	86–94% (for comparison with cytosol assays)	88–95%
Pertschuk et al.[117]	92% (for comparison with cytosol assays)	83%
King et al.[69]	75% (for comparison with cytosol assays)	98%
Reiner et al.[123]	96% (for comparison with cytosol assays)	73%
DeNegri et al.[83a]	71.4% (for comparison with immunoassay on cytosols)	86%
Sondergaard et al.[135a]	100% (for comparison with cytosol assays)	88.7%

Monoclonal Kit). Most encouraging is the documentation of successful histochemical localization of estrophilin in standard paraffin-embedded and formalin-fixed tissues.[18,132,133] Each of these methods relies in part on preincubation of the tissue slices with an enzyme reagent—either pronase, trypsin, or DNAase. Shintaku and Said reported success using paraffin sections after DNAase treatment.[133] Anderson et al. have favorably reported the use of trypsanized paraffin sections.[3] However, other laboratories have not been able to duplicate all of these results.[18] Our experience with the method of Shintaku and Said has also been less than satisfactory. Cheng et al. have performed a comparative analysis of five paraffin-based histochemical techniques for ER demonstration, and they advocate a method of their own elaboration that employs pronase pretreatment of the sections.[18] They obtained excellent results in a study of 27 breast cancers for which radioligand cytosol analyses of receptor content provided the standard for comparison with the paraffin histochemical technique. This pronase method, coupled with a biotinylated anti-rat Ig/avidin-alkaline phosphatase visualization technique, proved to be 100% sensitive and 89% specific for ER positivity in their study, when compared to cytosol assays.

Not only does the histochemical technique allow direct assessment of tumor cellularity and tissue viability, but it also permits assessment of tumor cell heterogeneity. That breast carcinomas are apparently heterogeneous in terms of cellular hormone receptor content has been frequently observed by those employing monoclonal histochemistry, whether in frozen or paraffin-embedded material.[18,108] The patterns of histochemical staining for ER fall roughly into four groups, as reported by Jensen, Greene, and DeSombre,[63] (an observation that has also been true in our laboratories). These patterns are summarized in Table 3.

The type of heterogeneity that is commonly seen is illustrated in Figure 2. Cells with positively stained nuclei are admixed with weakly stained or unstained ones. We have seldom seen striking geographic variation in the proportion of positively stained cells, except near the edges of paraffin sections or adjacent to foci of necrosis where nonspecific binding may be seen. It is important to exclude the regional variation that may result from differences in the fixation process, i.e., variable thicknesses and fixation times. Clearly, the choice of fixative is important for demonstration of estrogen receptor in the fixed state. Anderson et al. have shown that cross-linking fixatives (formaldehyde and glutaraldehyde) are superior to fixatives containing coagulating reagents (Carnoy's, Zenker's, Bouin's, and ethanol).[3] Work continues at this time

---

FIGURE 1 *(opposite page).* Illustrated are positive *(A)* and negative *(B)* monoclonal anti-estrophilin histochemical preparations in an immunoperoxidase system utilizing frozen sections of breast carcinomas. The nuclear localization of receptor protein can be seen in *A*, which illustrates a focus of comedo duct carcinoma and adjacent infiltrating duct carcinoma. In *B*, a pale counterstain highlights the nuclear outlines in an infiltrating duct carcinoma, which is unreactive with the monoclonal antibody reagent (Abbott ER-ICA, immunoperoxidase technique).

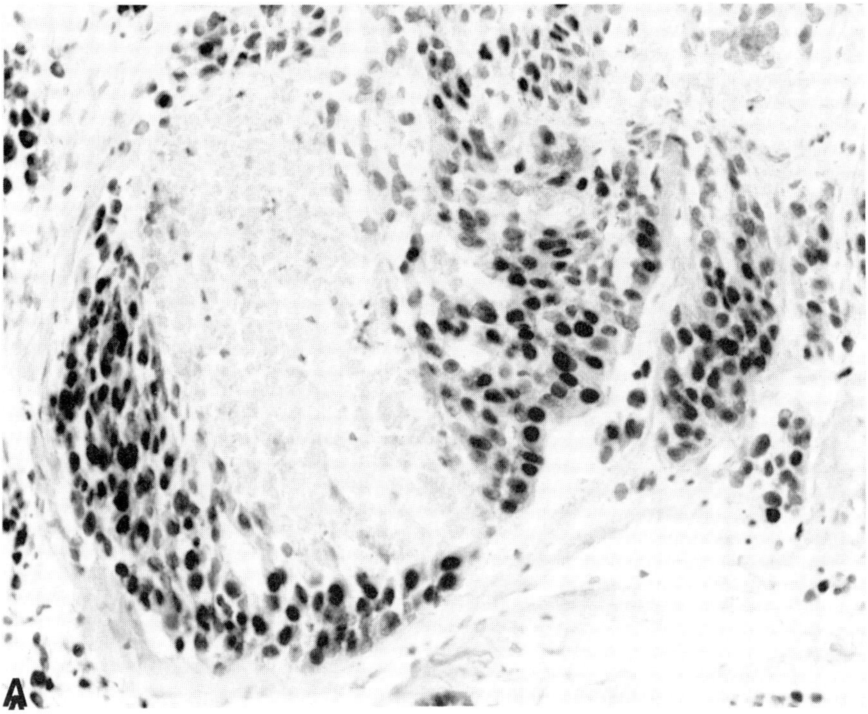
A

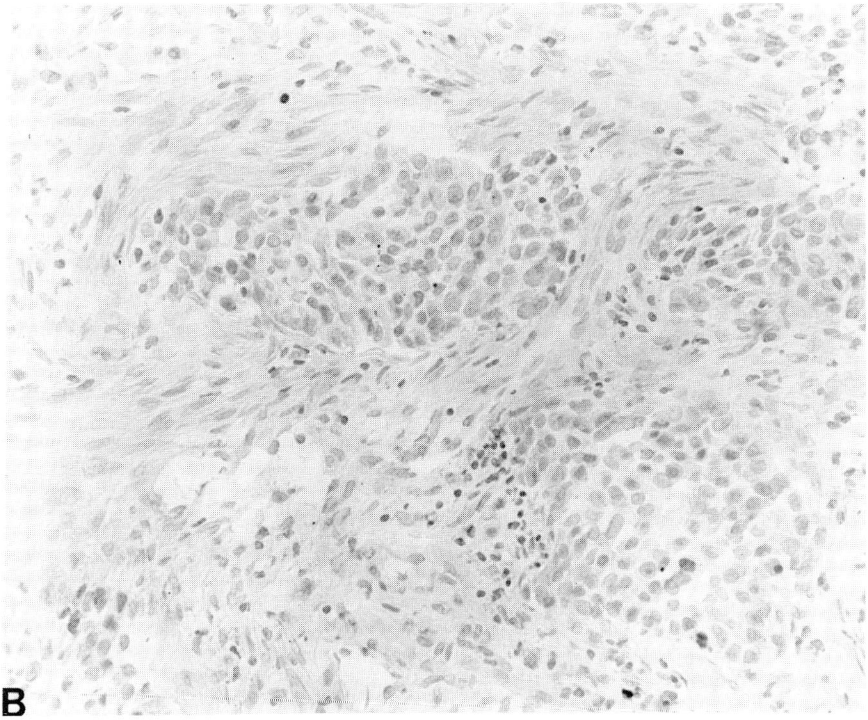
B

TABLE 3. Patterns of Histochemical Staining for ER

Pattern 0:	Receptor poor by cytosol techniques. No histochemical staining.
Pattern I:	Receptor poor by cytosol technique. Small population of histochemically positive cells, often weakly stained.
Pattern II:	Receptor rich by cytosol technique. Moderate-to-strong histochemical staining, but with many unstained cells.
Pattern III:	Receptor rich by cytosol technique. Moderate-to-strong staining of most or all cells.

define the optimal conditions for the immunohistochemical detection of steroid receptor proteins.[33]

Breast carcinomas frequently feature a mixture of cytologic and architectural patterns in different areas. These can be independently assessed for the presence of receptor protein using the histochemical technique. However, this would require more extensive sampling of lesions for receptor analysis than heretofore employed, and the clinical relevance of such data is speculative.

Samples of effusions and other cytologic preparations, such as touch preparations and smears, can be examined for ER content relatively easily.[83,122,123] We have found no difficulty in immunohistochemically examining carcinomas with large amounts of mucin production. In fact, a large study by Reiner et al. showed that using the immunohistochemical method, invasive lobular, mucoid, and tubular carcinomas were more frequently ER-positive than conventional ductal carcinomas. They also found that medullary carcinomas were more frequently ER-negative and that papillary carcinomas were more often ER-positive using the ER-ICA technique. Histologic grade also correlated well with ER status in their study. Similar results were obtained by Helin et al.[52]

A potential problem of monoclonal immunohistochemical methods for demonstrating ER receptor is their qualitative nature. Several studies employing cytosol analysis have provided evidence that a quantitative assessment of receptor content is advantageous, i.e., that the amount of ER receptor in the tumor is related to the likelihood of the hormonal responsiveness of breast carcinoma.[37,114] Some workers have addressed this issue by introducing in their histochemical analyses semi-quantitative assessments of the number of positively stained cells and the intensity of staining.[86,123] These methods remain relatively subjective and require substantial increase in labor by the microscopist. An alternative is now available, because computer-based photometry systems can be programmed to allow quantification of immunohistochemical staining. Such an adaptation has been reported by Bacus et al.

FIGURE 2 *(opposite page)*. *A* illustrates an infiltrating breast carcinoma which displays both estrogen-receptor positive and estrogen-receptor negative cells. This type of heterogeneity is commonly seen in preparations stained with monoclonal anti-estrophilin antibody (Abbot ER-ICA, immunoperoxidase technique). *B* illustrates a relatively paucicellular infiltrating lobular carcinoma in which stroma predominates over neoplastic cells. Most of the neoplastic cells show strong nuclear staining for estrogen receptor (Abbott ER-ICA, immunoperoxidase technique).

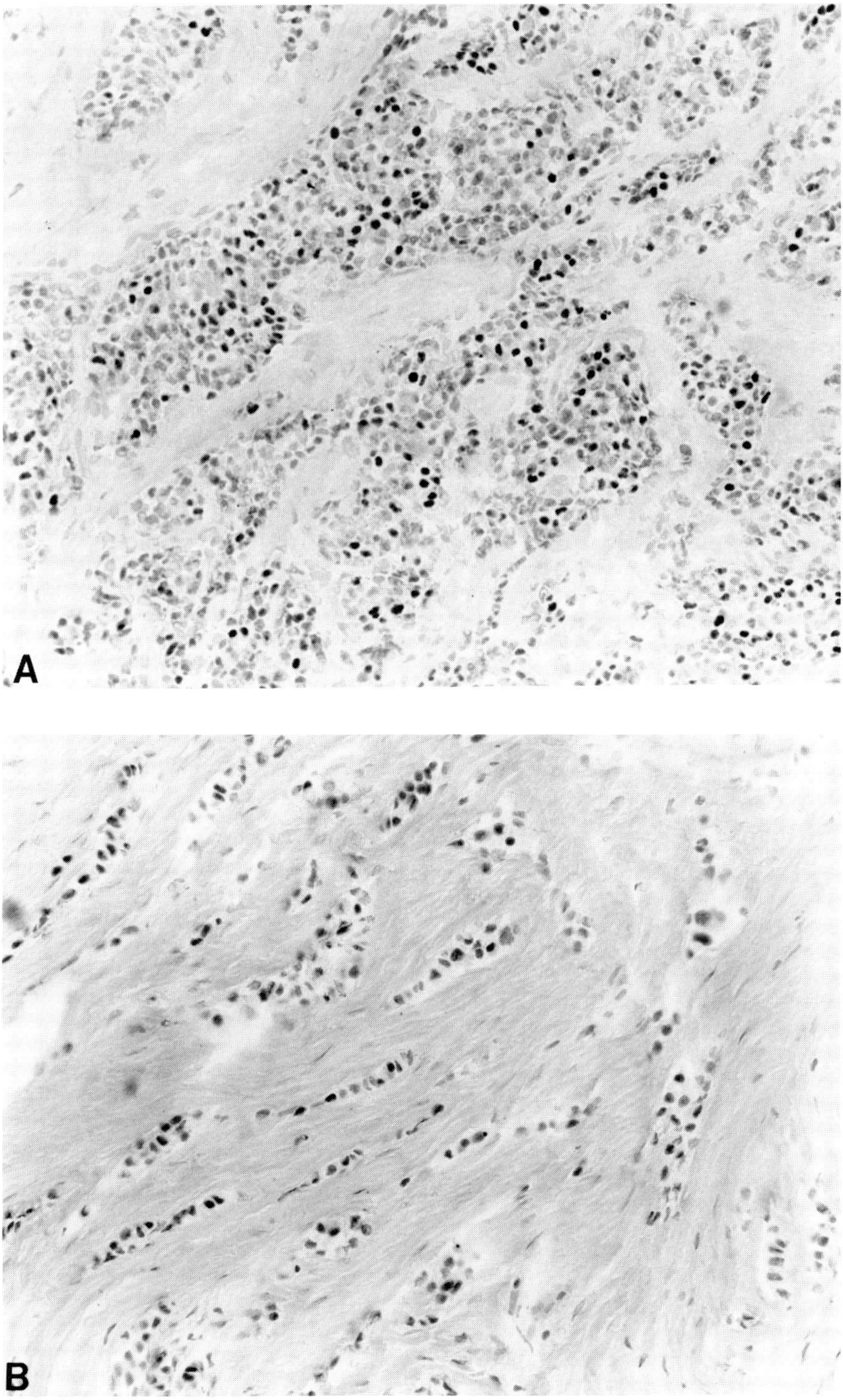
A
B

to be a specific and sensitive quantitative method for determining receptor status.[5] Using this monoclonal histochemical photometric technique, Bacus and colleagues were able to classify breast carcinoma specimens with 98% sensitivity and 100% specificity for ER content, when compared to the results of ER cytosol radioligand assays performed in parallel with the histochemistry. These photometric methods allow rapid quantification of ER by immunohistochemistry, but they require instrumentation that is costly. In this regard, El-Badawy et al. found that this cytophotometric system did not yield statistically significant differences from the results of ordinary or semiquantitative visual inspections, when compared to dextran-coated charcoal cytosol assays.[32a] Furthermore, cytophotometry of immunohistochemical preparations does not provide a direct measure of the molar concentration of the receptor, but rather a scaled value, QIC score or PNA (percentage of nuclear area immunopositivity), related to proportion and intensity of stained nuclear areas.[5,32a] Another image analysis system has recently been employed in an essentially similar manner to study both estrogen and progesterone receptors immunochemically stained in frozen sections of invasive breast carcinomas. A 93% concordance rate for ER and 90% concordance rate for PgR were demonstrated between the image analysis assessment of immunochemical preparations and traditional biochemical radioligand binding methods.[23,74]

It must be noted that the relevance to clinical decision making of the quantitative measures of estrogen and progesterone status in formalin-fixed tissues is uncertain. Although most laboratories and clinicians have adopted a cutoff of 10 fmol/mg for the dextran-coated charcoal cytosol binding assay, this number is not absolute, and other laboratories employ higher or lower thresholds. As cited above, some data suggest an intermediate rate of response to endocrine manipulations for patients who have "borderline positive" results in cytosol assays (3–19 fmol/mg protein). Other than in this borderline region, an absolute value for hormone receptor content probably carries little incremental value for patient prognosis over simply a positive or negative result. Furthermore, clinicians do not alter treatment based on the degree of positivity of the assay, given that they can rely on the positive versus negative classification. Thus, although it is necessary for assays to distinguish reliably between "positive" and "negative" results, the exact amount of positivity does not seem to correlate precisely with tumor behavior over a wide range. Unquantified immunocytochemistry procedures will likely be regarded as quite adequate if accurate "positive" and "negative" results can be supplied. In fact, a recent study by Pertschuk et al. suggests that immunocytochemistry may actually be *better than* dextran-coated charcoal assays in predicting endocrine responsiveness and prognosis in patients with breast cancer.[117a] This suggests that a new "gold standard" may evolve to replace the dextran-coated charcoal cytosol assay. In any event, a better definition of the threshold for a positive histochemical assay must await further direct correlations of this methodology with endocrine responsiveness of tumors. In the meantime, if a misclassification with the histochemical result occurs, it will most likely be a false negative in the borderline zone.[83a]

Numerous studies[3,18,33,112,125,140] have confirmed the close correlation between the determination of ER status by the conventional biochemical binding assay and the staining results of the immunohistochemical technique on formalin-fixed tissues. Indeed, many of the so-called "false positives" determined by the immunohistochemical technique have turned out to be "true positives" in retrospect. This is because the biochemical assay in these cases has often been inadequate, with sampling of non-neoplastic portions of the biopsy. In addition, some false positives by the DCC method have resulted from sampling of benign areas of breast epithelium.

The experience of Lewin and Binder in their large number of formalin-fixed specimens argues against a need for exact quantitation of ER status. The majority of their "positive" cases (those with a corresponding DCC value of > 10 fmol/mg) have more than 75% of tumor cells staining positive for the ER antibody. Similarly, the vast majority of their "negative" cases (DCC values < 10 fmol/mg) show less than 5% of tumor cells positive for ER antibody. Thus, analysis of their immunohistochemical data has not been fraught with difficulty or subjective interpretations. From a practical point of view, staining of more than scattered cells should be considered a positive result. The Children's Hospital of San Francisco experience is similar.

Very recently a monoclonal antibody reagent for detection of PgR has also become commercially available and is employed in the same manner for both cytosol and immunohistochemical assays. Several recent preliminary reports of successful immunostaining of tumor sections with a new progesterone receptor antibody have been published.[12,14,22,29a,83a] Masood et al.[83a] report sensitivity and specificity of the PgR immunohistochemical staining as 91% and 89% for frozen sections and 83% and 89% for paraffin sections, respectively, when compared to results of the dextran-coated charcoal assay. Berger et al. report a concordance rate of 84.3% between immunocytochemical and dextran-coated charcoal cytosol methods of determining progesterone receptor content.[5a]

Indirect Methods Employing Histochemistry

Because of the added difficulties of reserving frozen tumor tissue for biochemical steroid receptor assays of cytosols, there has long been an obvious premium on developing methods of assay that work on routinely handled paraffin-embedded tissue. For many years there were no adequate immunoreagents for directly identifying the estrogen and progesterone receptor molecules.* Although good monoclonal immunoreagents directed against the steroid receptors now exist, as discussed above, this is a comparatively recent development. Several earlier methods were proposed for measuring receptor indirectly, by histochemically assessing steroid ligand binding to tissue slices. This has been done both by immunochemistry employing **anti-estradiol antibodies** and by nonimmunological techniques employing **fluoresceinated estrogens** or **estrogen-protein complexes**. These methods were purported not

---

* Steroid receptors are notoriously labile proteins that were extremely difficult to purify, the first step in obtaining either polyclonal or monoclonal antisera to the receptor protein itself.

only to detect the receptor status of a breast carcinoma histochemically, but to do so in routinely processed paraffin-embedded material. With the recent availability of monoclonal immunochemical methods for detecting ER in paraffin sections, there has been a shift away from these earlier indirect techniques. Because of several serious problems with both anti-estradiol and fluoresceinated estrogen methods, we do not recommend their use at this time.

The best available evidence suggests that neither of the above indirect methods actually detects the estrogen-receptor protein.[17,92,95,144] High concentrations of estrogen are required, much higher than necessary to saturate the high affinity, low capacity binding of estrophilin.[17] The binding produced in these indirect assays is not saturable (as high affinity, low capacity binding of the true receptor molecules is known to be).[17,92,95] Furthermore, the estrogen bound to ER is probably inaccessible to anti-estradiol antibodies because of the phenomenon of clathrate binding (i.e., it is thought that the ER molecule "closes around" the bound estrogen, making it inaccessible to anti-estradiol antibodies).[95,144] Importantly, the pattern of staining of cells produced with these "indirect" methods does not fit the newer model of nuclear ER localization, that is, the staining is generally cytoplasmic rather than nuclear (Fig. 3). Finally, fluorescein and peroxidase conjugated estrogen reagents have a low affinity for ER and are contaminated with unconjugated estrogen [144].

Despite these problems, there is a body of literature that reports correlation of these indirect assays with the results of cytosol ER assays. These correlations are cited below. Because of the current availability of methods for direct immunohistochemical demonstration of the receptor proteins, which do not share the problems of the earlier "indirect" techniques, we think the methods of qualitatively assessing estradiol binding to paraffin tissue slices should be abandoned.

What correlation exists between various histochemical techniques for demonstrating ER or PgR and traditional cytosol assays? Do the histochemical methods predict endocrine therapy response?

Interestingly, despite the problems cited above, the literature reports some correlation of the results of indirect histochemical methods using estrogen ligands with those of traditional cytosol ER assays in as many as 60 to 90% of cases.[66,105,139] Less sanguine reports have also appeared.[28,87,110,116] As an example of the problems of these indirect histochemical methods of assessing steroid binding, the data of Cudahy may be cited. These workers found a 90% sensitivity rate for comparison with biochemical assay results, but, with large numbers of false positive histochemical assays, only a 7% sensitivity rate. These steroid ligand methods may be measuring a second lower affinity, but still specific binding site for estrogen in human breast cancer.[17,108,110,111] It has been speculated that these lower affinity binding sites may be induced by a mechanism that includes participation of the high affinity estrophilin nuclear protein. This hypothesis may provide an explanation for the empiric correlation some authors have reported between indirect ligand binding histochemical methods and biochemical cytosol receptor determinations.

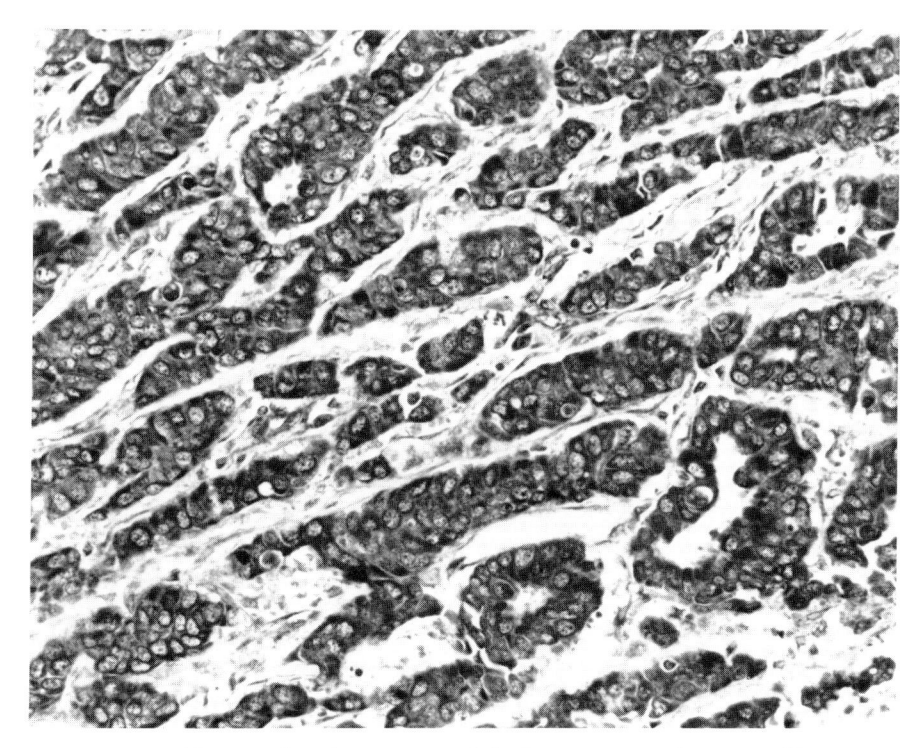

FIGURE 3. Infiltrating ductal carcinoma of the breast prepared as a paraffin section pre-incubated with polyestradiol phosphate (PEP) and stained with a polyclonal antiserum to PEP in an immunoperoxidase system (Ortho). Note the strong cytoplasmic staining of the neoplastic cells. The nuclei, counterstained with hematoxylin, show weaker staining for bound PEP. This result cannot be equated with estrogen receptor positivity (see text).

Monoclonal antibody histochemical assessment of breast cancer specimens for estrogen receptor has been shown to have excellent correlation with the results of traditional cytosol estrogen receptor analysis.[28,117,123] Sensitivity and specificity rates for comparison with traditional cytosol biochemical assays are both high (see Table 2). Instances in which the immunochemical method detects receptor visibly located in nuclei of the tumor cells, but in which traditional cytosol assays fail to show binding above thresholds for positivity, may often be false negatives by the cytosol method. This is especially credible if it can be shown that the specimen for cytosol analysis was deficient in viable neoplastic cells.

The best test of various methods of hormone receptor assay is to relate the results of the various methods to the subsequent clinical responses of patients undergoing endocrine adjuvant therapy. McClelland et al. showed immunohistochemical determination of receptor status to be an effective predictor of response to endocrine therapy.[88] Pertschuk, who has studied both the indirect histochemical methods using estrogen ligands and the direct immunohistochemical method employing anti-estrophilin monoclonal antibodies, found the latter technique superior in predicting hormone responsiveness of human breast carcinoma.[117,117a] McCarty found similar results.[86] However, Pertschuk et al. in an earlier study of estrogen and progestogen histochemical assays (performed before monoclonal antibody histochemistry was an available alternative), also demonstrated ability to predict response to endocrine therapies in 80% of 40 women studied by the ligand method.[118] Other authors did not demonstrate successful prediction of endocrine response by these indirect methods of ligand histochemistry.[85]

Given the results of comparative studies, should laboratories be using the monoclonal immunohistochemical or the cytosol methods for determination of ER-status?

All of the major studies comparing ER determination by the dextran-coated charcoal cytosol assay and the direct monoclonal immunohistochemical methods have shown very close correlation (88–100%) between the two different techniques. Moreover, several studies that have examined the discrepancies between the two procedures have concluded that the immunohistochemical method was in fact more sensitive and more specific. Park and Posey[112] and Thorpe[140] concluded that the immunohistochemical method was more accurate than the biochemical assay in their respective laboratories in identifying ER status in breast tumor cells. Clearly, until more studies are available on the accuracy of detection of receptors in formalin-fixed tissue, pathologists will need to submit specimens for biochemical assay results. Definitive prospective studies are in progress to correlate the immunohistochemical staining results with quantitation by biochemical assay and clinical patient outcome. It is very possible that after the results of these prospective studies are evaluated, the biochemical technique, with all of its inherent limitations, will be supplanted by histochemistry.

What are practical guidelines for the surgical pathologist in reserving tissue for ER/PgR assays and in employing histochemical techniques?

The major disadvantage of the cytosol-based techniques for demonstrating steroid receptors has been the requirement for frozen tissue. Until very recently, this was also a stumbling block for those employing the monoclonal antireceptor antibody histochemical technique, because methods employing monoclonals applicable to paraffin sections have been reported only recently and are certainly not in general use. A variety of pitfalls attend the requirement for fresh frozen specimens. Pending the disseminated use of paraffin histochemical assays for ER and PgR, the practicing pathologist will continue to encounter these problems. Our experience in evading these problems, often based on a history of misadventures, is summarized here.

Mammographically Directed Biopsies. As mammographic screening influences practice, the problems of handling needle-localized excisional biopsies of small breast lesions increasingly confront the surgical pathologist. In our laboratory we have evolved several guidelines for hormone receptor determinations on such small lesions. First, we do not reserve tissue for cytosol ER/PgR analysis from mammographically localized biopsies unless radiographic and gross examinations of the specimen reveal findings strongly indicative of an infiltrating carcinoma. This policy is based on the recognition that there is currently no known clinical significance of the receptor status of in-situ carcinomas, or of benign proliferative breast lesions. Sacrificing material from mammographically directed biopsies for cytosol hormone receptor assays, when the specimen does not contain a readily identifiable infiltrating carcinoma grossly, precludes an optimal histologic examination of a portion of the specimen. Foci of atypical hyperplasia, carcinoma in situ, or minimally invasive breast carcinoma may be obscured. It avails the patient nothing to have her diagnosis in doubt, with the remainder of the important biopsy tissue being homogenized for cytosol hormone receptor analysis. The availability of techniques for identifying receptors histochemically in paraffin-embedded material will allow the pathologist to circumvent reserving frozen tissue for analysis in equivocal circumstances, before a histologic diagnosis is known.

In Situ Vs. Invasive Disease. If the gross examination of the breast specimen is equivocal regarding in situ versus invasive disease, it is generally inappropriate to reserve frozen tissue for receptor studies. Performing a frozen section to aid in this assessment is often strategically unwise, because frozen section artifacts may preclude getting a good answer to the main question, "Is the neoplasm invasive?" If the carcinoma proves to be invasive on examination of permanent sections, immunohistochemical examination for ER is easily obtained. If the method is not available in the pathologist's own department, this can be done at a reference laboratory, with the convenience of merely mailing a paraffin block.

Small Carcinomas. Small, grossly typical infiltrating carcinomas frequently do not afford enough material to reserve frozen tissue for traditional cytosol assay. This is more commonly the case with the older biochemical cytosol assays that rely on radioligand binding than with monoclonal cytosol immunoassays. Roughly 250 milligrams of tumor tissue (a specimen equal to a quarter of a cubic centimeter in volume) will more than suffice for a cytosol assay of both ER and PgR, if the monoclonal antibody-based methods are employed. However, as noted above, it is not appropriate to sacrifice material that is likely to be needed for the diagnosis of cancer in order to perform steroid-binding assays. Cytologic scrapings or imprint preparations from the cut surface of small cancers are quite appropriate samples for the monoclonal histochemical receptor assay. However, we prefer to use immunohistochemistry on paraffin-embedded material for lesions that are less than 5 to 8 mm in greatest dimension.

Small Biopsies. Even if a carcinoma is large, the tumor sample available to the pathologist may be small (such as core needle biopsies or cytology specimens). There may or may not be sufficient neoplastic tissue to reserve a frozen specimen for cytosol steroid receptor assays. In some instances, obtaining material for a receptor determination may be the specific purpose of such a biopsy procedure (for example, a needle biopsy of a bone metastasis for ER and PgR determination). Generally a histologic or cytologic diagnosis is still required in such circumstances, and one of the strategies that conserves the material should be employed to document receptor status. Paraffin-section immunohistochemistry is ideal in such circumstances.

Unexpected Carcinoma. Occasionally the problem is not one of specimen size, but of a deceptively bland clinical or gross appearance of a breast lesion, which on permanent section turns out to be a carcinoma. It is a good practice to receive *all* breast specimens in the fresh state from the operating room and to cut each specimen promptly to make a gross appraisal. If a gross lesion is present, but its nature is uncertain, a cytologic smear made from the cut surface of the specimen and stained with rapid hematoxylin and eosin technique will usually allow recognition of a carcinoma. Alternatively, frozen section can also be employed in this circumstance, when the lesion is large enough that compromise of material for histologic diagnosis by permanent section is not a realistic concern. Again, paraffin section immunohistochemistry provides good back-up for determining ER status of carcinoma not detected grossly.

Causes of False Negative Receptor Assays. Another problem that sometimes arises is that of a false negative cytosol assay. A menstrual history and knowledge of hormonal therapy are necessary to interpret the results of traditional radioligand cytosol assays, because false negatives may be related to occupancy of the receptor binding sites by endogenous hormones or therapeutically administered hormones. As noted previously, the anti-estrogen tamoxifen is one agent that may interfere with such assays. Now that cytosol immunoassay techniques are replacing cytosol radioligand assays, this source of false negatives can be excluded from consideration, because the cytosol immunoassay does not depend on steroid ligand binding to the reactive site of the receptor. As noted above, anti-estrogens may actually increase the results of immunoassays because of conformational changes they induce in the receptor molecules, which expose additional antigenic sites.

However, other causes of false negative cytosol assays remain to be considered. These include small specimen size, delays in handling specimens that result in degradation of the receptor protein, and sampling errors related to necrosis or paucicellular tumors (in which most of the lesion is actually stroma, not neoplasm) (see Fig. 2B). These problems can be addressed in several ways. A traditional strategy has been to make a frozen section of the tumor tissue reserved for cytosol assay, or a section from the immediately adjacent portion of the breast lesion, to confirm that it is appropriately cellular and representative of the infiltrating cancer.[145] Another strategy, which we employ, is to perform a monoclonal histochemical assay whenever the cytosol assay is negative. If staining with a specific nuclear localization can be detected, this suggests that the cytosol assay may be a false negative result. Examination of the histology of the tumor may suggest a reason for such a false negative, such as a paucicellular sclerotic tumor.

Regarding specimen size for cytosol assay, the advantages claimed by some authors for small, putatively homogeneous samples[102] appear outweighed by sampling variation to be expected when only small amounts of breast tumors are assayed. We generally reserve 0.5 grams of tissue for ER/PgR analysis by cytosol immunoassay technique, and more if the lesion is large and grossly heterogeneous. Cellular areas and non-necrotic areas are obviously preferable for the sample, if they can be recognized grossly. When considering these issues of proper sampling for cytosol assays, it is again apparent how advantageous paraffin immunohistochemistry is for sampling widely or selectively.

The timeliness with which a frozen sample of breast carcinoma is reserved for hormone receptor analysis is also an important factor bearing on the false negative rate of radioligand cytosol assays (such as the common "dextran-coated charcoal technique"). The steroid receptor molecules' high-affinity binding of hormone degrades quickly in devitalized tissue at room temperatures.[102] In fact, Newsome et al. showed a significant drop in measurable receptor content, which occurred during the interval between open biopsy sampling of breast lesions and completion of mastectomy procedures.[102] Given this lability of the receptor, it is important to be prompt in reserving tissue snap frozen and stored in liquid nitrogen for those ER/PgR assays to be performed by biochemical cytosol techniques. A response time of 15 minutes or less should be the target for the pathologist. If tissue for steroid receptor assays is to be reserved from a mastectomy specimen, an intraoperative biopsy to remove tissue for assay is the optimal, if not standard, procedure to follow.

How does the development of immunoassays affect the need for rapid processing? Antigenicity of the receptor proteins is better preserved under adverse circumstances, including fixation, than is the receptor binding function itself. The authors are unaware of relevant studies that establish the antigenicity under various insults (such as storage at room temperature, thermal variation, et cetera) for frozen specimens which are to be analyzed for steroid receptors by cytosol immunoassays. We employ the same rapid response and storage for these frozen specimens as we were accustomed to using for biochemical cytosol assays of radioligand binding. Issues of tissue fixation for immunohistochemical determination of steroid receptors have been dealt with above.

In recognition of the lability of the steroid-binding capacity of the receptors, it is advisable to avoid admixture of foreign chemicals in samples of frozen tissue to be used for cytosol radioligand binding assays. Reports of difficulties induced by O.C.T. embedding compound should lead one to exercise care in excluding this material from the frozen samples.[49,96,97] Mordants, such as Bouin's solution, used to fix India ink to the margins of biopsy samples, should not be employed if the specimen is to provide a sample for receptor assay. We have not found India ink itself to be a problem, when simply painted on the margins of biopsy specimens. Now that cytosol *immunoassays* are in use by many laboratories, some of these precautions may be unnecessary, but we have found no reason to alter our practice of excluding foreign chemicals.

Record-keeping, Multiple Specimens, and Other Gremlins. Experience shows that pathologists on occasion simply forget to save frozen tissue from breast carcinomas, or mistakenly believe that the assay for steroid receptors has been performed on an earlier specimen, and thus do not reserve tissue. This is generally a problem related to communication and record-keeping, a problem that has been exacerbated as two-step surgical procedures for diagnosis and local control of breast carcinoma have begun to replace mastectomy based on frozen section diagnosis. The parsimonious pathologist, attempting to prevent repetition of a laboratory test at the time of mastectomy, may find that his department has reserved no tissue for receptor analysis, despite several opportunities.

In order to avoid this problem, we reserve tissue for receptor assay from *initial* biopsy specimens whenever possible, keep a log of these cases, and annotate the pathology reports to reflect the fact that tissue has been studied for receptor content. Whenever new gross specimens from breast cancer patients—whether from re-excisions, segmental mastectomies, modified mastectomies, or metastatic lesions—arrive in the cutting room, we review the patient's earlier pathology reports and our log to ensure that a sample of the tumor has been previously assayed for receptors. We also reserve a sample for receptor assay from metastatic or recurrent breast cancer if the lesion is biopsied after any substantial interval from the patient's original presentation, especially when there has been an intervening course of endocrine therapy. A system for maintaining records of receptor analyses can be easily computerized. When these precautions have failed, we analyze paraffin-embedded material by monoclonal immunohistochemistry.

Of course, frozen tissue may be reserved for hormone-receptor assay, and something may still go wrong in handling, transporting, or storing it. The problems are mainly those of frozen specimens in a warmer world, and every conceivable problem with refrigeration has at one time or another prevented cytosol receptor assays from being performed. The clinician's desire for a receptor assay often seems to be piqued by such adverse circumstances. A monoclonal immunohistochemical assay in paraffin section is clearly the method of choice in such circumstances. Since we believe monoclonal immunohistochemistry may soon come to replace cytosol assays as the routine method of receptor assay, we are certainly not bashful about employing this technique as an alternative to cytosol receptor studies in a pinch.

What is the role for steroid receptor assays in differential diagnosis?

The question of whether or not steroid receptor determination can prove useful in differential diagnosis usually arises in the context of the workup of a metastatic neoplasm of unknown primary origin. Sometimes the patient has a history of primary breast carcinoma or of multiple previous tumors. If there was a prior breast carcinoma, its receptor status may well be known to the pathologist. In any of these circumstances the pathologist may believe he can evaluate the diagnosis of metastatic breast carcinoma by simply determining whether or not there is ER or PgR in the metastasis.

The differential diagnostic value of steroid receptor analysis would be secure if these receptors had not been demonstrated in such a wide range of

TABLE 4. Estrogen Receptors in Neoplasms Other Than Breast Carcinoma

Gastric carcinoma[143]
Hepatocellular carcinoma[99,136]
Meningioma[136]
Lung carcinoma
Colonic carcinoma[136]
Melanoma[136]
Gynecomastia and male breast carcinoma[136]
Thymoma
Pancreatic carcinoma
Renal cell carcinoma[136]
Ovarian carcinoma[61,119,126,137,148]
Endometrial carcinoma[16,44,136,149]
Breast angiosarcoma[10]
Bone and soft tissue tumors[136,147]

human neoplasms other than breast carcinoma. The list of such reports presented in Table 4 does not purport to be exhaustive but illustrates the problem to be faced by anyone who wishes to employ receptor analysis in this diagnostic context, especially uncritically. Included in the list are neoplasms arising in organs not ordinarily regarded as sex steroid target tissues. Although some of these neoplasms have been found to contain receptors infrequently and only at low specific activities,[147] the low but measurable quantities of ER still overlap with the wide range of receptor concentrations seen in breast carcinomas. It is also important to remember that not all metastatic breast carcinomas will be ER positive, and that endometrial adenocarcinomas, ovarian epithelial tumors, melanomas, and renal cell carcinomas may contain substantial amounts of receptor protein and stain positively in immunohistochemical assays for ER and PgR. In many instances the reported experience with receptor assays is too limited to assess the frequency with which a particular type of carcinoma or sarcoma contains ER or PgR, and at what specific activities.

The current availability of paraffin immunohistochemical methods for demonstrating ER and PgR should soon lead to increased knowledge of the distribution of these receptors in various tumor types. The immunohistochemical method also allows comparison of the receptor status of a metastatic carcinoma and a purported earlier primary carcinoma, if archived blocks of the earlier carcinoma are available. Steroid ligand histochemistry may also have some residual application in this differential diagnostic context, although, as noted above, it is discredited as a method of assessing receptor status per se.

In practice, when used with discrimination, the estrogen receptor immunohistochemical stain is often a helpful differential diagnostic tool, especially when incorporated into a panel of appropriate histochemical and immunohistochemical tests. It may point to the origin of a metastatic focus when the usual battery of immunostains yields nonspecific results (as, for example, differentiating between metastatic lung versus colon versus breast carcinoma). The stain works adequately in decalcified tissue, and it is thus valuable in defining a metastatic lesion in the skeleton of a female patient. The finding of positive tumor cells by ER-immunohistochemistry at a metastatic site often dramatically alters a patient's prognosis and clinical treatment.

However, even a panel of tests may prove confusing. For example, a patient with a known prior ER-positive breast carcinoma might develop a late metastasis for which alternative diagnoses of metastatic renal cell carcinoma and melanoma are being considered. As noted above, both renal cell carcinoma and melanoma are neoplasms reported to contain ER on occasion. All of these lesions may also contain S100 protein and glycogen. Thus, a panel of tests that included receptor assay, PAS stains, and S100 immunochemistry would not necessarily discriminate among the possibilities being considered.

Do hormone receptor assays have practical clinical importance in the management of neoplasms other than breast carcinoma?

Attention increasingly focuses on female genital carcinomas as hormone receptor-containing neoplasms, the behavior of which may be predicted by receptor status or influenced by endocrine manipulations. Therefore, pathologists who routinely perform receptor studies of breast carcinomas will also be asked on occasion by their colleagues in gynecologic oncology to study ovarian or endometrial tumors for ER or PgR content.

Many studies have shown prognostic significance for steroid receptor determinations of endometrial[16,27,43,60,77,81] and ovarian[61,135] tumor specimens. Response to hormone manipulation therapy for these tumors is still being investigated,[16,31] although results are somewhat promising, especially for endometrial neoplasms. Variation in receptor content between primary ovarian carcinomas and metastases has been postulated to account for the relatively low rate of response of ovarian carcinoma patients to hormonal manipulative therapy, despite the fact that many such carcinomas do contain ER and PgR (often at low levels).[121] Other investigators have not shown this variation in receptor content for primary ovarian carcinomas and their metastases before and after chemotherapy.[126]

Just as for breast carcinoma, immunohistochemical determination of receptor status has been applied to ovarian and endometrial tumors.[12,98,119,138] For endometrial curettage specimens immunohistochemistry has the advantage of allowing specific study of neoplastic tissue, and not extraneous fragments of myometrium or non-neoplastic endometrium, which also contain receptors.[12,98] As a practical matter, determination of ER and PgR status for endometrial and ovarian carcinomas has not yet become adopted as a community standard of practice in pathology. Steroid receptor analysis for such carcinomas is often done on an ad hoc basis at present, often at the request of an interested clinician. The convenience of using paraffin-embedded material for analysis is obvious in that it does not require any change in pathologists' traditional handling of hysterectomy and oophorectomy specimens. The further question whether *quantification* of ER and PgR for endometrial and ovarian carcinomas is clinically useful enough to warrant a preference for quantitative cytosol assays has yet to be answered.

References

1. Alexieva-Figusch J, Van Putten WLJ, Blankenstein MA, et al: The prognostic value and relationships of patient characteristics, estrogen and progestin receptors, and site of relapse in primary breast cancer. Cancer 61:758–768, 1988.
2. Allegra JC, Barlock A, Huff KK, et al: Changes in multiple or sequential estrogen receptor determinations in breast cancer. Cancer 45:792–794, 1980.
3. Anderson J, Orntoft TF, Poulsen HS: Immunohistochemical demonstration of estrogen receptors (ER) in formalin-fixed, paraffin-embedded human breast cancer tissue by use of a monoclonal antibody to er. J Histochem Cytochem 36:1553–1560, 1988.
4. Andersen J, Orntoft T, Skovgaard Poulsen H: Semiquantitative estrogen receptor assay in formalin-fixed paraffin sections of human breast cancer tissue using monoclonal antibodies. Br J Cancer 53:691–694, 1986.
5. Bacus S, Flowers JL, Bacus JW, et al: The evaluation of estrogen receptor in primary breast carcinoma by computerized image analysis. Am J Clin Pathol 90:233–239, 1988.
5a. Berger U, Wilson P, Thethi S, et al: Comparison of an immunocytochemical assay for progesterone receptor with biochemical method of measurement and immunocytochemical examination of the relationship between progesterone and estrogen receptors. Cancer Res 49:5176–5179, 1989.
6. Bergeron C, Ferenczy A, Shyamala G: Distribution of estrogen receptors in various cell types of normal, hyperplastic, and neoplastic human endometrial tissues. Lab Invest 58:338–345, 1988.
7. Bicel P, Poulsen S, Andersen J: Estrogen receptor content and ploidy of human mammary carcinoma. Cancer 50:1771–1774, 1982.
8. Boccardo F, Rubagotti A, Bruzzi P, et al: Chemotherapy versus tamoxifen versus chemotherapy plus tamoxifen in node-positive, estrogen receptor-positive breast cancer patients: Results of a multicentric Italian study. J Clin Oncol 8:1310–1320, 1990.
9. Bonadonna G, Valagussa P, Zambetti M, et al: Milan adjuvant trials for stage I-II breast cancer. In Salmon SE (ed): Adjuvant Therapy of Cancer V. New York, Grune & Stratton, 1987, pp 211–221.
10. Brentani MM, Pacheco MM, Oshima CTF, et al: Steroid receptors in breast angiosarcoma. Cancer 51:2105–2111, 1983.
11. Brincker BH, Rose C, Rank F: Evidence of a castration-mediated effect of adjuvant cytotoxic chemotherapy in premenopausal breast cancer. J Clin Oncol 5:1771–1778, 1987.
12. Brustein S, Fruchter R, Greene GL, et al: Immunocytochemical assay of pregesterone receptors in paraffin-embedded specimens of endometrial carcinoma and hyperplasia: A preliminary evaluation. Modern Pathol 2:449–455, 1989.
13. Bur M, Chowdhary S: Estrogen and progesterone receptor immunohistochemistry in carcinoma in-situ of the breast with paraffin embedded sections (abstract). Lab Invest 60:13A, 1989.
14. Carpenter S, Kinsel L, Flowers J, et al: Comparison of two progesterone receptor specific antibodies in immunocytochemical analysis of human breast tumors (abstract). Lab Invest 60:15A, 1989.
15. Chabon AB, Goldberg JD, Venet L: Carcinoma of the breast: Interrelationships among histopathologic features, estrogen receptor activity, and age of the patient. Hum Pathol 14:368–372, 1982.
16. Chambers JT, MacLusky N, Eisenfield A, et al: Estrogen receptor and progestic receptor levels as prognosticators for survival in endometrial cancer. Gynecol Oncol 31:65–77, 1988.
17. Chamness GC, Mercer WD, McGuire WL: Are histochemical methods for estrogen receptor valid? J Histochem Cytochem 28:792–798, 1980.
18. Cheng L, Binder SW, Fu YS, et al: Demonstration of estrogen receptors by monoclonal antibody in formalin-fixed breast tumors. Lab Invest 58:346–353, 1988.
19. Chevallier B, Heintzmann F, Mosseri V, et al: Prognostic value of estrogen and progesterone receptors in operable breast cancer: Results of a univariate and multivariate analysis. Cancer 62:2517–2524, 1988.
20. Clark GM, McGuire WL: Progesterone receptors and human breast carcinoma. Breast Cancer Research Treat 3:157–163, 1983.
21. Clark GM, McGuire WL, Hubay CA, et al: Progesterone receptors as a prognostic factor in stage II breast cancer. N Engl J Med 309:1343–1347, 1983.
22. Colley M, Kommoss F, Bibbo M, et al: Estrogen and progesterone receptors and Ki-67 growth fraction in breast carcinoma: Quantitation of hormone receptors by image analysis and comparison with cytosolic methods (abstract). Lab Invest 60:19A, 1989.

23. Colley M, Kommoss F, Bibbo M, et al: Assessment of hormone receptors in breast carcinoma by immunocytochemistry and image analysis. II. Estrogen receptors. Anal Quant Cytol Histol 11:307–314, 1989.
24. Concolino G, Marocchi A, Conti C, et al: Human renal cell carcinoma as a hormone-dependent tumor. Cancer Res 38:4340–4344, 1978.
25. Contesso G, Mouriesse H, Friedman S, et al: The importance of histologic grade in long-term prognosis of breast cancer: A study of 1010 patients, uniformly treated at the Institut Gustave-Roussy. J Clin Oncol 5:1378–1386, 1987.
26. Corle DK, Sears ME, Olson KB: Relationship of quantitative estrogen-receptor level and clinical response to cytotoxic chemotherapy in advanced breast cancer: An extramural analysis. Cancer 54:1554–1561, 1984.
27. Creasman WT, Soper JT, McCarty KS Jr, et al: Influence of cytoplasmic steroid receptor content on prognosis of early stage endometrial carcinoma. Am J Obstet Gynecol 151:922–930, 1985.
28. Cudahy TJ, Boeryd BR, Franlund BK, et al: A comparison of three different methods for the determination of estrogen receptors in human breast cancer. Am J Clin Pathol 90:583–590, 1988.
29. DeGoeij FPM, Bosman FT, Berns EMJJ: Determination of steroid hormone dependency of tumours utilizing tissue sections. Survey of histochemical techniques and their application in surgical pathology. J Pathol 149:163–172, 1986.
29a. DeNegri F, Campani D, Sarnelli R, et al: Comparison of monoclonal immunocytochemical and immunoenzymatic methods for steroid receptor evaluation in breast cancer. Am J Clin Pathol 96:53–58, 1991.
30. DeSombre ER, Jensen EV: Estrophilin assays in breast cancer: Quantitative features and application to the mastectomy specimen. Cancer 46:2783–2788, 1980.
31. Dowle CS, Owainati A, Robins A, et al: Prognostic significance of the DNA content of human breast cancer. Br J Surg 74:133–136, 1987.
32. Dressler LG, Seamer LC, et al: DNA flow cytometry and prognostic factors in 1331 frozen breast cancer specimens. Cancer 61:420–427, 1988.
32a. El-Badawy N, Cohen C, De Rose PB, et al: Immunohistochemical estrogen receptor assay: Quantitation by image analysis. Mod Pathol 4:305–309, 1991.
33. Elias JM, Heimann A, Cain T, et al: Estrogen receptor localization in paraffin sections by enzyme digestion, repeated applications of primary antibody and immidazole. J Histotechnology 13:29–33, 1990.
34. Feldman JG, Pertschuk LP, Carter AC, et al: Histochemical estrogen binding: An independent predictor of recurrence and survival in stage II breast cancer. Cancer 57:911–916, 1986.
35. Fisher B, Costantino J, Redmond C, et al: A randomized clinical trial evaluating tamoxifen in the treatment of patients with node-negative breast cancer who have estrogen-receptor-positive tumors. N Engl J Med 320:479–484, 1989.
36. Fisher R, Neifeld J, Lippman M, et al: Oestrogen receptor in human malignant melanoma. Lancet ii:337–338, 1976.
37. Fisher B, Redmond C, Brown A, et al: Influence of tumor estrogen and progesterone receptor levels on the response to tamoxifen and chemotherapy in primary breast cancer. J Clin Oncol 1:227–241, 1983.
38. Fisher B, Redmond C, Dimitrov NV, et al: A randomized clinical trial evaluating sequential methotrexate and fluorouracil in the treatment of patients with node-negative breast cancer who have estrogen receptor-negative tumors. N Engl J Med 320:473–478, 1989.
39. Fisher B, Redmond C, Fisher ER, et al: Relative worth of estrogen or progesterone receptor and pathologic characteristics of differentiation as indicators of prognosis in node negative breast cancer patients: Findings from National Surgical Adjuvant Breast and Bowel Project Protocol B-06. J Clin Oncol 6:1076–1087, 1988.
40. Fisher ER, Redmond CK, Liu H, et al: Correlation of estrogen receptor and pathologic characteristics of invasive breast cancer. Cancer 45:349–353, 1980.
41. Fisher B, Redmond C, Poisson S, et al: Increased benefit from addition of adriamycin and cylophosphamide (AC) to tamoxifen (TAM, T) for positive-node, TAM-responsive postmenopausal breast cancer patients: Results from NSABP B-16 (abstract). Proceedings of ASCO 9:20, 1990.
42. Fisher B, Wickerham DL, Brown A, et al: Breast cancer estrogen and progesterone receptor values: Their distribution, degree of concordance, and relation to number of positive axillary nodes. J Clin Oncol 1:349–358, 1983.
43. Geisinger KR, Homesley HD, Morgan TM, et al: Endometrial adenocarinoma: A multiparameter clinicopathologic analysis including the DNA profile and the sex steroid hormone receptors. Cancer 58:1518–1525, 1986.

44. Geisinger KR, Marshall RB, Kute TE, et al: Correlation of female sex steroid hormone receptors with histologic and ultrastructural differentiation in adenocarcinoma of the endometrium. Cancer 58:1506–1517, 1986.
45. Glick JH, et al: National Institutes of Health consensus development conference statement: Adjuvant chemotherapy for breast cancer. September 9–11, 1985. CA-A Cancer Journal for Clinicians 36:42–47, 1986.
46. Gorski J, Welshons WV, Sakai D, et al: Evolution of a model of estrogen action. Rec Progress Hormone Res 42:297–329, 1986.
47. Greene GL, Nolan C, Engler JP, et al: Monoclonal antibodies to human estrogen receptor. Proc Natl Acad Sci (USA) 77:5115–5119, 1980.
48. Gross GE, Clark GM, Chamness GC, et al: Multiple progesterone receptor assays in human breast cancer. Cancer Res 44:836–840, 1984.
49. Hannah J, Anders K, Hall T, Fu Y: O.C.T. not a problem (letter to the editor). Am J Clin Pathol 83:404, 1985.
50. Hedley DW, Rugg CA, Gelber RD: Association of DNA index and S-phase fraction with prognosis of nodes positive early breast cancer. Cancer Res 47:4729–4735, 1987.
51. Helin HJ, Helle MJ, Kallioniemi O, et al: Immunohistochemical determination of estrogen and progesterone receptors in human breast carcinoma: Correlation with histopathology and DNA flow cytometry. Cancer 63:1761–1767, 1989.
52. Helin HJ, Markku JH, Kallioniemi O, et al: Immunohistochemical determination of estrogen and progesterone receptors in human breast carcinoma: Correlation with histopathology and DNA flow cytometry. Cancer 63:1761–1767, 1989.
53. Henderson IC: Adjuvant chemotherapy and endocrine therapy in patients with operable breast cancer. Cancer: Principles and Practice of Oncology Updates 1(3):1–14, 1987.
54. Henderson IC, Hayes DF, Parker LM, et al: Adjuvant systemic therapy for patients with node-negative tumors. Cancer 65:2132–2147, 1990.
55. Hiort O, Kwan PWL, DeLellis RA: Immunohistochemistry of estrogen receptor protein in paraffin sections: Effects of enzymatic pretreatment and cobalt chloride intensification. Am J Clin Pathol 90:559–563, 1988.
56. Holmes FA, Fritsche HQ, Loewy JW, et al: Measurement of estrogen and progesterone receptors in human breast tumors: Enzyme immunoassay versus binding assay. J Clin Oncol 8:1025–1035, 1990.
57. Horsfall DJ, Tilley WD, Orell SR, et al: Relationship between ploidy and steroid hormone receptors in primary invasive breast carcinoma. Br J Cancer 53:23–28, 1986.
58. Howanitz PJ, Howanitz JH, Skrodzki CA, et al: Protein method influences on calculation of tissue receptor concentration. Am J Clin Pathol 85:37–42, 1982.
59. Hull DF, Clark GM, Osborne CK, et al: Multiple estrogen receptor assays in human breast cancer. Cancer Res 43:413–416, 1983.
60. Ingram SS, Rosenman J, Heath R, et al: The predictive value of progesterone receptor levels in endometrial cancer. Int J Radiat Oncol Biol Phys 17:21–27, 1989.
61. Iverson OE, Skaarland E, Utaaker E: Steroid receptor content in human ovarian tumors: Survival of patients with ovarian carcinoma related to steroid receptor content. Gynecol Oncol 23:65–76, 1986.
62. Jensen EV, Greene GL, Closs LE, et al: Receptors reconsidered: A 20-year perspective. Recent Prog Horm Res 38:1–40, 1982.
63. Jensen EV, Greene GL, DeSombre ER: Immunochemical studies of estrogen receptors. In Cabot MC, McKeehan WL (eds): Mechanisms of Signal Transduction by Hormones and Growth Factors. New York, Alan R. Liss, 1987, pp 283–306.
64. Kallioniemi O, Blanco G, Alavaikko M, et al: Tumour DNA ploidy as an independent prognostic factor in breast cancer. Br J Cancer 56:637–642, 1987.
65. Kallioniemi O, Hietanen T, Mattila J, et al: Aneuploid DNA content and high S-phase fraction of tumor cells are related to poor prognosis in patients with primary breast cancer. Eur J Cancer Clin Oncol 23:277–282, 1987.
66. Katayama I, Shimizu M, Miura M, et al: Histochemical demonstration of endogenous estrogen in breast carcinomas: Biochemical and clinical correlation. Virchows Arch 402:353–359, 1984.
67. Kiang DT, Frenning DH, Goldman AI, et al: Estrogen receptors and responses to chemotherapy and hormonal therapy in advanced breast cancer. N Engl J Med 299:1330–1334, 1978.
68. Kiang DT, Kennedy BT: Factors affecting estrogen receptors in breast cancer. Cancer 40:1571–1576, 1977.
69. King WJ, DeSombre ER, Jensen EV, et al: Comparison of immunocytochemical and steroid binding assays for estrogen receptor in human breast tumors. Cancer Res 45:293–304, 1985.

70. King WJ, Greene GL: Monoclonal antibodies localize oestrogen receptor in the nuclei of target cells. Nature 307:745-747, 1984.
71. King WJ, Weigand RA: Estrogen receptor detection and measurement using monoclonal antibodies to human estrogen receptor. Pathologist (April):15-19, 1986.
72. Klinga K, Kaufmann M, Runnebaum B, et al: Distribution of estrogen and progesterone receptors on primary tumor and lymph nodes in individual patients with breast cancer. Oncology 39:337, 1982.
73. Klintenberg C, Stal O, Nordenskjold B, et al: Proliferative index, cytosol estrogen receptor and axillary node status as prognostic predictors in human mammary carcinoma. Breast Cancer Res Treat 7(Suppl):99-106, 1986.
74. Kommoss F, Bibbo M, Colley M, et al: I. Assessment of hormone receptors in breast carcinoma by immunocytochemistry and image analysis. II. Estrogen receptors. Anal Quant Cytol Histol 11:298-306, 1989.
75. Lacombe MJ, Delarue JC, Mouriesse H, et al: Human breast tumors: A comparison between the biochemical method of measuring estrogen and progesterone receptors and that of an immunohistochemical method. Gynecol Oncol 32:174-179, 1989.
76. Leclercq G, Bojar H, Goussard J, et al: Abbott monoclonal enzyme immunoassay measurement of estrogen receptors in human breast cancer. A European multicenter study. Cancer Res 46(Suppl):4233s-4236s, 1986.
77. Liao BS, Twiggs LB, Leung BS, et al: Cytoplasmic estrogen and progesterone receptors as prognostic parameters in primary endometrial carcinoma. Obstet Gynecol 67:463-467, 1986.
78. Lippman ME, Allegra JC, Thompson EB, et al: The relation between estrogen receptors and response rate to cytotoxic chemotherapy in metastatic breast cancer. N Engl J Med 298:1223-1228, 1978.
79. Magdelenat H, Merle S, Zajdela A: Enzyme immunoassay of estrogen receptors in fine needle aspirates of breast tumors. Cancer Res 46(Suppl):4265s-4267s, 1986.
80. Mansour EG, Gray R, Shatila AH, et al: Efficacy of adjuvant chemotherapy in high-risk node-negative breast cancer: An intergroup study. N Engl J Med 320:485-490, 1989.
81. Martin JD, Hahnel R, McCartney AJ, et al: The effect of estrogen receptor status on survival in patients with endometrial cancer. Am J Obstet Gynecol 147:322-324, 1983.
82. Martin PM, Berthois Y, Jensen EV: Binding of antiestrogens exposes an occult antigenic determinant in the human estrogen receptor. Proc Natl Acad Sci USA 85:2533-2537, 1988.
83. Masood S: Use of monoclonal antibody for assessment of estrogen receptor content in fine-needle aspiration biopsy specimen from patients with breast cancer. Arch Pathol Lab Med 113:26-30, 1989.
83a. Masood S, Dee S, Goldstein JD: Immunocytochemical analysis of progesterone receptors in breast cancer. Am J Clin Pathol 96:59-63, 1991.
84. Maynard PV, Davies CJ, Plamey RW, et al: Relationship between oestrogen-receptor content and histological grade in human primary breast tumours. Br J Cancer 38:745-748, 1978.
85. McCarty KS, Hiatt KB, Budwit DA, et al: Clinical response to hormone therapy correlated with estrogen receptor analyses. Arch Pathol Lab Med 108:24-26, 1984.
86. McCarty KS, Miller LS, Cox EB, et al: Estrogen receptor analyses: Correlation of biochemical and immunohistochemical methods using monoclonal antireceptor antibodies. Arch Pathol Lab Med 109:716-721, 1985.
87. McCarty KS Jr, Woodard BH, Nichols DE, et al: Comparison of biochemical and histochemical techniques for estrogen receptor analyses in mammary carcinoma. Cancer 46:2842-2845, 1980.
88. McClelland R, Berger U, Miller LS, et al: Immunocytochemical assay for estrogen receptor: Relationship to outcome of therapy with advanced breast cancer. Cancer Res 46(Suppl):4241s-4243s, 1986.
89. McDivitt RW, Stone KR, Craig RB, et al: A proposed classification of breast cancer based on kinetic information: Derived from a comparison of risk factors in 168 primary operable breast cancers. Cancer 57:269-276, 1986.
90. McGuire WL: Prognostic factors in primary breast cancer. Cancer Surveys 5:527-536, 1986.
91. McGuire WL: Estrogen receptor versus nuclear grade as prognostic factors in axillary node negative breast cancer (editorial). J Clin Oncol 6:1071-1072, 1988.
92. Mercer WD, Lippman ME, Wahl TM, et al: The use of immunocytochemical techniques for the detection of steroid hormones in breast cancer cells. Cancer 46:2859-2868, 1980.
93. Meyer JS, Rao BB, Stevens SC, et al: Low incidence of estrogen receptor in breast carcinomas with rapid rates of cellular replication. Cancer 40:2290-2298, 1977.
94. Moran RE, Black MM, Alpert L, et al: Correlation of cell-cycle kinetics, hormone receptors, histopathology, and nodal status in human breast cancer. Cancer 54:1856, 1984.

95. Morrow B, Leav I, DeLellis RA, et al: Use of polyestradiol phosphate and anti-17beta estradiol antibodies for the localization of estrogen receptors in target tissues: A critique. Cancer 46:2872–2879, 1980.
96. Muensch H, Maslow WC: Interference of O.C.T. embedding compound with hormone receptor assays. Am J Clin Pathol 82:89–92, 1984.
97. Muensch H, Maslow WC: Authors' reply—Depends on final concentration (letter to the editor). Am J Clin Pathol 83:404–405, 1985.
98. Mutch DG, Soper JT, Budwit-Novotny DA, et al: Endometrial adenocarcinoma estrogen receptor content: Association of clinicopathologic features with immunohistochemical analysis compared with standard biochemical methods. Am J Obstet Gynecol 157:924–931, 1987.
99. Nagasue N, Ito A, Yukaya H, et al: Estrogen receptors in hepatocellular carcinoma. Cancer 57:87–91, 1986.
100. National Cancer Institute Clinical Alert. National Cancer Institute, Bethesda, Maryland, May 16 and 18, 1988.
101. National Institutes of Health, Office of Medical Applications of Research. Consensus Conference: Adjuvant chemotherapy for breast cancer. JAMA 254:3461–3463, 1985.
101a. National Institutes of Health Consensus Development Conference Statement. Treatment of early stage breast cancer, June, 1990.
102. Newsome JF, Avis FP, Hammond JE, et al: Sampling procedures in estrogen receptor determinations. Ann Surg 193:549–552, 1981.
102a. Noguchi S, Miyauchi K, Imaoka S, et al: Comparison of enzyme immunoassay with dextran-coated charcoal method in the determination of progesterone receptor in breast cancer cytosols. Eur J Cancer Clin Oncol 24:1715–1719, 1988.
103. Nolvadex Adjuvant Trial Organization. Controlled trial of tamoxifen as single adjuvant agent in management of early breast cancer. Lancet i:836–840, 1985.
104. Nolvadex Adjuvant Trial Organization. Controlled trial of tamoxifen as single adjuvant agent in management of early breast cancer. Br J Cancer 57:608–611, 1988.
105. O'Connel M, Said JW: Estrogen receptors in carcinoma of the breast. A comparison of the dextran-coated charcoal, immunoflourescent, and immunoperoxidase techniques. Am J Clin Pathol 80:1–5, 1983.
106. Olszewski W, Darzynkiewicz Z, Rosen PP, et al: Flow cytometry of breast carcinoma. I. Relation of DNA ploidy level to histology and estrogen receptor. Cancer 48:980–984, 1981.
107. Olszewski W, Darzynkiewicz Z, Rosen PP, et al: Flow cytometry of breast carcinoma. II. Relation of tumor cell cycle distribution to histology and estrogen receptor. Cancer 48:985–988, 1981.
108. Osborne CK: Heterogeneity in hormone receptor status in primary and metastatic breast cancer. Sem Oncol 12:317–326, 1985.
109. Osborne CK, McGuire WL: The use of steroid hormone receptors in the treatment of human breast cancer: A review. Bulletin Cancer 66:203–209, 1979.
110. Panko WB, Mattioli CA, Wheeler TM: Lack of correlation of a histochemical method for estrogen receptor analysis with the biochemical assay results. Cancer 49:2148–2152, 1982.
111. Panko WB, Watson CS, Clark JH: The presence of a second specific estrogen binding site in human breast cancer. J Steroid Biochem 14:1311–1316, 1981.
112. Parl FF, Posey YF: Discrepancies of the biochemical and immunohistochemical estrogen receptor assays in breast cancer. Human Pathol 19:860–866, 1988.
113. Paridaens RJ, Leclercq G, Piccart MJ, et al: Comments on the treatment of breast cancer. Cancer Surveys 5:447–461, 1986.
114. Paridaens R, Sylvester RJ, Ferrazzi E, et al: Clinical significance of the quantitative assessment of estrogen receptors in advanced breast cancer. Cancer 46:2889–2895, 1980.
115. Parl FF, Wagner RK: The histopathological evaluation of human breast cancers in correlation with estrogen receptor values. Cancer 46:362–367, 1980.
116. Pascal RR, Santeusanio G, Sarrell D, Johnson CE: Immunohistologic detection of estrogen receptors in paraffin-embedded breast cancers: Correlation with cytosol measurements. Hum Pathol 17:370–375, 1986.
117. Pertschuk LP, Eisenberg KB, Carter AC, Feldman JG: Immunohistologic localization of estrogen receptors in breast cancer with monoclonal antibodies: Correlation with biochemistry and clinical endocrine response. Cancer 55:1513–1518, 1985.
117a. Pertschuk LP, Kim DS, Nayer K, et al: Immunocytochemical estrogen and progestin receptor assays in breast cancer with monoclonal antibodies: Histopathologic, demographic, and biochemical correlations and relationship to endocrine response and survival. Cancer 66:1663–1670, 1990.

118. Pertschuk LP, Tobin EH, Gaetjens E, et al: Histochemical assay of estrogen and progesterone receptors in breast cancer: Correlation with biochemical assays and patients' response to endocrine therapies. Cancer 46:2896–2901, 1980.
119. Press MF, Holt JA, Herbst AL, Greene GL: Immunocytochemical identification of estrogen receptor in ovarian carcinomas: Localization with monoclonal estrophilin antibodies compared with biochemical assays. Lab Invest 53:349–361, 1985.
120. Pritchard KI: Systemic adjuvant therapy for node-negative breast cancer: Proven or premature? Ann Intern Med 111:1–4, 1989.
121. Quinn MA, Rome RM, Cauchi M, et al: Steroid receptors and ovarian tumors: Variation within primary tumors and between primary tumors and metastases. Gynecol Oncol 31:424–429, 1988.
122. Redard M, Vassilakos P, Weintraub J: A simple method for estrogen receptor antigen preservation in cytologic specimens containing breast carcinoma cells. Diagnostic Cytopathol 5:188–193, 1989.
123. Reiner A, Spona J, Reiner G, et al: Estrogen receptor analysis on biopsies and fine-needle aspirates from human breast carcinoma: Correlation of biochemical and immunohistochemical methods using monoclonal antibodies. Am J Pathol 125:443–449, 1986.
124. Reiner A, Reiner G, Spona J, et al: Histopathologic characterization of human breast cancer in correlation with estrogen receptor status. A comparison of immunocytochemical and biochemical analysis. Cancer 61:1149–1154, 1988.
125. Riccobon A, Zoli W, Capucci A, et al: Radioligand-labelled binding assay and immunochemical assay for estrogen receptor in 115 human breast cancers. Tumori 74:167–170, 1988.
126. Richman CM, Holt JA, Lorincz MS, et al: Persistence and distribution of estrogen receptor in advanced epithelial ovarian carcinoma after chemotherapy. Obstet Gynecol 65:257–263, 1985.
127. Rosen PP, Medenez-Botet CJ, Nisselbaum JS, et al: Pathological review of breast lesions analyzed for estrogen receptor protein. Cancer Res 35:3187–3194, 1975.
128. Rosen PP, Menendez-Botet CJ, Urban JA, et al: Estrogen receptor protein (ERP) in multiple tumor specimens from individual patients with breast cancer. Cancer 39:2194–2200, 1977.
129. Rosner D, Lane WW: Node-negative minimal invasive breast cancer patients are not candidates for routine systemic adjuvant therapy. Cancer 66:199–205, 1990.
130. Said J, Shintaku IP: Detection of estrogen receptors with monoclonal antibodies in paraffin sections (letter to the editor). Am J Clin Pathol 90:120, 1988.
131. Schwartz PE, MacLusky N, Merino MJ, et al: Are cytosol estrogen and progestin receptors of prognostic significance in the management of epithelial ovarian cancers? Obstet Gynecol 68:751–753, 1986.
132. Shimada A, Kimura S, Abe K, et al: Immunochemical staining of estrogen receptor in paraffin sections of human breast cancer by use of monoclonal antibody: Comparison with that in frozen sections. Proc Natl Acad Sci (USA) 82:4803–4807, 1985.
133. Shintaku P, Said JW: Detection of estrogen receptors with monoclonal antibodies in routinely processed formalin-fixed paraffin sections of breast carcinoma. Am J Clin Pathol 87:161–167, 1987.
134. Skoog L, Humla S, Axelsson M, et al: Estrogen receptor levels and survival of breast cancer patients. A study on patients participating in randomized trials of adjuvant therapy. Acta Oncologicica 26:95–100, 1987.
135. Slotman BJ, Kuhnel R, Rao BR, et al: Importance of steroid receptors and aromatase activity in the prognosis of ovarian cancer: High tumor progesterone receptor levels correlate with longer survival. Gynecol Oncol 33:76–81, 1989.
135a. Sondergaard G, Pederson KO, Paulsen SM: Estrogen receptor analyses in breast cancer: Comparison of monoclonal immunohistochemical and biochemical methods. Eur J Cancer Clin Oncol 25:1425–1429, 1989.
136. Stedman KE, Moore GE, Morgan RT: Estrogen receptor proteins in diverse human tumors. Arch Surg 115:244–248, 1980.
137. Sutton GP, Senior MB, Strauss JF, et al: Estrogen and progesterone receptors in epithelial ovarian malignancies. Gynecol Oncol 23:176–182, 1986.
138. Tani E, Borregon A, Humla S, et al: Estrogen receptors in fine-needle aspirates from metastatic lesions of gynecologic tumors. Gynecol Oncol 32:365–367, 1989.
139. Taylor CR, Cooper CL, Kurman RJ, et al: Detection of estrogen receptor in breast and endometrial carcinoma by the immunoperoxidase technique. Cancer 47:2634, 1981.
140. Thorpe SM: Monoclonal antibody technique for detection of estrogen receptors in human breast cancer: Greater sensitivity and more accurate classification of receptor status than the dextran-coated charcoal method. Cancer Res 47:6572–6575, 1987.

141. Thorpe SM, Rose C: Oestrogen and progesterone receptor determinations in breast cancer: Technology and biology. Cancer Surveys 5:505–525, 1986.
142. Thorpe SM, Rose C, Rasmussen BB, et al: Steroid hormone receptors as prognostic indicators in primary breast cancer. Breast Cancer Res Treat 7(Suppl):91–98, 1986.
143. Tokunaga A, Nishi K, Matsukura N, et al: Estrogen and progesterone receptors in gastric cancer. Cancer 57:1376–1379, 1986.
144. Underwood JCE, Sher E, Reed M, et al: Biochemical assessment of histochemical methods for oestrogen receptor localisation. J Clin Pathol 35:401–406, 1982.
145. Van Netten JP, Algard FT, Coy P, et al: Estrogen receptor assay on breast cancer microsamples: Implications of percent carcinoma estimation. Cancer 49:2383–2388, 1982.
146. Vollenwieder-Zerargui L, Barrelet L, Wong Y, et al: The predictive value of estrogen and progesterone receptors' concentrations on the clinical behavior of breast cancer in women: Clinical correlation on 547 patients. Cancer 57:1171–1180, 1986.
147. Weiss SW, Langloss JM, Shmookler BM, et al: Estrogen receptor protein in bone and soft tissue tumors. Lab Invest 54:689–694, 1986.
148. Willcocks D, Toppila M, Hudson CN, et al: Estrogen and progesterone receptors in human ovarian tumors. Gynecol Oncol 16:246–253, 1983.
149. Zaino R, Satyaswaroop PG, Mortel R: The relationship of histologic and histochemical parameters to progesterone receptor status in endometrial adenocarcinomas. Gynecol Oncol 16:196–208, 1983.

Significance of DNA Content and Proliferative Rate of the Invasive Carcinoma Found in the Mammographically Directed Breast Biopsy

JAMES L. BENNINGTON, M.D.

From the Department of
 Anatomic Pathologic and
 Clinical Laboratories
California Pacific Medical
 Center, California Campus
San Francisco, California

Reprint requests to:
James L. Bennington, M.D.
Department of Anatomic
 Pathologic and Clinical
 Laboratories
California Pacific Medical
 Center, California Campus
P.O. Box 3805
San Francisco, CA 94119

RATIONALE FOR USING TUMOR GRADE AS A PROGNOSTIC INDICATOR

Among the features that characterize solid malignant neoplasms, three are of major importance in determining the clinical course of the patient with cancer. They are: (1) the predilection of the tumor for invasion; (2) the propensity of the tumor to metastasize; and (3) the rate of tumor cell proliferation. In general, the first two determine the likelihood of death from spread of the tumor, and the last, the duration of time to relapse and death. How these neoplastic properties are genetically controlled is poorly understood; however, clues to the behavior of a neoplasm are generally carried in its phenotype.

Pathologists routinely attempt to predict the future behavior of malignant neoplasms from morphologic features. *In the case of carcinoma of the breast, the tumor size, histologic type, nuclear grade, extent of glandular differentiation, mitotic activity, extent of necrosis, extent of vascular and perineural invasion, characteristics of tumor borders, extent of stromal elastosis, and nature of the cellular host response are all morphologic features that to one degree or another have been found to correlate with patient survival.*

There is no one established method of assigning a histologic tumor grade to invasive breast cancers, although a number of grading systems based on that of Bloom and Richardson[1] are widely used. Their method incorporates assessment of two features of tumor differentiation—**preservation of glandular architecture** (extent of tubule formation), and **degree of alteration of nuclear DNA content** (nuclear grade); and one feature of cell proliferation—**mitotic activity**.

In the hands of an expert, the grading system of Bloom and Richardson is highly reproducible and routinely provides useful prognostic information, particularly for those patients with negative axillary lymph nodes. However, there have been many contradictory reports regarding the prognostic utility of tumor grading because of problems with interobserver agreement. In a recent cooperative study,[2] which tested the level of agreement among 11 pathologists in the grading of 45 invasive breast cancers, it was found that interobserver agreement on each individual variable was very poor. For example, complete agreement on the assessment of nuclear grade was achieved in only one case (2%). Observations such as this have provided impetus to searching for reliable alternatives for predicting patient outcome.

RATIONALE FOR USING TUMOR DNA CONTENT AS A PROGNOSTIC INDICATOR

During the last few years considerable effort has been made to find genetic and biochemical markers that could be used to predict the behavior of cancers with greater accuracy than that obtained by histologic grading or the assessment of other established morphologic features. Because there is considerable evidence that malignant neoplasms have cytogenetic abnormalities, and because atypical features of the nucleus such as pleomorphism and hyperchromasia are known to be prognostically unfavorable findings, quantitative analysis of nuclear DNA was a prime candidate for evaluation. Many studies have shown that nuclear DNA content is substantially altered in most malignant neoplasms, and the extent of alteration carries prognostic significance for many tumor types.

The nuclear DNA content of tumor cells is generally expressed in terms of the **DNA index**, which is defined by the formula:

$$\text{DNA Index} = \frac{G_0G_1 \text{ Modal DNA of Tumor Cells}}{G_0G_1 \text{ Modal DNA of Normal (Diploid) Cells}}$$

For this calculation, the modal DNA values are obtained from histograms constructed from the plots of the number of cells detected per channel using flow cytometry (FCM) with cell suspensions, or the number of Feulgen-stained nuclei at various optical density levels detected in smears using static cytometry (SCM). Tumors with a DNA index of 1.0 ± 0.1 are usually regarded as nuclear DNA diploid, whereas those falling outside this range are regarded as nuclear DNA aneuploid. The term **ploidy** is used to refer to the state of a tumor as being nuclear DNA diploid or aneuploid.

Many authors make no attempt to go beyond identifying tumors as diploid or aneuploid; however, there is good evidence that within the group of cancers designated as aneuploid, there is a wide range of aggressiveness directly related to tumor DNA index. For example, tetraploid tumors, which have twice the nuclear DNA content of diploid tumors (DNA index = 2.0 ± 0.2), behave very much like diploid tumors, whereas other aneuploid tumors carry a much higher risk of recurrence and death, particularly those tumors with a DNA index > 2.2.

Further details on the prognostic significance of nuclear DNA content, alone or in combination with the cell proliferative rate of invasive breast cancers, are provided in subsequent sections of this article.

Some cancer-related chromosomal changes are relatively gross, i.e., deletions and replications of entire chromosomes. Others are associated with loss or gain of only small amounts of chromosomal material, or minor changes within a single chromosomal band too subtle to be detected by conventional flow or static cytometry. The accuracy of the cytometric methods used for nuclear DNA analysis is such that a gain or loss of the equivalent of one or more chromosomes is essential before deviation from the diploid level of nuclear DNA content can be readily detected.

Although benign breast tumors and some breast cancers have a diploid nuclear DNA content,[3-5] the majority of breast cancers are nuclear DNA aneuploid.[6] In a review of 18 published FCM studies on invasive breast cancers involving 4,315 patients, Visscher et al.[6] found that on the average 64% of the tumors studied were aneuploid.

RATIONALE FOR USING TUMOR PROLIFERATIVE RATE AS A PROGNOSTIC INDICATOR

The rate at which malignant tumor cells replicate, and the fraction of tumor cells participating in the proliferative process, are of considerable interest to oncologists for use in assessing patient prognosis and for guiding decisions on the use of various endocrine and cytotoxic agents for adjuvant endocrine and chemotherapy. Unfortunately, until relatively recently the only alternatives available for estimating the proliferative rate in breast cancers were: (1) to make sequential measurements of: (a) chest wall recurrences,[7] (b) images of invasive breast cancers seen in serial mammograms,[7b] and (c) images of metastatic cancer in the lung seen in serial chest radiograms[8]; or (2) to measure the thymidine labeling index (TLI), i.e., the percentage of cells in tumor specimens incorporating radioactively labeled thymidine into their nuclei during DNA synthesis.

Sequential measurement of the size of invasive breast cancers that have recurred in the chest wall, longstanding untreated primary breast cancers, or breast cancers that have already metastasized has little practical application in prospective patient care, because all of the above options for measuring the rate of tumor cell proliferation are limited to the patient with advanced disease. While TLI can be determined early in the course of a patient's disease, it is an expensive, time-consuming procedure, involves radioautography, requires use of a radioisotopic label, and requires either in vitro incubation of radioactively labeled thymidine with fresh viable tumor, or its administration to the patient before the tumor is removed. For these reasons, use of this method is generally limited to research applications.

Within the last several years, a number of excellent new methods for measuring the rate of cancer cell proliferation have become available. These methods are highly reproducible and overcome many of the limitations of the TLI method. They include: (1) estimation of the percentage of cells in DNA synthesis, referred to as the S-phase fraction (SPF) from: (a) flow cytometry data, and (b) quantitative immunochemical determination of the percentage of cells incorporating the nucleotide bromodeoxyuridine (BrdUrd), an analog of thymidine, into cell nuclei during DNA synthesis; and (2) estimation of the proliferative fraction of the tumor cell population by quantitative immunochemical determination of the percentage of cells staining positively for one of the proliferation-associated nuclear antigens.

Estimation of the percentage of cells falling between the G_0/G_1 and G_2/M peaks on flow cytometric histograms is frequently used to determine the SPF of the cell population being analyzed. In nonsynchronized cell populations without multiple aneuploid peaks, the SPF is a reliable indicator of cell proliferative activity. A diagram of the cell cycle and its components is shown in Figure 1. Figure 2 is a flow cytometric DNA histogram indicating the segments of the plot that correspond to the various cell cycle components.

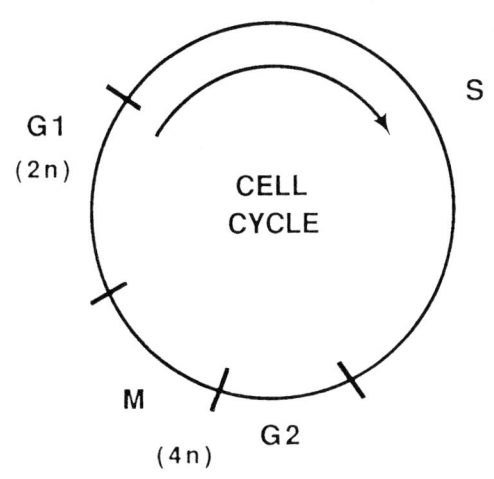

FIGURE 1. Diagrammatic representation of the mammalian cell cycle. Resting cells (G_0) and cells in the presynthetic phase (G_1) have a diploid chromosomal complement (2n). Cells in the postsynthetic phase (G_2) and in mitosis (M) have a tetraploid chromosomal complement (4n). Cells in the DNA synthesis phase (S) have intermediate values.

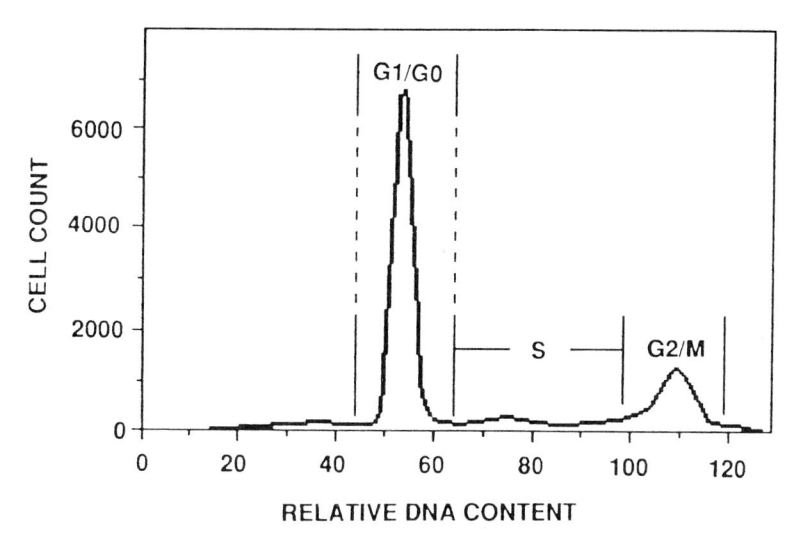

FIGURE 2. Nuclear DNA histogram of a diploid tumor. The first large peak corresponds to the relative DNA content of cells in G_0/G_1; the second smaller peak, to the cells in G_2/M; and the plateau between the two peaks, to the cells in S.

The percentage of cells incorporating BrdUrd into nuclei as determined by the peroxidase-antiperoxidase method using a monoclonal antibody to BrdUrd provides a measure of the size of the S-phase fraction, but without having to use a radioisotopic label. The major drawback of this method is that BrdUrd is not normally present in nuclear DNA. To be detected immunocytochemically in tissue sections, it must be either administered to the patient prior to surgical removal of the tumor, or a slice of fresh, viable tumor incubated with BrdUrd in vitro before tissue processing.

Immunochemical localization of proliferation-associated nuclear antigens, which appear in nuclei only during the non-resting phase of the cell cycle, also can be used to estimate proliferative rate.[9-13] The proliferation-associated nuclear antigen most extensively studied in invasive breast cancer is one that reacts with the Ki-67 monoclonal antibody. A distinct advantage of this method is its potential application to routine pathologic examination of breast cancers. It is not dependent on access to flow cytometry and can be performed in any laboratory experienced with immunocytochemistry. A disadvantage of the method is that the staining must be performed on frozen sectioned fresh tissue, because fixation renders the antigen nonreactive with the Ki-67 antibody.

Results obtained by the various methods for determining the proliferative component of a tumor cell population correlate with one another to various degrees. However, except for thymidine and BrdUrd labeling, which both directly measure the percentage of cells in a population engaged in DNA synthesis, these different methods do not give results that are directly interchangable.

SPF, determined by computerized analysis of FCM histograms, is highly correlated with TLI and is as effective in predicting patient outcome as TLI.

However, SPF values estimated by this method are generally higher than those obtained by TLI. This difference is due, in part, to contamination of the specimen with nuclear fragments (more frequently seen in preparations of disaggregated paraffin-embedded than in fresh tumor samples). The nuclear fragments may become aggregated or adherent to intact nuclei, producing artifacts in the S-phase region of the FCM histogram. Visscher et al.[6] reviewed the literature on attempted extraction of SPF values from FCM histograms of breast cancers. He found in these reports that an acceptable estimate could be obtained in 78% of the 3,460 tumors analyzed.

Immunocytochemical localization of the Ki-67-positive nuclear antigen provides an estimate of the proliferative fraction of a tumor cell population that is larger than that provided by TLI, BrdUrd labeling, or computer-derived estimates of SPF from nuclear DNA flow cytometry histograms. The reason for this difference is that the nuclear antigen detected by Ki-67 is expressed not only in S, but also the other non-resting phases of the cell cycle (G_1, G_2, and M). Therefore, the antigen is recognized by the Ki-67 antibody in a larger percentage of cells than is represented by cells in the S-phase. Estimates of the proliferative fraction based on immunochemical staining for PCNA/cyclin provide estimates that are closer to SPF, because this antigen is expressed almost exclusively in the S phase of the cell cycle.[13b]

The proliferative fraction of tumor cells in invasive breast cancers, as determined by the percentage of nuclei labeled by the Ki-67 antibody (KFS), is strongly correlated with the TLI,[14] BrdUrd labeling index,[15] and SPF extracted from FCM histograms.[16]

Tumor nuclear DNA content and rates of tumor cell proliferation have been studied extensively in relation to the prognosis of patients with invasive cancer of the breast. These studies have shown that nuclear DNA content and tumor cell proliferative rate correlate with several important prognostic variables for patients with invasive breast cancer. However, their clinical potential is far greater than as alternative prognostic indicators.

Each provides prognostic information independent of the other, and independent of other prognostic indicators. Furthermore, the predictive value of the two when used in combination is greater than that of either alone. In addition to their use in assessing prognosis, tumor nuclear DNA content and tumor rate of cell proliferation show considerable promise for guiding oncologists in deciding whether or not to use adjuvant endocrine therapy and chemotherapy with invasive breast cancer.

CORRELATION OF TUMOR NUCLEAR DNA CONTENT AND TUMOR PROLIFERATIVE RATE WITH ESTABLISHED PROGNOSTIC VARIABLES FOR PATIENTS WITH INVASIVE BREAST CANCER

Nuclear DNA Ploidy

Tumor Size. Two investigators have reported that preclinical invasive breast cancers detected by mammography are frequently diploid.[17,18] While a number of investigators have determined that small invasive breast cancers tend to be diploid and large invasive breast cancers aneuploid,[19-26] others have been unable to find any correlation between tumor size and nuclear DNA ploidy.[24,25,27-34]

Visscher et al.[6] compiled the findings on the relationship between tumor ploidy and tumor size reported in nine studies involving 2,554 patients with invasive breast cancer. He determined that the reported percentages of aneuploid tumors in relation to tumor size were: 59% (< 2 cm); 67% (2 ≤ 5 cm); and 72% (> 5 cm).

Early detection of clinically silent invasive breast cancers by mammography permits surgical removal of the cancer while it has a relatively small surface area, thus reducing the likelihood of cancer cells gaining access to lymphatic vessels. If indeed small invasive breast cancers were predominantly diploid, then early detection and treatment would further benefit patients by permitting removal of invasive breast cancers before they became aneuploid.

The last scenario seems unlikely, because the DNA index appears to be relatively stable during the life of a tumor,[35,36] and the relation between nuclear DNA ploidy and tumor size does not appear to be strong. The thesis that small, mammographically detected breast cancers are frequently diploid remains to be proved.

Lymph Node Metastases. The relation of DNA tumor ploidy to lymph node status in patients with invasive breast cancer is as uncertain as the relation of tumor ploidy to tumor size. Several authors have found that lymph node metastases at the time of diagnosis are more frequent among patients with aneuploid than patients with diploid invasive breast cancers,[20,21,25,37] whereas others[17,18,29,30,38,39] have found no such relationship. Visscher et al.[6] summarized the findings from 14 reported studies involving 3,739 patients on the relation between tumor nuclear DNA ploidy and frequency of axillary lymph node metastases. In this combined series, 55% of the lymph node-negative patients and 64% of the lymph node-positive patients had aneuploid breast cancers. Based on this relatively small difference in the frequency of axillary lymph node metastases between patients with diploid and aneuploid breast cancers, the relation between tumor ploidy and axillary lymph node status appears to be weak at best.

For patients with invasive breast cancer who are axillary lymph node-positive, there is a suggestion that the number of positive axillary lymph nodes increases in parallel with increasing tumor nuclear DNA aneuploidy.[18,19,21,26,32,41-43]

Distant Metastases. Although nuclear DNA ploidy of invasive breast cancers has not been shown to be strongly correlated with tumor size or with the likelihood of the patient developing axillary lymph node metastases, at least one investigator[25] has found a statistically significant association between the ploidy level of invasive breast cancers and the frequency of distant metastases. In a study of patients with invasive breast cancer followed for relatively long periods (11.5 to 13.3 years), Eskelinen et al.[25] found that 72% of the patients with aneuploid, but only 42% of the patients with diploid, tumors had developed distant metastases. These findings are consistent with the evidence that nuclear DNA ploidy is correlated with patient outcome, i.e., survival is greater for patients with diploid than aneuploid invasive breast cancers. This relation is discussed later in the section on "Tumor DNA Content as a Prognostic Indicator."

Tumor Stage. The construction of the WHO breast cancer staging system is based on the features of **primary tumor size, axillary lymph node status,** and the **presence or absence of distant metastases** at the time of diagnosis. As indicated in the earlier discussion, none of these three features individually has been correlated with tumor ploidy. Therefore, one would hardly expect tumor ploidy to correlate with these features in combination, i.e., tumor stage.

With the exception of Meckenstock,[44] investigators who have looked for an association between tumor ploidy and tumor stage[21,24,27,43] in patients with invasive breast cancer have been unable to find one. Erhard[24] specifically demonstrated that the prognostic information provided by tumor ploidy is completely independent of those features used for defining tumor stage in invasive breast cancers.

Tumor Type. The relatively few studies on nuclear DNA content of invasive breast cancers in relation to histologic type have shown, as might be expected, that well-differentiated breast cancers generally recognized as nonaggressive, e.g., tubular, papillary, and colloid carcinomas, are almost invariably diploid.[30,39,45,46] Surprisingly, in view of their generally aggressive behavior, invasive lobular carcinomas are predominantly diploid,[30] as are in situ lobular carcinomas.[47] In contrast, approximately 65% of invasive duct carcinomas and 80% of medullary and atypical medullary carcinomas are aneuploid.[30,39]

Tumor Grade. Most investigators[18,19,22,26-33,35,48-52] who have studied histologic grade in relation to the nuclear DNA content of invasive breast cancers have demonstrated a strong correlation between these two features. We are aware of only two studies in which no correlation between tumor ploidy and tumor histologic grade was found.[18,34]

As a rule, well-differentiated invasive breast cancers are predominantly diploid, and poorly differentiated invasive breast cancers are aneuploid. However, ploidy and tumor grade cannot be regarded as equivalents, because exceptions to this rule are common. These exceptions are clinically important, for they represent cases where aneuploid cancers are interpreted as Grade 1 and diploid cancers as Grade 3.

Owainati et al.[52] in a study of 280 invasive breast cancers graded according to the method of Bloom and Richardson[1] found that 22% of Grade 1 cancers turned out to be aneuploid, and 26% of Grade 3 cancers turned out to be diploid (Table 1). The combined results of six other studies lead to the same conclusion. In these studies 37% of Grade 1 tumors were aneuploid and 18% of Grade 3 tumors were diploid.[20,31,32,51,73]

The pathologist-assigned histologic grade and nuclear DNA content of invasive breast cancers are usually closely correlated. This should come as no

TABLE 1. Relation of Histologic Tumor Grades to Ploidy Among 280 Invasive Breast Cancers[52]

Ploidy	Grade 1	Grade 2	Grade 3
Diploid	38 (78%)	42 (41%)	33 (26%)
Aneuploid	11 (22%)	60 (59%)	96 (74%)
Total	49 (100%)	102 (100%)	129 (100%)

surprise, because two of the three components used in determining the histologic grade, i.e., nuclear grade and mitotic index, have been shown to be independently related to tumor nuclear DNA ploidy.

Nuclear grade. The nuclear grade of a breast cancer, determined by the pathologist, and its nuclear DNA content, measured cytometrically, are both representative of chromosomal complement. The major difference between the two methods is that the latter is more objective and quantifiable.

Mitotic rate. The proliferative rate of an invasive breast cancer, measured in terms of SPF and TLI, strongly correlates with nuclear DNA content. Diploid invasive breast cancers typically have low, and aneuploid breast cancers have high, proliferative rates. Uyterlinde et al.[33] found that 61% of invasive breast cancers with mitotic indices > 10 were aneuploid, but only 27% < 10. Baildam et al.[48] showed that tetraploid tumors were similar to diploid tumors in that both had relatively low mitotic counts. This was in marked contrast to aneuploid tumors that had high mitotic counts (Table 2).

These relationships have been documented by measurements of TLI,[32,53] SPF (by flow cytometry,[27-31,39,42,45,53-55] and static cytometry[56]), and tumor mitotic index.[32,46] We have found only one report where there was no correlation between tumor ploidy and SPF.[57]

The histogram in Figure 3 graphically demonstrates the interrelationship between tumor ploidy and proliferative rate. In this histogram the SPF values for 1,331 invasive breast cancers[43] are plotted separately for aneuploid and diploid tumors. While there is a broad range of SPF values for both aneuploid and diploid carcinomas, and the two ranges overlap, there is a distinct separation of their modal values.

Tumor Necrosis. Fisher et al.[58] found that the intrinsic tumor characteristics of **necrosis, differentiation,** and **size** were the three most important prognostic indicators for predicting the 5-year treatment failure in axillary lymph node-negative women with invasive breast cancer.

TABLE 2. Relation Between Tumor Nuclear DNA Content and Mitotic Activity in Invasive Breast Cancers[48]

Ploidy	Mitotic Score Low	Intermediate	High	N
Diploid	25 (41%)	13 (31%)	2 (18%)	40
Tetraploid	23 (38%)	14 (32%)	4 (36%)	41
Aneuploid	13 (21%)	42 (37%)	5 (46%)	33
Total	61 (100%)	42 (100%)	11 (100%)	114

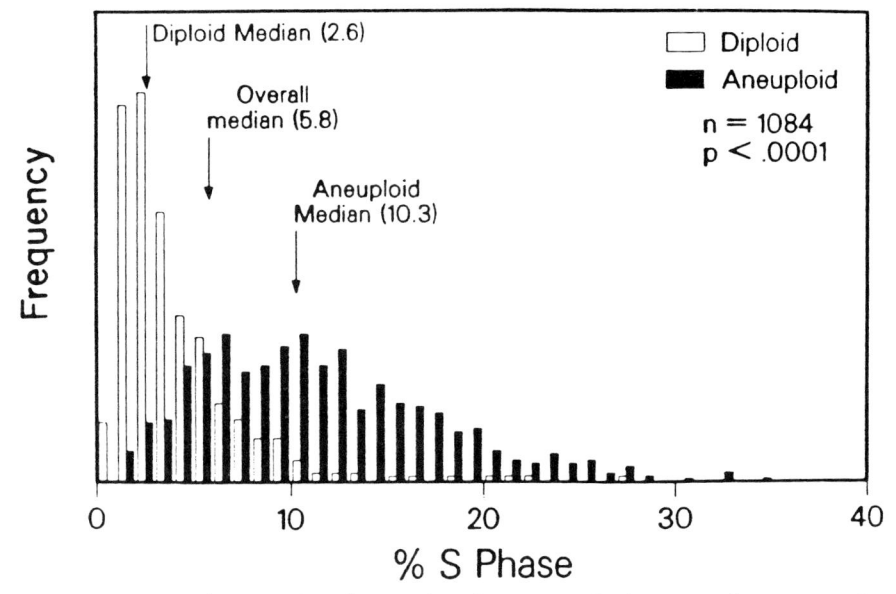

FIGURE 3. Distribution of S-phase values by tumor ploidy status. (From Dressler LG, et al: Cancer 61:420–427, 1988, with permission.)

Necrosis of the invasive component in breast cancers has been shown by two investigators to correlate with an aneuploid nuclear DNA content.[6,32] The most likely explanation for this association is that aneuploidy is a marker for rapid cancer cell proliferation, which favors tumor necrosis.

Intraparenchymal Lymphatic Invasion. The one report we have been able to find in which the presence of lymphatic vascular invasion was studied in relation to tumor ploidy showed no correlation between these two prognostic variables.[32] While the results of a single study are not conclusive, these findings are consistent with the observations of Fisher et al.,[59] who found that intraparenchymal lymphatic invasion, like tumor ploidy, is more closely related to the axillary lymph node status than survival for patients with invasive breast cancer.

Breast Cancer Hormone Receptor Protein Levels. It has been known for some time that poorly differentiated invasive breast cancers are more likely to be estrogen-receptor protein-negative than those that are well differentiated.[60-61] In view of the close correlation between tumor grade and tumor ploidy, a similar relation between tumor nuclear DNA ploidy and tumor hormone receptor protein levels could be predicted, and indeed has been found.

With only two exceptions,[30,32] investigators have reported that there is a strong correlation between tumor nuclear DNA ploidy and the steroid hormone receptor protein levels in invasive breast cancers.[22,23,29,31,38,41,43-45,48] Aneuploid breast cancers have been shown to have the lowest levels of

TABLE 3. Correlation Between DNA Index and Steroid Hormone Receptor Protein Status in Invasive Breast Cancers[48]

DNA Index	ER+	PR+
< 1.0	69%	55%
1.2–1.7	59%	52%
1.8–1.9	90%	58%
2.0	81%	62%
> 2.0	54%	35%

estrogen and progesterone receptor proteins, whereas tetraploid and near-tetraploid tumors, followed by diploid and hyperdiploid tumors, have the highest levels[48] (Table 3).

Age/Menopausal Status. The relation of a patient's age and menopausal status to the ploidy status of her invasive breast cancer is a much-debated issue. Aneuploidy has been reported as being more frequent in the invasive breast cancers of older[3,19,20,46,62] and postmenopausal women than in younger and premenopausal women.[19,20,27,54] However, aneuploidy has also been reported as higher in the breast cancers of pre- than postmenopausal women[63] and has also been reported as having no relation to menopausal status.[21,28,29,35,37,43,51,64]

Visscher at el.[6] summarized the results from five studies involving 1,025 women with invasive breast cancers. They determined that there was no difference in the reported frequency of aneuploid tumors with respect to menopausal status. In this series, 58% of the invasive breast cancers in premenopausal women and 57% in postmenopausal women were aneuploid.

In view of these conflicting reports, it would appear that if either the patient's age, menopausal status, or both are related to the ploidy of invasive breast cancers, the association is not a strong one.

Tumor Cell Proliferative Rate

Tumor Size. As with tumor ploidy, the rate of cell proliferation in invasive breast cancers does not seem to be related to the size of the primary tumor. A weak correlation of a high SPF,[32] and a strong correlation of a high TLI,[65] with large breast cancers have been reported. However, other investigators have found no association between tumor size and SPF,[28–31] TLI,[32,66] or the percentage of cells staining positively for Ki-67.[67]

Lymph Node Status. The impact of proliferative rate on the frequency of axillary lymph node metastases in invasive breast cancers has not been established. One investigator[27] has reported that axillary lymph node metastases occur more frequently with high (above median) than with low SPF invasive breast cancers. However, three investigators[6,21,29] have found only a weak association, and two investigators[20,32] no association, between SPF levels and lymph node status. Studies using TLI[65,66,68] and the percentage of Ki-67-positive cells[67,69,70] have also failed to show a relation between tumor proliferative rate and the frequency of lymph node metastasis.

It may well be that the impact of proliferative rate is significant in diploid invasive breast cancers. Dressler[71] found a statistically significantly higher mean SPF in axillary lymph node-positive than lymph node-negative patients with diploid breast cancers. However, he could find no difference between the mean SPF levels of lymph node-positive and lymph node-negative patients with aneuploid breast cancers.

Distant Metastases. There is relatively little published data on the rate of breast cancer cell proliferation in relation to the likelihood of distant metastases. In one study Kallioniemi[29] found that patients with breast cancers with SPF values below the median had fewer distant metastases than did patients with breast cancers with SPF values above the median. We have found no reports on the association between either TLI or percent of Ki-67-positive cells and the presence or absence of distant metastases.

Tumor Stage. Most investigators have been unable to demonstrate a relation between the rate of breast cancer cell proliferation and tumor stage, although both Meckenstock[44] and Kallioniemi et al.[70] observed a tendency for SPF values to rise with increasing cancer stage. This tendency was more pronounced for diploid than for aneuploid invasive breast cancers.

We are not aware of any published data on the association of TLI and tumor stage. In the one report where Ki-67 staining of tumor cells[67] was studied in relation to tumor stage, no correlation was found.

Tumor Type. Each individual histologic type of invasive breast cancer appears to have a fairly characteristic rate of cell proliferation as measured by SPF[45,60,70] and TLI.[72] The rates of tumor cell proliferation are highest for medullary and atypical medullary carcinomas, intermediate for duct carcinomas (all grades combined) and lobular carcinomas, and are lowest for adenoid cystic, papillary, tubular, and mucinous carcinomas of the breast.

Tumor Grade. Many studies have demonstrated that the rate of tumor cell proliferation, as measured by SPF,[6,29,31,32,35,39,45,73] TLI,[14,65-67,68,74] and percentage of cells with Ki-67-positive nuclei[14,65-67,74,75] in invasive breast cancers correlate closely with tumor histologic grade. When duct carcinomas of the breast are stratified by histologic grade, Grade 3 tumors have the highest rates, Grade 2 tumors intermediate rates, and Grade 1 tumors the lowest rates of cell proliferation, as measured in terms of SPF.[39] This relationship holds true irrespective of ploidy status. Typically for both diploid and aneuploid breast cancers, an increase in tumor grade is associated with increasing SPF.[39]

These results are not at all surprising. Mitotic activity, one measure of the rate of tumor cell proliferation, figures prominently in most methods for determining the histologic grade of invasive breast cancers and has been shown to parallel proliferative activity as measured by TLI,[16,49,67,68] the percentage of cells in S-phase,[46] and the percentage of cells staining with Ki-67.[16,67,69]

Tumor Necrosis. As indicated in the discussion in the preceding section on tumor necrosis in relation to tumor ploidy, the rate of cell proliferation would be expected to correlate with tumor necrosis, if indeed the postulate is correct that tumor necrosis occurs as a result of a tumor cell population expanding so rapidly that it outgrows its own blood supply. Whatever the underlying mechanism, several investigators have observed that in invasive breast cancers the rate of cell proliferation, as measured by SPF[32,49] and TLI,[65] is directly related to the extent of tumor necrosis.

Intraparenchymal Lymphatic Invasion. Tumor nuclear DNA ploidy is poorly correlated with intraparenchymal lymphatic invasion and the same is true for the rate of breast cancer cell proliferation. The few published studies on this subject report no strong association between either SPF[32] or TLI[65] with intraparenchymal lymphatic invasion. The only hint of relationship is found in a report where a weak correlation of TLI with lymphatic invasion[32] was observed.

Breast Cancer Hormone Receptor Protein Levels. With few exceptions, investigators have found that rapidly proliferating breast cancers, whether measured in terms of SPF,[28,32,35,38,39,43,50,73,76] TLI,[53,65-67,77] or percentage of cells staining for Ki-67,[53,65,67,75] have low or no measurable steroid hormone (estrogen and progesterone) receptor protein levels. This is in marked contrast to slowly proliferating breast cancers that typically have positive estrogen receptor and progesterone receptor protein levels.

The distribution of SPF values in invasive breast cancers, stratified by tumor estrogen and progesterone receptor protein status, as reported by Dressler et al.,[43] is shown in Figure 4.

Menopausal Status. Invasive breast cancers in premenopausal patients tend to have higher rates of cell proliferation, as measured by SPF,[28,39,43,64] TLI,[66,67,77] and the percentage of cells staining with Ki-67,[66,67] than those in postmenopausal patients. In Silverstrini's series,[76] the reported median TLI of

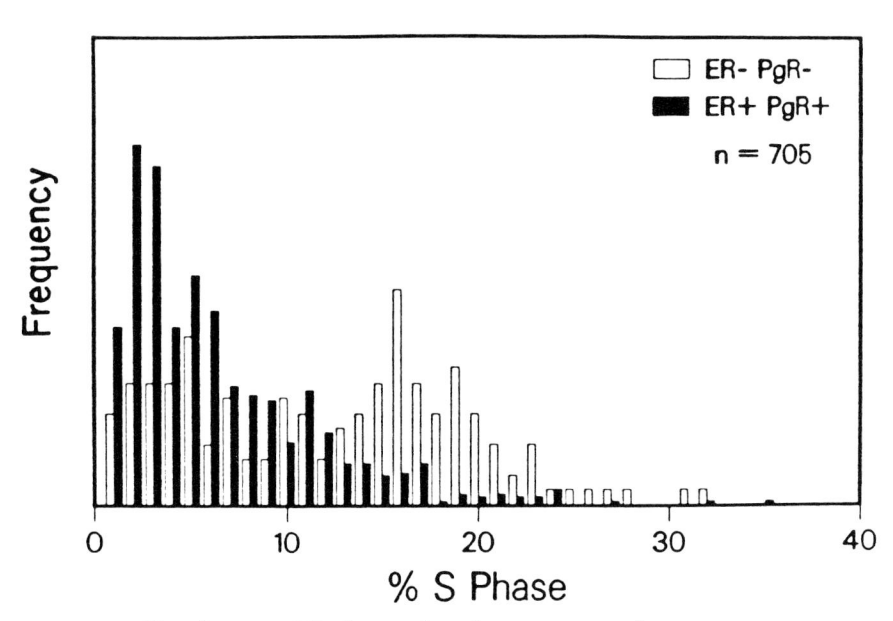

FIGURE 4. Distribution of S-phase values by estrogen and progesterone receptor protein status. (From Dressler LG, et al: Cancer 61:420–427, 1988, with permission.)

invasive breast cancer cells was twice as high for premenopausal as it was for postmenopausal patients.

The finding that invasive breast cancers have higher rates of tumor cell proliferation in premenopausal than in postmenopausal women is consistent with the observation that high-grade invasive duct cancers, which are associated with high rates of cell proliferation, are more common in premenopausal than in postmenopausal women.

TUMOR DNA CONTENT AND TUMOR PROLIFERATIVE RATE AS PROGNOSTIC INDICATORS

Tumor DNA Content

DNA Ploidy. The overall patient survival rate[22,23,27,31,40,53,62,70,78,79,80] and the disease-free survival rate[19,21,23,31,37,40–42,52] are better for patients with diploid than for patients with aneuploid invasive breast cancers. Furthermore, tumor nuclear DNA content is an independent prognostic indicator for patients with invasive breast cancer.[23,26,30,46,70] This holds true for both axillary lymph node-negative[22,26,40,46,78] and axillary lymph node-positive[22,23,26,27,40,42] patients, and persists for follow-up periods that range up to 12.5 years[27,64,57] (Table 4).

There are a relatively small number of reports in which investigators have been unable to demonstrate a relationship between tumor nuclear DNA ploidy status and patient outcome.[19,30,52,81]

DNA Index. Conventionally, most authors have defined those malignant neoplasms characterized by a nondiploid nuclear DNA content as aneuploid. However, the DNA index, which like DNA ploidy is an independent prognostic indicator,[70] contains more information than just ploidy status. Relatively recently it has been shown that the risk of recurrence for patients with tetraploid invasive breast cancers (DNA Index of 2.0 ± 0.2), which in the past have been regarded as aneuploid, is much lower than the risk of recurrence for patients with other aneuploid (hyperdiploid and hypertetraploid) breast cancers.[70]

Patients with aneuploid (nontetraploid) breast cancers have a much greater risk of recurrence and death than patients with either diploid or tetraploid cancers. This difference in risk rises with increasing DNA index. The risk of death for patients with hypertetraploid (DNA index > 2.2) invasive breast cancers has been estimated to be 3–5 times, and from hyperdiploid

TABLE 4. Overall Survival Rates for Patients with Aneuploid and Diploid Breast Cancers

Follow-up (Years)	Diploid	Aneuploid
4[57]	87%	61%
5[70]	89%	60%
8[70]	75%	51%
12.5[27]	67%	35%

TABLE 5. Survival Rates for Patients with Invasive Breast Cancer by DNA Index and DNA Class

DNA Index	DNA Class	8 Years[70]	12.5 Years[27]
1	Diploid	75%	67%
1.1–1.8	Hyperdiploid	50%	35%
1.8–2.2	Tetraploid	58%	40%
>2.2	Hypertetraploid	40%	0%

(DNA index > 1.1 ≤ 1.8) to be 2–3 times that for patients with diploid invasive breast cancers.[64]

Survival figures for patients with invasive breast cancer, for each of the four nuclear DNA categories described above, have been reported from two large studies[27,70] in which the patients were followed for relatively long periods. A summary of these results is provided in Table 5.

The importance of considering tetraploid breast cancers separately from other aneuploid (nondiploid) breast cancers also has been demonstrated by Fallenius.[26] He also showed that lymph node status, considered in combination with tumor nuclear DNA content (expressed as tumors being diploid, tetraploid, or aneuploid), provides even greater accuracy in predicting both 5- and 10-year disease-free patient survival (Table 6).

Tumor Proliferative Rate

Numerous studies on the clinical significance of the proliferative rate of invasive breast cancers, measured by SPF[29,31,41,52,57,78] and TLI[65,66,68,82] have shown that there is a strong correlation between the proliferative rate of breast cancers and patient survival.

Most investigators have found that SPF is not only highly correlated with patient survival, but is a statistically significant independent prognostic indicator for patients with invasive breast cancer,[5,7,29–31,41,68,70,78,83] including those patients with axillary lymph node-negative cancers.[30] Clark et al.[78] found that SPF was a highly reliable predictor of recurrence, primarily in axillary lymph node-negative patients with diploid invasive breast cancers. A relatively small number of investigators[27,30] have reported that the rate of cancer cell proliferation does not appear to be an independent prognostic variable.

TABLE 6. The 5-Year and 10-Year Disease-free Survival Rates for Patients with Invasive Breast Cancer in Relation to Tumor Ploidy and Axillary Lymph Node Status[26]

Lymph Node Status	5-Year	10-Year
Negative		
Diploid	100%	95%
Tetraploid	76%	73%
Aneuploid	65%	58%
Positive		
Diploid	86%	76%
Tetraploid	57%	45%
Aneuploid	33%	31%

Stal et al.,[64] Klintberg et al.,[84] and Hedley et al.[31] found that for patients with Stage I and II invasive breast cancers, a high SPF was predictive for recurrence, but SPF was less powerful as a prognostic indicator and appeared to lose statistical significance as an independent variable when allowance was made for its correlation with tumor grade,[64,82] tumor size, and the patient's lymph node status.[29,64]

TLI, however, is both strongly associated with disease-free survival[68] and has been shown to be a stage-independent prognostic indicator.[68,76,83,85] Four-year to 6-year relapse rates of 21–26% are reported for patients with low TLI, and 50–52% for patients with high TLI.[65,66,68]

Tumor Nuclear DNA Content and Tumor Proliferative Rate Combined

Kallioniemi et al.[70] performed flow cytometry on 308 invasive breast cancers and extracted from the resulting DNA histogram features for evaluation of prognostic significance, including: DNA ploidy type, DNA index, size and number of aneuploid peaks, and the percentages of cells in S-phase and G_2/M. Using multivariate linear regression analysis, they determined that the DNA index and SPF were each powerful independent prognostic indicators for patients with both diploid and aneuploid invasive breast cancers.

Although the DNA index is an independent prognostic indicator, the percentage of cells in S-phase helped to further define patient prognosis within groups of nuclear DNA diploid and aneuploid cancers. Kallioniemi et al.[70] were able to identify three combinations of DNA histograms and SPF values that corresponded to favorable, intermediate, and unfavorable patient prognosis. The combination of tumor DNA content and SPF was more powerful as a prognostic indicator than DNA ploidy, DNA index, or SPF alone.

The Type I combination, defined as diploid DNA content and low SPF ($< 7\%$), was associated with a 90% 8-year cumulative patient survival. The Type III combination, defined as DNA index > 2.20 (irrespective of SPF) or an aneuploid DNA index < 2.20 and SPF $> 12\%$, was associated with a poor short-term and a 50% 8-year cumulative patient survival. The Type II combination, defined as diploid DNA index and high SPF ($= > 7\%$) or aneuploid DNA index and low SPF, was associated with an intermediate survival rate (Fig. 5).

TUMOR RESPONSE TO ENDOCRINE AND CHEMOTHERAPY IN RELATION TO PLOIDY AND RATES OF CELL PROLIFERATION

Response to Endocrine Therapy

To date, there have been only two reports on the relation of tumor DNA ploidy to the response of invasive breast cancers to endocrine therapy. No difference in the response by either diploid or aneuploid invasive breast cancers to endocrine therapy was found by Stuart-Harris et al.[86] However, Baildam et al.[48] reported that on tamoxifen therapy, patients with tetraploid

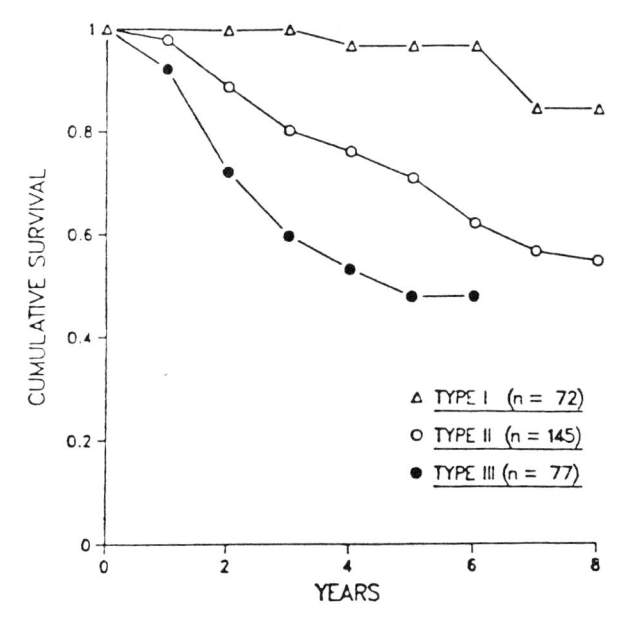

FIGURE 5. Survival for patients with Stage I–III invasive breast cancer in relation to DNA histogram type. Type I: DNA diploid tumors, SPF < 7%; Type III: DNA aneuploid tumors, SPF > 12% or DNA aneuploid (DNA Index > 2.2); Type II: All other tumors. (From Kallioniemi O-P, et al: Cancer 62:2183–2190, 1988, with permission.)

and near-tetraploid invasive breast cancers survived longer and remained remission-free longer than patients with aneuploid invasive breast cancers.

Response to Chemotherapy

In a large series of pre- and postmenopausal women with axillary lymph node-positive invasive breast cancer, Hedley et al.[31] showed that with adjuvant chemotherapy and endocrine therapy the disease-free survival was somewhat longer for patients with diploid-low SPF tumors than for patients with either aneuploid or high SPF tumors.

Remvikos et al.[87] were unable to show any correlation between tumor nuclear DNA ploidy and response to adjuvant cytotoxic chemotherapy (cyclophosphamide and 5-fluorouracil) among 60 premenopausal patients with previously untreated, lymph node-negative, invasive breast cancer. However, they did find a strong correlation between response to chemotherapy and SPF.

In Remvikos et al.'s study, all 12 patients with an SPF > 10% showed a demonstrable clinical regression; 6 with a complete remission on treatment with adjuvant cytotoxic chemotherapy. Six of 13 patients with low SPF (< 5%) had a definite response (46%), with only 1 complete remission; while 21 of 25 patients (84%) with an intermediate SPF (5 ≤ 10%) responded, including 6 with complete remissions. Similar results were reported by Bonadonna et al.,[88] who found that lymph node-negative patients with rapidly proliferating (high TLI) invasive breast cancers were more likely to respond to cytotoxic chemotherapy with cyclophosphamide, methotrexate, and 5-fluorouracil than patients with slowly proliferating (low TLI) invasive breast cancers.

SUMMARY

As described earlier in this issue (Bennington J, *"Impact of mammographic screening on the size and relative frequency of invasion of invasive breast cancer seen at Children's Hospital, 1975–1988,"* pp 11–21), the introduction of routine mammography has the potential to substantially reduce the average size of breast cancers removed surgically in screened populations.

Unfortunately, detection and removal of an invasive breast cancer while it is still relatively small does not guarantee the patient protection from developing metastases. As many as 20–24% of patients with invasive breast cancers that are 5–10 mm,[89,90] and 14–28% of patients with invasive breast cancers that are < 5 mm in diameter,[90-92] develop axillary lymph node metastases.

Adjuvant endocrine therapy and chemotherapy have been shown in several studies to prolong the disease-free survival for both pre- and postmenopausal, axillary lymph node-negative women with invasive breast cancer.[93-96] Absent sufficiently reliable indicators to accurately predict which axillary lymph node-negative patients are most likely to develop metastases, many oncologists have chosen to offer adjuvant chemotherapy to all breast cancer patients, irrespective of lymph node status.

Better prognostic discriminants are essential in order to develop an approach to treatment that will spare those axillary lymph node-negative patients not destined to develop metastases the unnecessary costs and the morbidity of prophylactic chemotherapy. This need is as great for women with small, mammographically detected breast cancers as it is for women with large, clinically diagnosed breast cancers.

Tumor nuclear DNA content and **tumor cell proliferative rate** are prime candidates for use as predictors of distant metastases in axillary lymph node-negative patients with invasive breast cancer. The rationale for selecting nuclear DNA content and proliferative rate for evaluation, the extent to which they correlate with other predictors of patient outcome, and their potential as prognostic indicators, individually and in combination, are reviewed in this article.

An increase in chromosomal material produced by cancer-related cytogenetic changes is manifested morphologically at the light microscopic level by nuclear hyperchromasia, nuclear pleomorphism and abnormal chromatin distribution. At the biochemical level it is manifested by an increase in nuclear DNA content.

The pathologist routinely incorporates into the pathology report of invasive breast cancer an assessment of the degree of cytogenetically-induced nuclear changes in the form of a tumor grade. Because tumor grade has been shown to be a reliable prognostic indicator under the right conditions, the cost of which is negligible, tumor grading is widely used. However, tumor grading has a number of inherent limitations, most notably poor interobserver agreement. By contrast, nuclear DNA measurements made by flow or static cytometry are quantitative and highly reproducible, but relatively expensive.

The mitotic index, one indicator of cell proliferation, has been shown to have prognostic significance, and along with nuclear grade, has been incorporated into the Bloom and Richardson method for histologic grading of breast cancers.[1] Because of the practical limitations of mitotic counting, a number of quantitative methods have been developed for determining the percentages of tumor cells in the various proliferative phases of the cell cycle. They include: thymidine labeling, BrdUrd labeling, extraction of S-phase fractions (SPF) from flow cytometric histograms, and immunocytochemical demonstration of proliferation-associated nuclear antigens such as those detected by Ki-67 and PCNA/Cyclin antibodies.

Typically, one of the first steps in evaluating a feature for its potential as a prognostic indicator is to establish whether or not it shows any correlation with other features known to have prognostic significance. In this article, we have reviewed the findings of many investigators who have studied tumor nuclear DNA content and the rate of tumor cell proliferation in relation to tumor features, which historically have been found to be useful prognostic indicators for patients with invasive breast cancer. They include: **tumor size, tumor histologic grade, tumor histologic type, tumor stage, extent of tumor necrosis, tumor steroid hormone receptor protein content,** and **patient age and menopausal status**.

Five of the prognostic indicators—tumor size, tumor stage, tumor extension to intraparenchymal lymphatics, axillary lymph node status, and metastasis to distant sites—show no strong association with either tumor nuclear DNA content or tumor proliferative rate. The remaining five prognostic indicators, all are strongly correlated with tumor cell proliferative rate and two also with tumor nuclear DNA content (Table 7).

Tumor nuclear DNA content and tumor cell proliferative rate are both highly correlated with a number of established prognostic indicators for patients with invasive breast cancer, and each is a useful prognostic indicator in its own right. Nuclear DNA content of invasive breast cancers, expressed in terms of ploidy, effectively distinguishes patients with a good chance for survival (patients with diploid cancers) from those with a poor chance of survival (patients with aneuploid cancers) (see Table 4).

TABLE 7. Prognostic Indicators for Patients with Invasive Breast Cancer That Are Strongly Correlated with Either Tumor DNA Ploidy or Proliferative Rate

	DNA Content	Proliferative Rate
Tumor Type	−	+
Tumor Grade	+	+
Tumor Necrosis	−	+
ER, PR Content	+	+
Age, Menopausal Status	−	+

TABLE 8.[70] Relative Risk of Death for Patients with Invasive Breast Cancer for the Four DNA Classes

DNA Class	Relative Risk of Death
Diploid	1.0
Tetraploid	1.1
Hyperdiploid	2–3
Hypertetraploid	3–5

By stratifying aneuploid invasive breast cancers (DNA index > 1.1) into three groups—**tetraploid cancers** (DNA index = 2.0 ± 0.2), **hyperdiploid cancers** (DNA index = > 1.1–1.8), and **hypertetraploid cancers** (DNA index > 2.2), the measurement of nuclear DNA provides even greater power as a predictor of patient survival (see Table 5). The relative risk of death for patients with invasive breast cancer, calculated according to the Cox proportional hazard model after eliminating the effects of primary tumor size and nodal status, for each of the four DNA classes is shown in Table 8.

The proliferative rate of invasive breast cancers shares with tumor nuclear DNA content the attributes of being highly correlated with patient survival and being an independent prognostic indicator. What is unique about tumor cell proliferative rate is that it appears to reliably predict response to chemotherapy. Recently both Remvikos[87] and Bonadonna et al.[88] reported that premenopausal women with rapidly proliferating invasive breast cancers exhibited a striking response to adjuvant cytotoxic chemotherapy; many of these patients experienced complete remissions.

Nuclear DNA content and SPF are each excellent prognostic indicators but individually cannot provide the diagnostic accuracy of nuclear DNA content in combination with SPF, axillary lymph node status, or estrogen receptor protein level. Any of the combinations of: (1) tumor nuclear DNA content plus SPF, (2) tumor nuclear DNA content plus patient axillary lymph node status, and (3) tumor nuclear DNA content plus tumor estrogen receptor protein level can predict an 8- to 10-year survival rate with an accuracy of 90% or greater (Table 9).

With any luck, some combination of nuclear DNA, tumor cell proliferative rate, and one or more additional prognostic variables will be identified that further improves prognostic accuracy. As the level of prognostic accuracy rises, the risk-benefit ratio increasingly favors not giving chemotherapy to patients who are in the most prognostically favorable group.

TABLE 9. Percent 8-Year Survival for Patients with Invasive Breast Cancer According to Tumor Nucler DNA Content in Combination with Tumor SPF, Lymph Node Status, and Tumor Estrogen Receptor Protein Content

	SPF Level[70]		Lymph Node Status[26]*		ER Status[40]	
	High	Low	Pos	Neg	Pos	Neg
Diploid	—	90%	86%	95%	91%	53%
Aneuploid	50%	—	33%	65%	53%	51%

* 10-year survival.

Pending resolution of whether or not some other combination of prognostic variables provides more information, it seems reasonable to perform analysis of tumor nuclear DNA content, tumor cell proliferative rate, and tumor steroid hormone receptor protein levels routinely on all invasive breast carcinomas, other than those listed below.

It is doubtful that there is anything to gain by performing nuclear DNA analysis on invasive breast carcinomas that are: (1) of a histologic type known to carry an excellent prognosis (papillary, adenoidcystic, colloid, or tubular), (2) pure lobular (almost invariably diploid in spite of being aggressive), or (3) pure medullary (almost invariably aneuploid in spite of not being highly aggressive). Tumor cell proliferative rate may well be useful in evaluating the metastatic behavior of invasive lobular and medullary carcinomas; however, I am not aware of any studies that address this issue.

References

1. Bloom HG, Richardson WW: Histological grading and prognosis of breast cancer. A study of 1409 cases of which 359 have been follwed up for 15 years. Br J Cancer 11:359–377, 1957.
2. Gilchrist KW, Kalish L, Gould VE, et al: Interobserver reproducibility of histopathological features in stage II breast cancer. An ECOG study. Breast Cancer Treat Rep 5:3–10, 1985.
3. Spyratos F, Briffod M, Gentil A, et al: Flow cytometric study of DNA distribution in cytopunctures of benign and malignant breast lesions. Anal Quant Cytol Histol 9:486–494, 1987.
4. Levack PA, Mullen P, Anderson TJ, et al: DNA analysis of breast tumor fine needle aspirates using flow cytometry. Br J Cancer 56:643–646, 1987.
5. Uccelli R, Caugi A, Forte D, et al: Flow cytometrically determined DNA content of breast carcinoma and benign lesions. Correlations with histopathologic parameters. Tumor 72:171–177, 1986.
6. Visscher DW, Zarbo RJ, Greenwald KA, Crissman JD: Prognostic significance of morphologic parameters and flow cytometric DNA analysis in carcinoma of the breast. In Rosen PP, Fechner RE (eds): Pathology Annual, Vol. 25. East Norwalk, CT, Appleton and Lange, 1990, pp 171–210.
7. Pearlman AW: Breast cancer—Influence of growth rate on prognosis and treatment evaluation. A study based on mastectomy scar recurrences. Cancer 38:1826–1833, 1976.
7a. Lundgren B: Observations on growth rate of breast carcinomas and its possible implications for lead time. Cancer 40:1722–1725, 1977.
8. Ingleby H, Moore L: Periodic roentgenographic studies of growing human mammary cancers. Cancer 9:749–752, 1956.
9. Gerdes J, Schwab U, Lemke H, Stein H: Production of a mouse monoclonal antibody reactive with a human nuclear antigen associated with proliferation. Int J Cancer 31:13–20, 1983.
10. Freeman JW, McRorie DK, Busch RK, et al: Identification and partial purification of a nucleolar antigen with a molecular weight of 145,000 found in a broad range of human cancers. Cancer Res 46:3593–3598, 1986.
11. Heck MMS, Earnshaw WC: Topoisomerase II. A specific marker for cell proliferation. J Cell Biol 103:2569–2581, 1986.
12. Clevenger CV, Epstein AL, Bauer KD: Modulation of the nuclear antigen p105 as a function of cell-cycle progression. J Cell Physiol 130:336–343, 1987.
13. Ogata K, Kurki P, Celis JE, et al: Monoclonal antibodies to nuclear protein (PCNA/cyclin) associated with DNA replication. Exp Cell Res 168:475–486, 1987.
13a. Kurki P, Vanderlaan M, Dolbeare F, et al: Expression of proliferating cell nuclear antigen (PCNA)/cyclin during the cell cycle. Exp Cell Res 166:209–219, 1986.
14. Kamel OW, Franklin WA, Ringus JC, Meyer JS: Thymidine labeling index and Ki-67 growth fraction in lesions of the breast. Am J Pathol 134:107–113, 1989.
15. Sasaki K, Matsumura K, Tsuji T, et al: Relationship between labeling indices of Ki-67 and BrdUrd in human malignant tumors. Cancer 62:989–993, 1988.
16. Isola JJ, Helin HI, Helle MJ, et al: Evaluation of cell proliferation in breast carcinoma: Comparison of Ki-67 immunohistochemical study, DNA flow cytometric analysis, and mitotic count. Cancer 65:1180–1184, 1990.

17. Hatschek T, Fagerberg G, Stal O, et al: Cytometric characterization and clinical course of breast cancer diagnosed in a population-based screening program. Cancer 64:1074–1081, 1989.
18. Kallioniemi O-P, Karkkainen A, Auvinen O, et al: DNA flow cytometric analysis indicates that many breast cancers detected in the first round of mammographic screening have low malignant potential. Int J Cancer 42:697–702, 1988.
19. Dowle CS, Owainati A, Robins A, et al: Prognostic significance of the DNA content of human breast cancer. Br J Surg 74:133–136, 1987.
20. Thorud E, Fossa DS, Vaage S, et al: Primary breast cancer. Flow cytometric DNA pattern in relation to clinical and histopathological characteristics. Cancer 57:808–811, 1986.
21. Ewers SB, Langstrom E, Baldetorp B, Killander D: Flow-cytometric DNA analysis in primary breast carcinomas and clinicopathological correlations. Cytometry 5:408–419, 1984.
22. Harvey J, De Klerk N, Berryman I, et al: Nuclear DNA content and prognosis in human breast cancer: A static cytophotometric study. Breast Cancer Res Treat 9:101–109, 1987.
23. Cornelisse CJ, Van de Velde RJ, Caspers AJ, et al: DNA ploidy and survival in breast cancer patients. Cytometry 8:225–234, 1987.
24. Erhardt KY, Auer GU: Mammary carcinoma. Comparison of nuclear DNA content of in situ and infiltrative components. Anal Quant Cytol 9:263–267, 1987.
25. Carpenter R, Gibbs N, Matthews J, Cooke T: Importance of cellular DNA content in pre-malignant breast disease and pre-invasive carcinoma of the female breast. Br J Surg 74:905–906, 1987.
26. Fallenius AG, Franzen SA, Auer GU: Predictive value of nuclear DNA content in breast cancer in relation to clinical and morphologic factors. A retrospective study of 227 consecutive cases. Cancer 62:521–530, 1988.
27. Eskelinen MJ, Pajarinen P, Collan Y, et al: Relationship between DNA ploidy and survival in patients with primary breast cancer. Br J Surg 76:830–834, 1989.
28. Kute TE, Muss HB, Hopkins M, et al: Relationship of flow cytometry results to clinical and steroid receptor status in human breast cancer. Breast Cancer Res Treat 6:113–121, 1985.
29. Kallioniemi O-P, Hietanen T, Mattila J, et al: Aneuploid DNA content and high S-phase fraction of tumor cells are related to poor prognosis in patients with primary breast cancer. Eur J Cancer Clin Oncol 23:277–282, 1987.
30. Muss HB, Kute TE, Case LD, et al: The relation of flow cytometry to clinical and biologic characteristics in women with node negative breast cancer. Cancer 64:1894–1900, 1989.
31. Hedley DW, Rugg CA, Gelber RD: Association of DNA index and S-phase fraction with prognosis of nodes positive early breast cancer. Cancer Res 47:4729–4735, 1987.
32. McDivitt RW, Stone KR, Craig RB, et al: A proposed classification of breast cancer based on kinetic information: Derived from a comparison of risk factors in 168 primary operable breast cancers. Cancer 57:269–276, 1986.
33. Uyterlinde AM, Schipper NW, Baak JPA: Comparison of extent of disease and morphometric and DNA flow cytometric prognostic factors in invasive ductal breast cancer. J Clin Pathol 40:1432–1436, 1987.
34. Bedrossian CW, Raber M, Barlogie B: Flow cytometry and cytomorphology in primary resectable breast cancer. Anal Quant Cytol 3:112–116, 1981.
35. Raber MN, Barlogie B, Latreille J, et al: Proliferative activity and estrogen receptor content in human breast cancer. Cytometry 3:36–41, 1982.
36. Auer G, Fallenius AG, Erhardt KY, Sundelin B: Progression of mammary adenocarcinomas as reflected by nuclear DNA content. Cytometry 5:420–425, 1984.
37. Hedley DW, Rugg CA, Ng AB, Taylor IW: Influence of cellular DNA content on disease-free survival of stage II breast cancer patients. Cancer Res 44:5395–5398, 1984.
38. Horsfall DJ, Tilley WD, Orell SR, et al: Relationship between ploidy and steroid hormone receptors in primary invasive breast cancer. Br J Cancer 53:23–28, 1986.
39. Moran RE, Black MM, Albert L, Straus MJ: Correlation of cell-cycle kinetics, hormone receptors, histopathology and nodal status in human breast cancer. Cancer 54:1586–1590, 1984.
40. Ballare C, Bravo AI, Laucella S, et al: DNA synthesis in estrogen receptor-positive human breast cancer takes place preferentially in estrogen receptor-negative cells. Cancer 64:842–848, 1989.
41. Klintenberg C, Wallgren A, Bjelkenkrantz, et al: DNA distribution, cytosol estrogen receptors and axillary lymph nodes as prognostic predictors in breast carcinoma. ACTA Radiol Oncol 24:253–258, 1984.
42. Coulson PB, Thornwaite JT, Wooley TW, et al: Prognostic indicators including DNA histogram type, receptor content and staging related to human breast cancer patient survival. Cancer Res 44:4187–4196, 1984.

43. Dressler LG, Seamer LC, Owens MA, et al: DNA flow cytometry and prognostic factors in 1331 frozen breast cancer specimens. Cancer 61:420–427, 1988.
44. Meckenstock G, Bojar H, Hort W: Differentiated DNA analysis in relation to steroid receptor status, grading, and staging in human breast cancer. Anticancer Research 7:749–754, 1987.
45. Olszewki W, Darzynkiewicz Z, Rosen PP, et al: Flow cytometry of breast carcinoma. I. Relation of DNA ploidy level to histology and estrogen receptor. Cancer 48:980–984, 1981.
46. Taylor IW, Musgrove EA, Friedlander ML, et al: The influence of age on DNA ploidy levels of breast tumors. Eur J Cancer Clin Oncol 19:623–628, 1983.
47. Ludwig AS, Okagaki T, Richert RM, Lattes R: Nuclear DNA content of lobular carcinoma in situ of the breast. Cancer 31:1553–1560, 1973.
48. Baildam AD, Zaloudik J, Howell A, et al: DNA analysis by flow cytometry, response to endocrine treatment and prognosis in advanced carcinoma of the breast. Br J Cancer 55:553–559, 1987.
49. McDivitt RW, Stone KR, Meyer JS: A method for dissociation of viable human breast cancer cells that produces flow cytometric kinetic information similar to that obtained by thymidine labeling. Cancer Res 44:2628–2633, 1984.
50. Bichel P, Poulsen HS, Andersen DJ, Karrison T: Estrogen receptor content and ploidy of human mammary carcinoma. Cancer 50:1771–1774, 1982.
51. Jakobsen A, Poulsen HS, Madsen EL, et al: Ploidy level of human breast carcinoma. Relation to histopathologic features and hormone receptor content. Acta Radiol Oncol 23:103–107, 1984.
52. Owainati AAR, Robins RA, Hinton C, et al: Tumour aneuploidy, prognostic parameters and survival in primary breast cancer. Br J Cancer 55:449–454, 1987.
53. Gerdes J, Pickartz H, Brotherton J, et al: Growth factors and estrogen receptors in human breast cancers as determined in situ with monoclonal antibodies. Am J Pathol 129:486–492, 1987.
54. McGuire WL: Prognostic factors for recurrence and survival in human breast cancer. Breast Cancer Res Treat 10:5–9, 1987.
55. Lykkesfeldt AE, Balslev I, Christensen IJ, et al: DNA ploidy and S-phase fraction in primary breast carcinomas in relation to prognostic factors and survival for premenopausal patients at high risk for recurrent disease. Acta Oncologica 27:749–756, 1988.
56. Stal O, Klintenberg C, Franzen G, et al: A comparison of static cytofluorometry and flow cytometry for the estimation of ploidy and DNA replication in human breast cancer. Breast Cancer Res Treat 7:15–22, 1986.
57. Meyer JS, Coplin MD: Thymidine labeling index, flow cytometric S-phase measurement, and DNA index in human tumors: Comparison and correlations. Am J Clin Pathol 89:586–595, 1988.
58. Fisher ER, Redmond C, Fisher B: Pathologic findings from the National Surgical Adjuvant Breast Project (Protocol no. 4). VI. Discriminants for five-year treatment failure. Cancer 46:908–918, 1980.
59. Fisher ER, Sass R, Fisher B, et al: Pathologic findings from the National Surgical Adjuvant Breast Project (Protocol no. 4). X. Discriminants for tenth-year treatment failure. Cancer 53:712–723, 1984.
60. Fu YS, Maksem JA, Hubay CA, et al: The relationship of breast cancer morphology and estrogen receptor protein status. In Fenoglio CM, Wolff MW (eds): Progress in Surgical Pathology, Vol. 3. New York, Masson, 1981.
61. McCarty KS, Barton TK, Fetter BF, et al: Correlation of estrogen and progesterone receptors with histologic differentiation in mammary carcinoma. Cancer 46:2851–2858, 1980.
62. Hedley DW, Friedlander ML, Taylor IW: Application of DNA flow cytometry to paraffin-embedded archival material for the study of aneuploidy and its clinical significance. Cytometry 6:327–333, 1985.
63. Abandowitz RM, Ow KT, Hardy D, et al: Relationship between flow cytometric parameters, steroid receptors, and menopausal status in breast cancers. Oncology 44:24–29, 1987.
64. Stal O, Wingren S, Carstensen J, et al: Prognostic value of DNA ploidy and S-phase fraction in relation to estrogen receptor content and clinicopathological variables in primary breast cancer. Eur J Cancer Clin Oncol 25:301–309, 1989.
65. Meyer JS, Prey MU, Babcock DS, McDivitt RW: Breast carcinoma cell kinetics, morphology, stage, and host characteristics. A thymidine labeling study. Lab Invest 54:41–51, 1986.
66. Gentil C, Sanfilippo O, Silvestrini R: Cell proliferation and its relationship to clinical features and relapse in breast cancers. Cancer 48:974–979, 1981.
67. McGurrin JF, Doria MI, Dawson PJ, et al: Assessment of tumor cell kinetics by immunohistochemistry in carcinoma of breast. Cancer 59:1744–1750, 1987.
68. Tubiana M, Pejovic MJ, Renaud A, et al: Kinetic parameters and the course of the disease in breast cancer. Cancer 47:937–943, 1981.

69. Marchetti E, Querzoli P, Marzola A, et al: Assessment of proliferative rate of breast cancer by Ki-67 monoclonal antibody. Modern Pathology 3:31–35, 1990.
70. Kallioniemi O-P, Blanco G, Alavaikko M, et al: Improving prognostic value of DNA flow cytometry in breast cancer by combining DNA index and S-phase fraction. Cancer 62:2183–2190, 1988.
71. Dressler LG, Seamer L, Owens MA, et al: Evaluation of a modeling system for S-phase estimation in breast cancer flow cytometry. Cancer Res 47:5294–5302, 1987.
72. Meyer JS, McDivitt RW, Stone KR, et al: Practical breast carcinoma cell kinetics: Review and update. Breast Cancer Res Treat 4:79–88, 1984.
73. Feichter GE, Mueller A, Kaufmann M, et al: Correlation of DNA flow cytometric results and other prognostic factors in primary breast cancer. Int J Cancer 41:823–828, 1988.
74. Gerdes J, Lelle RJ, Pickertz H, et al: Growth fractions in breast cancers determined in situ with monoclonal antibody Ki-67. J Clin Pathol 39:977–980, 1986.
75. Helin ML, Helle MJ, Helin HJ, Isola JJ: Proliferative activity and steroid receptors determined by immunochemistry in adjacent frozen sections of 102 breast cancers. Arch Pathol Lab Med 113:854–857, 1989.
76. Silvestrini R, Daidone R, Gasparini G: Cell kinetics as a prognostic marker in node-negative breast cancer. Cancer 56:1982–1987, 1985.
77. McDivitt RW, Stone KR, Craig RB, Meyer JS: A comparison of human breast cancer cell kinetics measured by flow cytometry and thymidine labeling. Lab Invest 52:287–291, 1985.
78. Clark GM, Dressler LG, Owens MA, et al: Prediction of relapse or survival in patients with node-negative breast cancer by DNA flow cytometry. N Engl J Med 320:627–633, 1989.
79. Barlogie B, Raber MN, Schumann J, et al: Flow cytometry in clinical cancer research. Cancer Res 43:3982–3997, 1983.
80. Friedlander ML, Hedley DW, Taylor IW: Clinical and biological significance of aneuploidy in human tumors. J Clin Pathol 37:961–974, 1984.
81. Keyhani-Rofagha S, O'Toole RV, Farrar WB, et al: Is DNA ploidy an independent prognostic indicator in infiltrative node-negative breast adenocarcinoma. Cancer 65:1577–1582, 1990.
82. Tubiana M, Pejovic MJ, Chavaudra G, et al: The long-term prognostic significance of the thymidine labelling index in breast cancer. Int J Cancer 33:441–445, 1984.
83. Meyer JS, Friedman MS, McCrate MM, Bauer WC: Prediction of early course of breast carcinoma by thymidine labeling. Cancer 51:1879–1886, 1983.
84. Klintenberg S, Stal O, Nordenskjold B, et al: Proliferative index, cytosol estrogen receptor and axillary node status as prognostic predictors in human mammary carcinomas. Breast Cancer Res Treat 7(Suppl):S99–S106, 1986.
85. Meyer JS, Lee JY: Relationships of S-phase fraction of breast carcinoma in relapse to duration of remission, estrogen receptor content, therapeutic responsiveness, and duration of survival. Cancer Res 40:1980–1986, 1980.
86. Stuart-Harris R, Hedley DW, Taylor IW, et al: Tumor ploidy, response and survival in patients receiving endocrine therapy for advanced breast cancer. Br J Cancer 51:573–576, 1985.
87. Remvikos Y, Beuzeboc P, Zajdela N, et al: Correlation of pretreatment proliferative activity of breast cancer with response to cytotoxic chemotherapy. J Natl Cancer Inst 81:1383–1387, 1989.
88. Bonadonna G, Valagussa P, Tancini G, et al: Current status of Milan adjuvant chemotherapy trials for node-positive and node-negative breast cancer. NCI Monogr 1:45–49, 1986.
89. Fisher B, Slack NH, Bross JD: Cancer of the breast: Size of neoplasm and prognosis. Cancer 24:1071–1080, 1969.
90. Nemoto T, Vana J, Bedwanni RN, et al: Management and survival of female breast cancer: Results of a national survey by the American College of Surgeons. Cancer 45:2917–2924, 1980.
91. Carter CL, Allen C, Henson DE: Relation of tumor size, lymph node status, and survival in 24,740 breast cancer cases. Cancer 63:181–187, 1989.
92. Kern WH, Mikkelsen WP: Small carcinomas of the breast. Cancer 28:948–955, 1971.
93. Fisher B, Redmond C, Dimitrov NV, et al: A randomized clinical trial evaluating sequential methotrexate and fluoracil in the treatment of patients with node-negative breast cancer who have estrogen-receptor-negative tumors. N Engl J Med 320:473–478, 1989.
94. Fisher B, Constantino J, Redmond C, et al: A randomized clinical trial evaluating tamoxifen in the treatment of patients with node-negative breast cancer who have estrogen-receptor-positive tumors. N Engl J Med 320:479–484, 1989.
95. Mansour EG, Gray R, Shatila AH, et al: Efficacy of adjuvant chemotherapy in high-risk node-negative breast cancer: An intergroup study. N Engl J Med 320:485–490, 1989.
96. The Ludwig Breast Cancer Study Group: Prolonged disease-free survival after one course of perioperative adjuvant chemotherapy for node-negative breast cancer. N Engl J Med 320:491–496, 1989.

Breast Biopsies: The Content of the Surgical Pathology Report

ONSI W. KAMEL, M.D.
MICHAEL R. HENDRICKSON, M.D.
RICHARD L. KEMPSON, M.D.

From the Department of
  Pathology
Stanford University Medical
  Center
Stanford, California

Reprint requests to:
Richard L. Kempson, M.D.
Department of Pathology
Stanford University Medical
  Center
300 Pasteur Drive
Stanford, CA 94305

The current approach to breast cancer detection and treatment has evolved dramatically over recent years because of the increasing use of mammography to detect non-palpable breast lesions and because excisional biopsy (lumpectomy) combined with radiation therapy and axillary dissection has been shown to be effective local therapy for invasive carcinoma. In the context of these developments, the role of the surgical pathologist in evaluating and reporting breast cancer specimens has become more important. The pathologist must not only diagnose carcinoma in a given patient, but must also document a set of morphologic features that have been shown to be important in determining prognosis and guiding therapy.

Current breast cancer management requires adequate local cancer control (surgery with or without radiation therapy) and may require systemic adjuvant therapy (chemotherapy and/or antiestrogen therapy). Certain of the morphologic features discussed are predictive of an increased risk for local failure and are used to guide local treatment; other features are predictive of systemic disease and may be used by oncologists to arrive at chemotherapy treatment decisions, particularly for patients with negative lymph nodes. The latter group of patients represents a major therapeutic challenge because 30% of surgically

TABLE 1. Pathologic Features Considered Important Enough in the Management of Patients with Carcinoma of the Breast That Should Be Included in Every Pathology Report

---

Breast excision specimens
   Diagnosis, to include histologic type of invasive carcinoma
   Grading features
     Nuclear grade (1,2,3)
     Tubule formation (1,2,3)
     Mitotic index (1,2,3)
   Composite histologic grade
   Size of invasive carcinoma
   Type of ductal carcinoma in situ (DCIS)
   Extent of DCIS associated with invasive ductal carcinoma
   Size of DCIS (in the absence of invasive carcinoma)
   Excisional biopsy margins
   Blood vessel and lymphatic involvement (including dermal lymphatic involvement)
Lymph node specimens
   Number of lymph nodes involved
   Documentation of micrometastases
   Extension of tumor in perinodal soft tissue

---

treated, node-negative patients will relapse and die from their disease and therefore are likely to benefit from adjuvant therapy, whereas 70% are cured by surgery alone and do not need adjuvant therapy. The morphologic features discussed in this paper can help identify those node-negative patients who are most likely to fail, as well as those who are at so little risk to fail that chemotherapy may not be warranted. While numerous prognostic variables have been investigated, the features we discuss are the ones we think have been shown to provide sufficiently useful information to be included routinely in every pathology report (Table 1). Documentation of these features may be incorporated into the gross and histologic evaluation of the breast specimen at little or no added cost to the patient.

In addition to these morphologic features, there are a number of new and relatively costly biologic techniques currently under investigation to determine their value as predictors of outcome for patients with breast carcinoma. Some of these new procedures have been shown to be predictive of clinical outcome, but, in our opinion, none has yet clearly been demonstrated to provide sufficient independent information over and above that obtained by traditional histologic methods to warrant the expense of its routine use. Because this situation may change in the future as more clinicopathologic studies are reported, these new techniques are briefly discussed. The following discussion focuses on specimens containing infiltrating ductal carcinoma, infiltrating lobular carcinoma, and in situ carcinoma of both lobular and ductal types.

THE DIAGNOSIS OF INVASIVE CARCINOMA

The histologic diagnosis of invasive breast carcinoma is usually straightforward; however, certain problems confront the surgical pathologist with sufficient frequency to warrant further discussion.

TABLE 2. Breast Carcinomas of Low Malignant Potential

1. Tubular carcinoma[3,33]
2. Invasive cribriform carcinoma[39]
3. Medullary carcinoma[43,54]
4. Pure mucinous carcinoma[7,42]
5. Invasive papillary carcinoma[17]
6. Adenoid cystic carcinoma[41,44,56]
7. Secretory carcinoma[51]

The first is the recognition that infiltrating ductal (usual type) carcinoma represents no more than 70–75% of all infiltrating carcinomas of the breast, and lobular carcinoma no more than 5–10%. Within the remaining infiltrating carcinomas, there is a group that has a significantly better prognosis than ordinary infiltrating ductal (usual type) carcinomas. These carcinomas, which we designate "carcinomas of low malignant potential," are listed in Table 2. Enumeration and discussion of the criteria required for the diagnosis of each of these carcinomas are beyond the scope of this article; however, it is important to recognize their existence and to adhere to the criteria required for their diagnosis, because clinicopathologic studies report excellent relapse-free survival and overall survival (particularly for patients with histologically negative nodes), to the extent that adjuvant chemotherapy generally is not warranted for the treatment of the great majority of patients harboring these lesions.

Second, identification of early stromal invasion in the setting of comedo carcinoma in situ frequently causes diagnostic problems, because the in situ ductal process often extends into contiguous ramifying terminal ducts and lobular units. The resulting histologic pattern may simulate infiltrating carcinoma. Moreover, in situ comedo carcinoma *without* invasion is regularly associated with a granulation tissue stromal reaction of the type found in invasive carcinoma. Careful examination of several levels of the paraffin block may help in the evaluation of this type of lesion. We insist on jagged infiltration of carcinoma cells beyond the confines of lobules before interpreting suspicious areas as definite evidence of stromal invasion. Sometimes, one cannot be certain whether invasion is present or not, and this uncertainty should be expressed in the surgical pathology report using such terms as "suspicious for invasion" or "early microinvasion cannot be excluded." However, these statements should be reserved for the truly equivocal cases, because inclusion of such statements in the pathology report will usually result in an axillary lymph node dissection, an operation not routinely performed for in situ comedo carcinoma of small size.

Third, infiltrating lobular carcinoma may present a set of diagnostic problems because of certain architectural and cytologic features. There are four described patterns of infiltrating lobular carcinoma: (1) the classic type in which the neoplastic cells are present in a single file arrangement, often with a targetoid distribution around lobules; (2) the solid pattern characterized by neoplastic cells arranged in sheets or irregular nests; (3) an alveolar pattern that is marked by rounded or circumscribed aggregates of neoplastic cells; and (4) the mixed type, featuring a mixture of two or more of the preceding patterns.[10a] The classic pattern of infiltrating lobular carcinoma can be easily missed because small foci of the relatively small, bland neoplastic cells may be mistaken for stromal fibroblasts or histiocytes. For this reason, particularly careful evaluation of the stroma is required whenever lobular carcinoma in situ or atypical lobular hyperplasia is present in a specimen. Distinguishing minimal microscopic infiltration from foci of lobular carcinoma in situ can be a problem, because in some instances it is difficult to be sure whether or not the neoplastic cells are confined to lobular units, ducts, or, particularly, foci of sclerosing adenosis. We require the presence of neoplastic cells away from such structures before making a diagnosis of invasive carcinoma. The diagnostic problem that most often arises in the solid pattern of infiltrating lobular carcinoma is distinction from lymphoma. This is especially the case when fixation and processing of the tissue is suboptimal. Cytologic features may be helpful in making this distinction. Mucin stains are not completely reliable because rare diffuse, large cell, signet-ring lymphomas with PAS-positive diastase-resistant material have been described. Immunohistochemical markers against leukocyte common antigen and cytokeratins will nearly always resolve cases that are difficult to distinguish on histologic grounds. Finally, small foci of the alveolar pattern of infiltrating lobular carcinoma may be misinterpreted as an in situ process. The absence of a lobular architecture and the disregard for the normal breast architecture help to distinguish this pattern of infiltrating lobular carcinoma from lobular carcinoma in situ.

HISTOLOGIC AND NUCLEAR GRADE

Several large studies, including the National Surgical Adjuvant Breast Project (NSABP), have documented the prognostic importance of the grade of invasive carcinoma independent of nodal status.[10,11,18,19,22,32] In particular, nuclear grade has proven to be an independent variable for identifying the subset of node-negative patients at highest risk to fail after surgical therapy.[22,32] We think only infiltrating ductal carcinomas should be graded. We identify the other types of carcinomas by name and indicate the expected behavior. For example, while tubular carcinoma could be considered a grade I (well-differentiated) invasive carcinoma, it is current practice to designate it as tubular carcinoma and to indicate in the pathology report that it is a low-grade, well-behaving neoplasm. Data or references that describe its clinical behavior may be provided.

Ideally, a grading scheme should be easy to use, reasonably reproducible, and should have been clinically validated. Moreover, it should have been shown to provide sufficient prognostic and therapeutic information to warrant the expenditure of time required to learn the system and employ it reliably. Pathologists should employ a grading scheme with explicit criteria in order to ensure reproducibility. Several grading schemes have been proposed for infiltrating carcinoma. The two most widely used (both of which are based on

TABLE 3. Scarff-Bloom-Richardson Grading Scheme for Breast Cancer

Category	Points 1	Points 2	Points 3
Tubule formation	Marked	Moderate	Little to absent
Nuclear pleomorphism	Slight	Moderate	Marked
Mitoses (#/10 hpf)	<10	10–19	≥ 20

Histologic grade is determined as follows:
Grade I (well differentiated) = 3–5 points
Grade II (moderately differentiated) = 6–7 points
Grade III (poorly differentiated) = 8–9 points

Refs. 12, 32.

the scheme of Bloom and Richardson[2]) are the Scarff-Bloom-Richardson grading scheme (Table 3), which has been widely used in Europe,[12,32] and the NSABP[19] grading scheme (Table 4). Both assess the degree of tubule (ductule) formation and nuclear grade; however, only the Scarff-Bloom-Richardson system incorporates mitotic index into grading criteria. The chief consequence of adding mitotic index as a grading criterion is to diminish the number of tumors assigned to the poorly differentiated category.

We use the Scarff-Bloom-Richardson grading scheme because it results in a more even distribution of invasive carcinomas among the three grades than does the NSABP scheme, and because we think mitotic rate provides a good assessment of the biologic aggressiveness of a ductal carcinoma. As mentioned, the Scarff-Bloom-Richardson system evaluates three morphologic parameters: (1) degree of tubule formation, (2) nuclear grade, and (3) mitotic rate (Table 3). Points are assigned to each category. In the assessment of degree of tubule formation, 1 point is given when the majority of the tumor is composed of well-formed ducts with clearly visible lumens, 2 points when a moderate amount of the tumor is composed of such ducts, and 3 points when little to no tubule formation is present and the tumor cells grow predominantly in sheets and cords. In evaluating nuclear grade, an assessment is made of the variability in size and shape of the nuclei (Table 5). Tumors in which the constituent cell nuclei are regular and show little variation are given 1 point, tumors containing cells with nuclei with moderate variability are given 2 points, and tumors whose cells demonstrate marked variation in the size and shape of nuclei are given 3 points. In the mitotic count category, 1 point is given for < 10 mf/10 hpf,

TABLE 4. Breast Cancer Grading Scheme Employed in the National Surgical Adjuvant Breast Project*

Degree of Tubule Formation	with	Nuclear Grade	equals	Histologic Grade
Pure or marked		1, 2, or 3		I
Slight, moderate		1, 2, or 3		II
Absent		1		II
Absent		2,3		III

* Ref. 19.

TABLE 5. Criteria for Assessing the Nuclear Grade of Invasive Carcinoma of the Breast

Low nuclear grade (I)
Nuclei are small and spherical
Nuclear-to-cytoplasmic ratio is low
Nucleoli are inconspicuous
Chromatin is delicate
Nuclear membranes are uniformly thin
Little variability between nuclei

High nuclear grade (III)
Nuclei are enlarged, some greatly enlarged
Nuclear/cytoplasmic ratio is high
Nucleoli are prominent
Chromatin is coarse and clumped
Nuclear membranes are unevenly thickened
Variability in nucler size and shape is prominent

Intermediate nuclear grade (II)
Nuclear features are intermediate between those of low-grade and high-grade

Modified from Gilchrist et al: Breast Cancer Res Treat 5:3–10, 1985.

2 points for 10–19 mf/10 hpf, and 3 points for > 20 mf/10 hpf. A total of 9 points is possible, with 9 representing the most anaplastic neoplasm. The overall grade is determined as follows: grade I (well-differentiated), 3–5 points; grade II (moderately differentiated), 6–7 points; and grade III (poorly differentiated), 8–9 points. The grading is based on evaluation of the invasive component only. Nuclear grade and mitotic counts are determined from the most anaplastic areas of the tumor. This grading scheme that is designated as the "histologic grade" is semiquantitative, reproducible, and of proven prognostic significance.

In addition to the information provided by histologic grade, nuclear grade taken by itself has been identified as a very powerful factor in determining the prognosis of large numbers of node-negative breast cancer patients (Table 6). In fact, two large clinical trials[22,32] that investigated the prognostic value of

TABLE 6. Prognostic Value of Nuclear Grade in Patients with Invasive Breast Carcinoma and Histologically Negative Lymph Nodes

Reference	Total No. of Patients	Follow-up (yrs)	Outcome	Survival		No. of Patients	p Value
Fisher et al.[22]	950	8	OS	NG: good poor	86% 64%	(580) (370)	<.01
Connolly et al.[10]	261	7	MFS	NG: 1 & 2 3	92% 79%	(107) (154)	<.01
le Doussal et al.[32]	650	3	MFS	Combined 1 NG & MI: 2 3 4 5	100% 98.5% 93.7% 88% 78%	(21) (72) (152) (263) (142)	< .01

OS = overall survival; MFS = metastasis-free survival; NG = nuclear grade only; MI = mitotic index several clinical and pathological variables (using multivariate analysis based on the Cox regression model) have found nuclear grade to be the single most important independent predictor of overall survival[22] and metastasis-free survival[32] for node-negative patients. Because nuclear grade is an important factor in predicting the clinical course of patients with node-negative invasive carcinoma[22,32] and because it is an important piece of information for the oncologist considering adjuvant therapy for the treatment of a node-negative patient, we think nuclear grade should be included and separately identified in the pathology report. We report the final histologic grade in the diagnosis line of our pathology reports and indicate the score for tubule formation, nuclear grade, and mitotic counts in the body of the report, so that the nuclear grade can be obtained by the clinician.

SIZE OF NEOPLASM

Although lymph node status is established as the most important predictor of treatment failure, the size of an infiltrating carcinoma is independently significant within patient groups stratified by the number of positive nodes.[4,10,18,19] The NSABP data at 5 and 10 years of follow-up have continued to show the importance of tumor size, with lesions less than 2 cm faring significantly better (when controlled for nodal status).[18,19] A recent report from the Surveillance, Epidemiology and End Results (SEER) Program of the National Cancer Institute on more than 24,000 breast cancer cases also has confirmed the prognostic significance of tumor size independent of nodal status.[4] Data from this study, shown in Table 7, clearly identify tumor size as an important factor in patient outcome. For example, over 96% of the 5,728 node-negative patients with carcinomas less than 2 cm were alive at the end of the follow-up period. If routine adjuvant therapy had been employed, 96% of the patients would have received unnecessary therapy. These data emphasize the absolute necessity of accurately recording the size of breast carcinomas unambiguously in the pathology report. The prosector at the time of frozen section or in the cutting room has this responsibility. If the tumor is removed in pieces, this important prognostic information may be lost unless the specimen can be reconstructed. Tumor size may be reported by providing measurements of the three dimensions of the tumor or by providing a single measurement that represents the tumor's greatest dimension with a statement

TABLE 7. Five-Year Breast Cancer Survival According to Tumor Size and Lymph Node Status in 24,470 Breast Cancer Cases

Tumor Size	All Cases % Survival	(No)	Negative % Survival	(No)	1-3+ % Survival	(No)	≥ 4+ % Survival	(No)
< 2.0 cm	91.3	(8,319)	96.3	(5,728)	87.4	(1,767)	66.0	(824)
2–5 cm	79.8	(13,723)	89.4	(6,927)	79.9	(3,622)	58.7	(3,174)
> 5.0 cm	62.7	(2,698)	82.2	(809)	73.0	(630)	45.5	(1,259)

Ref. 4.

TABLE 8. Postsurgical Treatment Pathological Classification (UICC–AJC*)[†]

Primary tumor (T)
- T0 No evidence of primary tumor
- T1 ≤ 2 cm
  - i < 0.5 cm
  - ii 0.5–0.9 cm
  - iii 1.0–1.9 cm
- T2 2–5 cm
- T3 > 5 cm
- T4 Direct extension into chest wall or skin (any tumor size)

Nodal involvement (N)
- N0 Histologically uninvolved axillary lymph nodes
- N1 Mobile, histologically involved axillary lymph nodes
  - i Micrometastatic (< 0.2 cm)
  - ii Metastasis (> 0.2 cm) in 1–3 lymph nodes
  - iii Metastasis to four or more lymph nodes
  - iv Extension of metastasis beyond lymph node capsule
  - v Any involved node > 2 cm in diameter
- N2 Fixed axillary lymph nodes
- N3 Involved clavicular nodes or edema of arm

* International Union Against Cancer–American Joint Commission.
[†] Modified from Henderson IC, et al: Cancer of the breast. In Devita VT, Hellman S, Rosenberg SA (eds): Cancer: Principles and Practice of Oncology, 3rd ed. Philadelphia, J.B. Lippincott, 1989.

defining the measurement being provided (e.g., "2.5 cm in greatest dimension"). The size of the primary tumor is an important factor in the Postsurgical Treatment Pathological Classification developed by the International Union Against Cancer and the American Joint Commission (Table 8). We routinely indicate the greatest dimension of the tumor in the diagnosis line of our reports.

It is particularly important to accurately identify and measure invasive carcinomas measuring 1 cm or less in greatest dimension, because patients with such carcinomas and negative lymphs nodes have an excellent prognosis. A recent study by Rosner and Lane[44a] reported 91% disease-free survival and 96% overall survival at 7 years in a group of 91 patients with invasive breast carcinoma measuring 1 cm or less and histologically negative axillary nodes. Interestingly, all five relapses were among patients with poorly differentiated tumors and histologic or nuclear grading would have identified them.

The terms "minimally invasive" and "microinvasive" carcinoma both have been used to describe small carcinomas, usually less than 0.5 cm. To us, "microinvasive" denotes the very earliest invasion limited to no more than a few fields of invasion as detected by microscopy. We do not use the term "minimally invasive" carcinoma; rather we give the size of the invasive component if it is greater than microinvasive. Unfortunately, the implications of microinvasion are not definitely known, but the data available from at least one large study of patients with slightly larger than microinvasive but less than 0.5 cm carcinomas indicate survival is greater than 99%.[4]

Recording the size of the area of involvement of an in situ ductal carcinoma is important, even when an infiltrating component is not present, because the size of the pure intraductal carcinoma predicts for occult invasion elsewhere in the breast, residual multifocal lesions after excision, and occult lymph node metastases. These three adverse findings are extremely rare when the in situ carcinoma involves an area less than 2.5 cm.[30] Because the size (extent) of ductal carcinoma in situ may well have therapeutic implications for the type of therapy that is selected, the size of an in situ carcinoma always should be determined and recorded whenever the lesion is grossly recognizable. If the lesion is not grossly identified (as is often the case with non-comedo in situ carcinoma), an estimate of size based on its presence in the histologic sections should be provided. A more complete discussion of the clinical implications and current treatment strategies for ductal carcinoma in situ is provided in the article on in situ proliferative epithelial lesions of the breast (p. 87).

TYPE OF DUCTAL CARCINOMA IN SITU

Documentation of the histologic-type of ductal carcinoma in situ (DCIS) should be provided whenever a diagnosis of DCIS is reported, particularly if an invasive component is not present. This suggestion is primarily the result of recent studies that indicate the comedo-type of ductal carcinoma in situ has a more ominous natural history than the cribriform and micropapillary types.[31,47] The definitional features of comedo DCIS are ducts lined by cytologically malignant cells, often stratified, with central necrosis of tumor cells. The cells in comedo-type in situ carcinoma have striking nuclear enlargement, and they demonstrate considerable nuclear pleomorphism, frequent mitotic figures (some of which may be abnormal), and prominent nucleoli. They may grow in solid sheets around the duct or they may form cribriform spaces. Thymidine labeling studies have shown the cells of comedo DCIS to have a higher proliferative rate than other DCIS types.[35] In addition, the cells in comedo DCIS lesions express the Neu oncogene more frequently than do cells in the other types of DCIS.[52]

Lesions with cytologic and architectural features intermediate between comedo and cribriform in situ carcinoma will be encountered. In comparison with comedo carcinoma, these intermediate lesions have cells with smaller nuclei and less conspicuous nucleoli, and mitoses are more difficult to find. However, the nuclei are larger and more abnormal than those found in the usual cribriform lesions. Moreover, the nuclear membranes are more irregular, chromatin is less even and often clumped, and nuclear pleomorphism is readily apparent in the intermediate lesion. We use the expression "in situ carcinoma intermediate between comedo and cribriform types" when we report such lesions.

Lagios et al. have shown in a recent study of small (< 25 mm) DCIS lesions treated by tylectomy (lumpectomy) alone that DCIS of the comedo type is associated with a significant incidence of local recurrence. In that study, 19% (seven of 36) of patients who had DCIS with high-grade nuclear morphology and comedo-type necrosis developed recurrence; only one of ten patients with intermediate-grade DCIS developed a local recurrence; and none of the 33 patients with DCIS of the micropapillary/non-necrotic cribriform type and low-grade nuclear morphology developed a local recurrence.[31]

Silverstein et al. have more recently reported on the local treatment of 208 intraductal carcinomas and have confirmed that the great majority of patients who develop a recurrence following local treatment for DCIS are those with comedo-type DCIS in the initial biopsy.[47] Therefore, the type of in situ carcinoma has prognostic implications and may well have therapeutic importance. Care should be taken to follow the definitions for classifying the type of in situ carcinoma.

EXTENT OF DUCTAL CARCINOMA IN SITU ASSOCIATED WITH INVASIVE DUCTAL CARCINOMA

With the increasing use of excisional biopsy combined with radiation therapy for local treatment of infiltrating carcinoma,[14] there has been a search for morphologic features that would predict for local failure.[23,28,45,46,55] One such feature that has been identified is the extent of ductal carcinoma in situ associated with an infiltrating ductal carcinoma. The initial reports evaluating the relationship between the extent of ductal carcinoma in situ and the incidence of local recurrence originated from the Joint Center for Radiation Therapy in Boston.[23,45,46] In brief, infiltrating ductal carcinomas treated by excisional biopsy and radiation therapy associated with extensive intraductal carcinoma (EIC) were shown to have a significantly lower 5-year local control rate than those without EIC (77% vs. 99%, p = .001).[45] EIC is defined as intraductal carcinoma comprising greater than 25% of the area delimited by the infiltrating tumor *and* intraductal carcinoma of any extent outside the margin of the infiltrating tumor, regardless of whether it is in breast parenchyma near the infiltrating carcinoma or remote from it. The difference in local control increased even more when nuclear grade or mitotic rate were taken into account. Tumors with EIC and high nuclear grade had a 61% local control probability, compared to 96% for tumors without these features (p < .001).[45]

In a subsequent study, these investigators examined breast specimens from patients with infiltrating ductal carcinoma who were selected for re-excision of the tumor site prior to radiotherapy, because of extensive intraductal carcinoma (EIC) in the primary excision specimen or microscopic infiltrating carcinoma at or close to the margins in the initial excision. Residual carcinoma was more frequent in patients with EIC than those without (88% vs. 48%, p = .002). Interestingly, the nature of the residual tumor differed between the two groups. Residual carcinoma in patients with EIC was often widespread and composed predominantly of intraductal carcinoma, whereas residual tumor in patients without EIC consisted of only scattered microscopic foci of infiltrating and/or intraductal carcinoma. The authors concluded that this finding may explain the increased risk for local recurrence in patients with EIC treated without re-excision of the tumor site before radiotherapy.[46]

A recent report from the Institut Curie in Paris has largely confirmed the results of the Boston group.[55] This study examined 434 patients with infiltrating ductal carcinoma who were treated with limited surgery and radiation therapy and then followed for a median of 103 months. The investigators

TABLE 9. Pathologic Features Predictive of Increased Risk for Local Failure Following Lumpectomy (Excisional Biopsy) and Radiation Therapy

1. Positive excision margins[28,45,55]
2. Extensive intraductal carcinoma (EIC)[28,45,55]
3. High nuclear grade[45]
4. High histologic grade[28]
5. Angiolymphatic space involvement[55]
6. Major mononuclear cell reaction[28]

found three pathologic predictors of local recurrence: (1) incomplete surgical excision of infiltrating carcinoma ($p < .001$); (2) lymphatic invasion ($p < .02$); and (3) the presence of an extensive in situ component ($p < .03$). Their definition of extensive intraductal carcinoma was very similar to that of Schnitt and associates. In yet another study, Kurtz et al. have reported that EIC (as defined by Schnitt et al.), histologic grade, and a major mononuclear cell reaction were significant predictors of risk for local recurrence by Cox multivariate analysis in a group of 496 clinical stage I–II patients with breast carcinoma.[28] Thus, extensive intraductal carcinoma has been confirmed by three independent studies as a predictor for an increased risk of local recurrence following lumpectomy and radiation therapy (Tables 9 and 10).

Given these data and the increasing number of patients choosing breast conservation therapy, it seems important that pathologists report the extent of intraductal carcinoma in excisional biopsy specimens. For tumor confined to the area of infiltrating carcinoma, the categories for quantitating extent of DCIS as proposed by Schnitt et al. are as follows: absent, $< 25\%$, 25–50%, and $> 50\%$. The presence or absence of intraductal carcinoma outside the confines of the main tumor is also important to report. Patients with this latter feature *and* with DCIS comprising $> 25\%$ of the main tumor mass fulfill the criteria for extensive intraductal carcinoma.

EXCISIONAL BIOPSY MARGINS

It has been shown by several investigators that local tumor control is significantly better when the tumor has been completely excised, as determined by examination of excision margins (Table 10).[1,28,45,55] Given this information, it is the pathologist's responsibility to provide an indication of the adequacy of

TABLE 10. Prognostic Value of Extensive Intraductal Carcinoma and Positive Excision Margins for Increased Risk for Local Treatment Failure in Patients with Invasive Breast Cancer Treated by Lumpectomy and Radiation Therapy

Reference	No. of Patients	Clinical Stage	Follow-up (yrs)	Local Failure Overall	EIC+/EIC−	EM+/EM−
Schnitt et al.[45]	255	I, II	5	7%	23%/1%	36%/8%
Zafrani et al.[55]	434	I, II	10	13%	23%/5%	24%/9%
Kurtz et al.[28]	496	I, II	5	12%	18%/8%	23%/6%

EIC = extensive intraductal carcinoma; EM = excision margins.

excision. The gross evaluation of excisional breast specimens is often a complex task for which several methods have been described.[5,9] The approach will vary somewhat depending on the particular specimen and from laboratory to laboratory; however, certain basic guidelines have gained general acceptance. We think all excisional breast specimens that are received in one piece should be inked on their external (marginal) surface. The ink can be kept from seeping into the specimen when it has been incised by applying only the necessary amount of ink with the use of a cotton-tipped, wooden applicator stick (instead of pouring ink onto the specimen or dunking the specimen in ink). Painting the specimen with Bouin's solution (which acts as a mordant) followed by blotting allows the ink to fix to the specimen. After this process, the specimen can be cut for further gross examination, frozen section, or selection of tissue for receptor studies.

The size of the specimen, the size and gross features of the carcinoma, and the apparent proximity of the lesion to the specimen margins should be documented in the gross description. The report of the microscopic findings should indicate the status of inked margins: involved or uninvolved, by DCIS or infiltrating carcinoma, focally or extensively. If, when viewed microscopically, tumor is close to, but not at, the inked margins, either an estimate or an exact measurement of the distance from ink can be provided.

BLOOD VESSEL AND LYMPHATIC INVOLVEMENT

Although there is some uncertainty regarding the significance of angiolymphatic tumor involvement, a number of studies have shown an increased risk for distant metastases when intralymphatic or vascular tumor emboli are present.[37,53] The large study of the NSABP demonstrated that lymphatic involvement in the vicinity of the dominant tumor mass is related to nodal status but not independently to failure.[19] Investigators at the Institut Curie in Paris have reported a strong trend for lymphatic invasion to be correlated with local recurrence in patients treated by lumpectomy.

Several factors may contribute to the conflicting reports of the significance of vascular invasion by tumor. First, there is the well-known difficulty of distinguishing vascular space involvement from artifactual separation of stroma away from nests of invasive and intraductal carcinoma, a phenomenon that gives the false impression that such nests are in vascular spaces. Secondly, the location of foci of vascular invasion may be of great importance, because it is well known that breast carcinomas with dermal lymphatic permeation are those clinically recognized as the prognostically dismal "inflammatory carcinomas." Microscopic dermal lymphatic involvement, even in the absence of clinical "inflammatory carcinoma," is an important feature to be be identified, because patients with this finding have a clinical course similar to those patients who present with microscopically confirmed, clinical "inflammatory carcinoma."[32b] We consider it useful to report the presence or absence of unequivocal angiolymphatic involvement by tumor cells along with an indication of the location of involvement: confined to the main tumor mass, outside the main tumor mass and/or within dermal lymphatics. We use the term "angiolymphatic space" when it is not possible to distinguish small vessels from lymphatics. We define angiolymphatic space involvement as the presence of a cluster of tumor cells within a space that is clearly lined by endothelial cells. Adherence of the tumor cells to the endothelial lining and association of tumor cells with a fibrin thrombus are features that help to confirm angiolymphatic space involvement. We have not found immunohistochemistry (i.e., anti-factor VIII) to be helpful; however, a recent report claims that immunohistochemistry identified 40% of vascular space invasion that would have been missed by routine histologic examination.[32a] If there is uncertainty whether tumor cells are in vascular spaces or not, we report that uncertainty.

LYMPH NODE STATUS

Pathologic lymph node status remains the most powerful predictor of treatment failure.[13,19] The most useful groupings have been found to be those patients with: (a) negative nodes, (b) 1 to 3 involved nodes, (c) 4 to 6 involved nodes, (d) 7 to 12 involved nodes, and (e) 13 or more involved nodes (Table 11). Note that there is now evidence that further stratifying patients with more than 3 nodes involved is prognostically useful. This emphasizes the need for adequate axillary dissections, thorough pathologic examination of resulting specimens, and accurately counting the number of lymph nodes involved. Examining just a few lymph nodes is unsatisfactory even if, for example, the first 4 lymph nodes contain carcinoma. Extension of carcinoma outside the lymph nodes into the axillary fat should be recorded because this is an adverse prognostic finding.[15]

The axillary tail from a modified radical mastectomy or from an axillary dissection procedure is divided into high and low lymph node groups by dividing the specimen into two roughly equal portions after removal from the breast. These divisions are primarily for the purpose of convenience, because it has been shown that the level of axillary node involvement does not provide additional prognostic information once the number of lymph nodes involved is known.[49a]

Patients with micrometastasis, defined as disease in which the largest nodal metastasis is less than 2 mm in maximum dimension, have at least short-term survival similar to patients with negative lymph nodes, although treatment

TABLE 11. Nodal Status and Treatment Failure (10 Years)

Status	No. of Patients	Failure
Negative	279	20%
1–3 positive	160	47%
4+ positive	175	71%
4–6 positive	65	59%
7–12 positive	55	69%
13+ positive	55	87%

Ref. 19.

failure rates are somewhat higher for the former group. In patients with micrometastases less than or equal to 1.3 mm, survival and treatment failure rates are similar to those of patients without nodal metastases.[16] Typically micrometastatic disease involves one low axillary lymph node, although a few such lymph nodes may be encountered. If any node contains foci of tumor greater than 2 mm in the aggregate, the case should be assigned to the "usual" metastatic carcinoma group, and all lymph nodes should be counted as involved whether the metastatic foci are greater or less than 2 mm. Levels of the paraffin block are indicated whenever a micrometastasis is found in a lymph node to be certain other foci of carcinoma are not present in that lymph node.

More data must be gathered before the long-term prognostic significance of micrometastases is known. Until that time, we advocate careful documentation of micrometastases when they are all that is found in the axillary dissection, with specific notation of the number and size of the foci that have been discovered. The presence of axillary lymph node involvement by carcinoma has been incorporated into the Postsurgical Treatment Pathological Classification (Table 8).

HORMONE RECEPTOR STATUS

Hormone receptor status may be considered a biochemical reflection of the differentiation of breast carcinoma. It is not surprising, then, that the estrogen receptor (ER) status of breast carcinoma correlates with certain histopathologic and biologic features and conveys information regarding prognosis and response to treatment. Estrogen receptor-negative tumors more often are poorly differentiated and exhibit high nuclear grade and necrosis, features rarely present in ER-positive tumors. Moreover, ER-positive tumors generally have a lower proliferative activity (as determined by thymidine labeling index,[38] Ki-67 growth fraction[34] and flow cytometry[29]) than ER-negative carcinomas and are diploid more often than ER-negative tumors.[38]

Tissue should be routinely submitted for receptor studies whenever a biopsy specimen is found to contain a suspicious mass lesion of sufficient size (0.5 cm or larger) to allow for both tissue diagnosis and for receptor analysis. Smaller lesions are submitted entirely for diagnosis. Moreover, we do not submit tissue from mammographically detected needle-localized breast biopsy specimens unless they contain an obvious mass lesion greater than 0.5 cm. Frozen section diagnosis is often used by us to determine if tissue needs to be submitted for receptor analysis.

Hormone receptor status is usually determined by the radioimmunoassay technique, so the results are not usually incorporated into the surgical pathology report. Antibodies active in frozen tissue have been produced against the ER protein. We have not used this antibody, because if frozen tissue is available, we think the radioimmunoassay technique should be used, since this method has been employed extensively in clinical trials and the clinical significance of the quantitative data derived by this technique is well understood. An antibody that is reported to identify ER protein in paraffin-embedded tissue is available, but we do not currently use it because a negative result may not be reliable. It is possible this can be overcome by insisting on positive normal breast tissue in the same section before reporting a negative result. If receptor status is determined immunohistochemically, we think the results and the interpretation should be a part of the surgical pathology report. A more detailed review of hormone receptors in breast cancer is provided in another article in this issue (p. 103–134).

FUTURE DIRECTIONS

The morbidity and expense of currently available adjuvant therapy combined with the increasing percentage of patients with minimal disease (and low relapse rates) continue to fuel efforts to identify more reliable prognostic features than those described above. Advances in cancer biology and molecular engineering have supplied oncologists with many sophisticated techniques that show promise of providing a more direct measure of the intrinsic biologic aggressiveness of breast cancers. These techniques include the identification of growth factors, growth factor receptors, oncogene expression, DNA ploidy, proliferation rate, and, most recently, an enzyme-induced lysosomal protease, cathepsin D.[50] The methods that have received greatest attention include the thymidine labeling index, amplification of the Neu oncogene, and flow cytometry to assess proliferation rate and DNA ploidy.

The thymidine labeling index, which measures the fraction of tumor cells in the S-phase (DNA synthesis phase) of the cell cycle, is an established tool for determining the proliferative activity of a tumor. This index has been well documented as a prognostic determinant in breast cancer; however, technical aspects of the method have limited its widespread use.[26,48] Amplification of the Neu oncogene by tumor cells also has been reported to be a prognostic variable.[49] This technique is laborious, time consuming, and requires a relatively large amount of tissue. In our opinion it should be regarded as a research tool at present.

Flow cytometric determination of proliferative activity (S-phase fraction) and DNA ploidy probably has been publicized most widely as a method that provides prognostic information for patients with breast cancer, particularly those with negative lymph nodes. The method is easier to perform than the aforementioned techniques and fresh, frozen, or paraffin-embedded tissue may be employed.[53] Recently, Clark and colleagues[6] reported node-negative patients with aneuploid tumors to have a significantly lower disease-free survival than patients with diploid tumors (74% vs. 88%; $p = .02$). Moreover, patients having diploid tumors with high S-phase had a worse prognosis than diploid tumors with low S-phase (70% vs. 90%; $p = .007$). While some authors have reported findings similar to Clark et al., other investigators have failed to confirm these findings.[22a] Muss et al.[36] found neither ploidy nor S-phase to be significantly associated with time to relapse. In addition, ploidy was not significantly associated with overall survival and S-phase was only of borderline significance. Keyhani-Rofagha et al.[27] investigated the predictive value of DNA content for long-term survival in patients with node-negative, infiltrating ductal carcinoma and found that ploidy analysis did not show independent prognostic value for patient survival at 10 years.

While flow cytometry is potentially useful, its clinical utility for the individual patient is at least controversial at present.[25,40a] Large clinical trials to determine whether flow cytometry provides information not available by other methods, particularly tumor grade, are needed and apparently are underway. Moreover, we think several refinements of the method, including standardization and quality control, are required before this tool achieves routine clinical use. Until that time, we do not think that flow cytometry, a relatively expensive method, is required for each patient with breast carcinoma. This seems particularly true for the node-negative patient whose invasive carcinoma is detected only by mammography. Such carcinomas are almost always of such small size that death from disease can be expected in less than 5% of patients, and many of those 5% can be detected by nuclear grading.[4] A review of DNA content and the proliferative rate of invasive breast carcinoma that reaches a different conclusion is presented elsewhere in this issue (p. 137–160). If flow cytometry is performed, we think reporting and interpretations should be done by the pathologist, ideally as a part of the surgical pathology report.

THERAPEUTIC IMPLICATION OF INVASIVE BREAST CARCINOMA

Two important questions for the patient with infiltrating lobular or ductal carcinoma of the breast are, to a great extent, answered by pathologic examination of the primary excision specimen: (1) What is the most effective method for local tumor control, i.e., mastectomy vs. lumpectomy combined with radiation therapy and lymph node dissection? (2) Will a particular node-negative patient benefit from adjuvant chemotherapy?

In addressing the first question, several clinical aspects, including the size and location of the lesion, the size of the breast, and the desires of the patient, must be considered. As more women continue to choose breast conservation therapy for the local control of invasive carcinoma, it has become increasingly important to identify the group of patients at increased risk for local failure. Overall, the local control of invasive breast carcinoma provided by lumpectomy and radiation therapy is quite good, approaching 90% (Table 10). It has been shown, however, that the presence of extensive intraductal carcinoma or positive excision margins identifies a group of women at increased risk for local failure. The data indicate that approximately 25–30% of patients with positive excision margins and approximately 20–25% of patients with extensive intraductal carcinoma, treated by lumpectomy and radiation therapy, will develop a local recurrence, in contrast to a recurrence rate of 5–10% in the absence of these features. In addition, there are data that suggest that the presence of other features, such as high nuclear grade in the setting of extensive intraductal carcinoma, places a patient at an even greater risk for local recurrence.[45] It has been recommended, therefore, that patients with invasive breast carcinoma at an increased risk for local recurrence be offered re-excision prior to radiation therapy (for those who desire breast conservation) or mastectomy. Extensive intraductal carcinoma (EIC) and positive excision margins are currently the only features that have been confirmed by different independent studies to place a patient at significantly increased risk for local recurrence.

The question of whether or not to provide adjuvant chemotherapy to node-negative patients is one of the most controversial questions in breast cancer management today. Currently, approximately 50% of newly diagnosed breast cancer patients have histologically negative nodes, and this percentage is expected to increase. Although 70% of node-negative patients are cured by local therapy, recent studies have indicated that, as a group, node-negative patients have an improved relapse-free survival following adjuvant therapy. This prompted the National Cancer Institute to issue a clinical alert recommending consideration of adjuvant therapy for all node-negative patients.[8] Many oncologists are reluctant to implement this recommendation, for this would result in the unnecessary treatment of 70% of node-negative patients. Oncologists are therefore looking to the particular features of a patient's cancer to decide whether a node-negative patient is likely to benefit from adjuvant therapy.

There is now sufficient information available from several large clinical studies to allow for a reasonable prediction of the behavior of node-negative breast carcinoma based on a set of morphologic features. In particular, nuclear grade appears to be the single most important predictor of overall survival and metastasis-free survival in node-negative patients. Approximately 90% of node-negative breast cancer patients with tumors of low nuclear grade are cured by surgery alone (Table 5). Node-negative patients with tumors of high nuclear grade have an overall survival of approximately 65% and a metastasis-free survival rate of approximately 80%; it is this group of patients that is most likely to benefit from adjuvant chemotherapy. In addition, histologic grade and tumor size are strongly associated with patient outcome and help to define categories of behavior in node-negative breast cancer; for example, patients with well-differentiated (low grade) carcinomas less than 2 cm probably do not need adjuvant therapy.

Current management for patients with breast cancer, more than any time in the past, requires a team approach involving surgery, radiology, pathology, radiation therapy, and oncology. The pathologist's responsibility is to carefully examine the specimen and report all the information that is known to bear on prognosis and may be needed to make therapeutic decisions. The check list we use is provided in Table 1. These features can be routinely incorporated into the surgical pathology report with little or no extra cost to the patient. Until new methods aimed at predicting biologic behavior of breast carcinoma are found to be superior or found to provide information not available from morphology and receptor status, we think complete morphologic evaluation of breast cancer specimens as outlined in this review is critical to ensure the best therapy for each patient with carcinoma of the breast.

Acknowledgment

The authors thank Mrs. Kelley Ramey for preparation of the manuscript.

References

1. Amalric R, Santamaria F, Robert F, et al: Conservation therapy of operable breast cancer—Results of five, ten and fifteen years in 2,216 consecutive cases. In Harris JR, Hellman S, Silen W (eds): Conservative Management of Breast Cancer. Philadelphia, J.B. Lippincott, 1983.
2. Bloom HJG, Richardson WW: Histological grading and prognosis in breast cancer. A study of 1,409 cases of which 359 have been followed for 15 years. Br J Cancer 11:359–377, 1957.
3. Carstens PHB, Greenberg RA, Francis D, Lyon H: Tubular carcinoma of the breast. A long term follow-up. Histopathology 9:271–280, 1985.
4. Carter CL, Allen C, Hensen DE: Relation of tumor size, lymph node status and survival in 24,470 breast cancer cases. Cancer 63:181–187, 1989.
5. Carter D: Margins of "lumpectomy" for breast cancer. Hum Pathol 17:330–332, 1986.
6. Clark GM, Dressler LG, Owens MA, et al: Prediction of relapse or survival in patients with node-negative breast cancer by DNA flow cytometry. N Engl J Med 320:627–633, 1989.
7. Clayton F: Pure mucinous carcinoma of the breast: Morphologic features and prognostic correlates. Hum Pathol 17:34–38, 1986.
8. Clinical alert from the National Cancer Institute. May 18, 1988. Breast Cancer Res Treat 12:3–5, 1988.
9. Connolly JL, Schnitt SJ: Evaluation of breast biopsy specimens in patients considered for treatment by conservative surgery and radiation therapy for early breast cancer. Pathol Ann 23:1–23, 1988.
10. Connolly JL, Schnitt S, Silver B, et al: Prognostic factors in node-negative (N–) breast cancer patients (abstract). Lab Invest 62:22A, 1990.
10a. Dixon JM, Anderson TJ, Page DL, et al: Infiltrating lobular carcinoma of the breast. Histopathology 6:149–161, 1982.
11. Contesso G, Mouriesse H, Friedman S, et al: The importance of histologic grade in long-term prognosis of breast cancer: A study of 1,010 patients, uniformly treated at the Institut Gustave-Roussy. J Clin Oncol 5:1378–1386, 1987.
12. Elston CW, Gresham GA, Rao GS, et al: The cancer research campaign (King's/Cambridge) trial for early breast cancer: Clinico-pathological aspects. Br J Cancer 45:655–668, 1982.
13. Fisher B, Bauer M, Wickerham L, et al: Relation of number of axillary nodes to the prognosis of patients with primary breast cancer: An NSABP update. Cancer 52:1551–1557, 1983.
14. Fisher B, Redmond C, Poisson R, et al: Eight-year results of a randomized clinical trial comparing total mastectomy and lumpectomy with or without irradiation in the treatment of breast cancer. N Engl J Med 320:822–828, 1989.
15. Fisher ER, Gregorio RM, Redmond S, et al: Pathologic findings from the National Surgical Adjuvant Breast Project (protocol no. 4): II. The significance of extranodal extension of axillary metastases. Am J Clin Pathol 65:439–444, 1976.
16. Fisher ER, Palekar A, Rockette H, et al: Pathologic findings from the National Surgical Adjuvant Breast Project (protocol no. 4): V. Significance of axillary nodal micro- and macrometastases. Cancer 42:2032–2038, 1978.
17. Fisher ER, Palekor AS, Redmond C, et al: Pathologic findings from the National Surgical Adjuvant Breast Project (protocol no. 4). VI. Invasive papillary cancer. Am J Clin Pathol 73:313–322, 1980.
18. Fisher ER, Redmond C, Fisher B: Pathologic findings from the National Surgical Adjuvant Breast Project (protocol no. 4): VI. Discriminants for 5-year treatment failure. Cancer 46:908–918, 1980.
19. Fisher ER, Sass R, Fisher B: Pathologic findings from the National Surgical Adjuvant Project for Breast Cancers (protocol no. 4): X. Discriminants for tenth year treatment failure. Cancer 53:712–723, 1984.
20. Fisher ER, Sass R, Fisher B, et al: Pathologic findings from the National Surgical Adjuvant Breast Project (protocol no. 6). II. Relation of local breast recurrence to multicentricity. Cancer 57:1717–1724, 1986.
21. Fisher ER, Sass R, Bernard F, et al: Pathologic findings from the National Surgical Adjuvant Breast Project. Correlations with concordant and discordant estrogen and progesterone receptors. Cancer 59:1554–1559, 1987.

22. Fisher ER, Redmond C, Fisher B, et al: Pathologic findings from the National Surgical Adjuvant Breast and Bowel Projects (NSABP). Prognostic discriminants for 8-year survival for node-negative invasive breast cancer patients. Cancer 65:2121–2128, 1990.
22a. Frierson HF: Ploidy analysis and S-phase fraction determination by flow cytometry of invasive adenocarcinomas of the breast. Am J Surg Pathol 15:358–367, 1991.
23. Harris JR, Connolly JL, Schnitt SJ, et al: The use of pathologic features in selecting the extent of surgical resection necessary for breast cancer patients treated by primary radiation therapy. Ann Surg 201:164–169, 1985.
24. Hutter RVP: The influence of pathologic factors on breast cancer management. Cancer 46:961–976, 1980.
25. Ingle JN: Assessing the risk of recurrence in breast cancer. N Engl J Med 322:329–331, 1990.
26. Kamel OW: Adjuvant therapy for breast cancer [correspondence]. N Engl J Med 319:445, 1988.
27. Keyhani-Rofagha S, O'Toole RN, Farrar WB, et al: Is DNA ploidy an independent prognostic indicator in infiltrative node-negative breast adenocarcinoma? Cancer 65:1577–1582, 1990.
28. Kurtz JM, Jacquemier J, Almaric R, et al: Risk factors for breast recurrence in premenopausal and postmenopausal patients with ductal cancers treated by conservation therapy. Cancer 65:1867–1878, 1990.
29. Kute TE, Muss HB, Anderson D, et al: Relationship of steroid receptor, cell kinetics and clinical status in patients with breast cancer. Cancer Res 41:3524–3529, 1981.
30. Lagios MD, Westdahl PR, Margolin FR, Rose MR: Duct carcinoma in situ. Relationship of extent of noninvasive disease to the frequency of occult invasion, multicentricity, lymph node metastases, and short-term treatment failures. Cancer 50:1309–1314, 1982.
31. Lagios MD, Margolin FR, Westdahl PR, Rose MR: Mammographically detected duct carcinoma in situ. Frequency of local recurrence following tylectomy and prognostic effect of nuclear grade on local recurrence. Cancer 63:618–624, 1989.
32. le Doussal V, Tubiana-Hulin M, Hacene K, et al: Nuclear characteristics as indicators of prognosis in node negative breast cancer patients. Breast Cancer Res Treat 14:207–216, 1989.
32a. Lee AKC, DeLellis PA, Silverman ML, et al: Prognostic significance of tumoral lymphatic and blood vessel invasion in node negative carcinoma of the breast. J Clin Oncol 8:1457–1465, 1990.
32b. Lucas FV, Perez-Mesa C: Inflammatory carcinoma of the breast. Cancer 41:1595–1605, 1978.
33. McDivitt RW, Boyce W, Gersell D: Tubular carcinoma of the breast: Clinical and pathological observations concerning 135 cases. Am J Surg Path 6:401–411, 1982.
34. McGurrin JF, Doria MI, Dawson PJ, et al: Assessment of tumor cell kinetics by immunohistochemistry in carcinoma of breast. Cancer 59:1744–1750, 1987.
35. Meyer JS: Cell kinetics of histologic variants of in situ breast carcinoma. Breast Cancer Res Treat 7:171–180, 1986.
36. Muss HB, Kute TE, Case LD, et al: The relation of flow cytometry to clinical and biologic characteristics in women with node negative primary breast cancer. Cancer 64:1894–1900, 1989.
37. Nime FA, Rosen PP, Thaler HT, et al: Prognostic significance of tumor emboli in intramammary lymphatics in patients with mammary carcinoma. Am J Surg Path 1:25–30, 1977.
38. Osborne CK: Receptors. In Harris JR, Hellman S, Henderson IC, Kinne DW (eds): Breast Diseases. Philadelphia, J.B. Lippincott, 1987, pp 210–232.
39. Page DL, Dixon JM, Anderson TJ, et al: Invasive cribriform carcinoma of the breast. Histopathology 7:525–536, 1983.
40. Page DL, Anderson TJ: Diagnostic Histopathology of the Breast. Edinburgh-New York, Churchill-Livingstone, 1987.
40a. Page DL: Prognosis and breast cancer. Recognition of lethal and favorable prognostic types. Am J Surg Pathol 15:334–349, 1991.
41. Peters GN, Wolf M: Adenoid cystic carcinoma of the breast. Report of 11 new cases: Review of the literature and discussion of biologic behavior. Cancer 52:680–686, 1982.
42. Rasmujssen BB, Rose C, Christensen I: Prognostic factors in primary mucinous carcinoma. Am J Clin Pathol 87:155–160, 1987.
43. Ridolfi RL, Rosen PP, Port A, et al: Medullary carcinoma of the breast. A clinicopathologic study with 10 year follow-up. Cancer 40:1365–1385, 1987.
44. Ro JY, Silva EG, Gallager HS: Adenoid cystic carcinoma of the breast. Hum Pathol 18:1276–1281, 1987.
44a. Rosner D, Lane WW: Node-negative minimal invasive breast cancer patients are not candidates for routine systemic adjuvant therapy. Cancer 66:199–205, 1990.
45. Schnitt SJ, Connolly JL, Harris JR, et al: Pathologic predictors of early local recurrence in stage I and II breast cancer treated by primary radiation therapy. Cancer 53:1049–1057, 1984.

46. Schnitt SJ, Connolly JL, Khettry U, et al: Pathologic findings on re-excision of the primary site in breast cancer patients considered for treatment by primary radiation therapy. Cancer 59:675–681, 1987.
47. Silverstein MJ, Waisman JR, Gamagami P, et al: Intraductal carcinoma of the breast (208) cases. Clinical factors influencing treatment choice. Cancer 66:102–108, 1990.
48. Silvestrini R, Daidone MG, Gasparini G: Cell kinetics as a prognostic marker in node-negative breast cancer. Cancer 56:1982–1987, 1985.
49. Slamon DJ, Clark GM, Wong SG, et al: Human breast cancer: Correlation of relapse and survival with amplification of the HER-2/neu oncogene. Science 235:177–182, 1987.
49a. Smith JA, Gamez-Araujo J, Gallager HS, et al: Carcinoma of the breast: Analysis of total lymph node involvement versus level of metastasis. Cancer 39:527–532, 1977.
50. Tandon AK, Clark GM, Chamness GC, et al: Cathepsin D and prognosis in breast cancer. N Engl J Med 322:297–302, 1990.
51. Tavassoli FA, Norris HJ: Secretory carcinoma of the breast. Cancer 45:2404–2413, 1980.
52. van de Vijver MJ, Peterse JL, Mooi WJ, et al: Neuprotein overexpression in breast cancer. Association with comedo-type ductal carcinoma in situ and limited prognostic value in stage II breast cancer. N Engl J Med 319:1239–1245, 1988.
53. Visscher DW, Zarbo RJ, Greenawald KA, Crissman JD: Prognostic significance of morphological parameters and flow cytometric DNA analysis in carcinoma of the breast. Pathol Ann 24:171–210, 1990.
54. Wargotz ES, Silverberg SG: Medullary carcinoma of the breast. Hum Pathol 19:1340–1346, 1988.
55. Zafrani B, Vielh P, Fourquet A, et al: Conservative treatment of early breast cancer: Prognostic value of the ductal in situ component and other pathological variables on local control and survival. Eur J Cancer Clin Oncol 25:1645–1650, 1989.
56. Zaloudek C, Ortel YC, Orenstein JM: Adenoid cystic carcinoma of the breast. Am J Clin Pathol 81:292–307, 1984.

Index

Entries in **bold face** type indicate complete chapters.

Absolute risk, definition of, 67
Adjuvant chemotherapy, value of, 176
Age/menopausal status, and ploidy, 147
Aneuploid, 139
Aneuploid cancer, survival and, 150
Angiolymphatic tumor involvement, 172–173
Anti-estradiol antibodies, 120
Apocrine hyperplasia, 72
Apocrine metaplasia, 72
Atypical ductal hyperplasia, 73–76, 78
  as a marker, 68
Atypical hyperplasia, 73–76
  clinical implications, 76
Atypical lobular hyperplasia, 73–76
  as a marker, 68

Bilateral total mastectomy, for lobular carcinoma in situ, 17
Biopsy, needle guided, for mammographically identified breast lesions, **1–10**
Biopsy specimen, gross examination of, 56
  handling of, 122–126
  processing of, 29, 31, 37
    fixation, 31, 37
    sampling, 29, 31
  unfixed, marking margins of, 55–56
  with small invasive carcinoma, case study of, 57–62
Blood vessel involvement, by tumor, 172–173
Bloom and Richardson grading system, 138, 165
Blunt duct adenosis, 72
Breast biopsy, containing invasive carcinoma, handling of, 54–56
  containing small invasive carcinoma, case study of, 57–62
  processing of, **51–64**
  pathologic examination of, **23–45**
    procedures for, 24–25
  processing of, **47–49**
  sources of interpretive error in evaluation of, 39–42
  surgical pathology report of, **161–180**
  tissue processing for, **23–45**
Breast cancer, *See* Breast carcinomas
Breast carcinomas, behavior of, 137–138
  clinically occult mammographically identified, features of, 2–4
  current management of, 176–177
  infiltrating, 163
    size of, 167–169

Breast carcinomas *(Cont.)*
  invasive, absolute risk of, 66–67
    axillary lymph node metastases and, 19
    mammographic screening and, 19–20
    mammography and, 15
    precursor lesions and, 68
    relative risk of, 66–67
  lobular, 163–164
    patterns of, 163–164
  low risk, 163
  mammographic screening of, **11–21**
  NIH Guidelines for, 106
  steroid receptor status of, after treatment, 111
    over time, 110–111
  therapeutic implications of, 176–177
  tumor size and, 19–20
  unexpected, 123–124

Calcifications, in breast mass, 3
Cancer, *See* Breast carcinomas
Carcinomas of low malignant potential, 163
Chemotherapy, adjuvant, rationale for, 52
  prognostic indicators and, 53–54
  steroid receptors and, 106–107
  tumor response to, vs. tumor ploidy, 153–154
Clinging carcinoma of Azzopardi, 78
Cytosol assay, 104
Cytosol monoclonal immunoassay, 112–113
  false negative, 124–125
  of small carcinomas, 123
  vs. histochemical techniques, 113, 121

DNA classes, survival and, 151
  relative risk of death and, 156
DNA content, *See also* Tumor DNA content
  and proliferation rate, correlation with prognostic variables, 142–150
  significance of, 137–160
  as a prognostic indicator, 138–139
DNA index, 138–139, 156
  as a prognostic indicator, 150–151
  S-phase fraction and, 152
  survival and, 151
DNA ploidy, as a prognostic indicator, 150–151
Dextran-coated charcoal assays, vs. immunohistochemistry techniques, for steroid receptor protein assays, 110–119
Diagnosis, in pathology report, 45
Diploid cancers, 139, 156
  histogram of, 141
  survival and, 150

183

Index

Duct carcinoma in situ, 76–89
  as a precursor lesion, 68
  associated with invasive ductal carcinoma, extent of, 170–171
  comedo type, 78, 80, 82–83, 84, 169–170
    clinical implications of, 86–87
  cribriform type, 77–78, 79, 169–170
    vs. ductal epithelial hyperplasia, 80
Duct carcinoma in situ,
  frequency of, 14
  grade of, 87
  histologic types of, 77
  intermediate type, 169
  micropapillary type, 77–78, 80–81
  noncomedo type, clinical implications of, 82, 84, 86
  pathology report of, 88
  progression of, 18
  removal of, 17–19
  size of, 87
  size of focus of, 18
  solid type, 82, 84–85
  treatment of, 88–89
  type of, 169–170
  vs. atypical ductal hyperplasia, 74, 75
  vs. lobar carcinoma in situ, 92
Ductal epithelial hyperplasia, florid, 73, 74–75
  mild, 72
  moderate, 73
  vs. cribriform DCIS, 80

Endocrine therapy, tumor response to, histochemical techniques and, 121
  vs. tumor ploidy, 152–153
Epithelial hyperplasia, 72
Estrogen-protein complexes, 120
Estrogen receptor assays, 104–128
  See also Steroid receptors
  cytosol vs. immunohistochemical methods, 122
  in management of breast cancer, 104–108
    in situ carcinoma, 108
    prognosis, 104–105
    response to therapy, 105–106
    treatment decisions, 106–108
  in other neoplasms, 127
Estrogen receptor content, determination of, 111–113
Estrogen receptor immunohistochemical stain, 127
Estrogen receptor protein analysis, 57, 62
  monoclonal antibody histochemical assessment of, 121
  patterns of histochemical staining for, 116
Estrogen receptor protein status, determination of, 122
Estrophilin, 113, 114
Excisional biopsy, local failure following, 170–171
  margins of, 171–172
Extensive intraductal carcinoma, 170

Faxitron industrial x-ray unit, 24, 55
Fibroadenoma, handling biopsy specimen of, 55
  hyalinized degeneration in, 3
Fibrocystic change, definition of, 69
  vs. fibrocystic disease, 69
Fixation, of biopsy specimen, 31, 37
Flow cytometry, 175–176
Fluoresceinated estrogens, 120
Frozen section examination, 27, 29, 48
  criteria for, 55
Frozen tissue, reserving of, for steroid receptor assays, 122–126

Grading, of infiltration carcinomas, 164–167

Histochemical techniques, reserving tissue for, 122–126
Histogenesis, vs. histologic appearance, 68–69
Histologic appearance, vs. histogenesis, 68–69
Hook wire, localization with, 5–6
Hormone receptor protein analysis, preparation of biopsy specimen for, 57
Hormone receptors, See Steroid hormone receptor assays and Steroid hormone receptor proteins
Hyperdiploid cancers, 156
Hyperplasia, 72–76
Hypertetraploid cancers, 156

In situ carcinoma, intermediate type, 169
  steroid receptors and, 108
  vs. invasive carcinoma, determination of, 123
In situ proliferative epithelial lesions, **65–102**
  morphologic continuum of, 66
Intracystic papillary carcinoma, 94–97
Intraductal papillary carcinoma, 94–97
Intraoperative breast biopsy specimen radiogram, interpretation of, 25–27
  documentation of, 25, 27
  microcalcific lesions, 25
  soft tissue abnormalities, 25
Invasive breast carcinoma, diagnosis of, 162–164
  See also Breast carcinoma
  in breast biopsy, handling of, 54–56
  nuclear grade of, 164–165
    criteria for, 166
  relative risk of, 66–67
  small, case study of, 57–62
    processing of biopsy of, **51–64**
  vs. in situ carcinoma, determination of, 123

Juvenile papillomatosis, 98
J-wire localization film, 41

Lobular carcinoma in situ, 89–94
  as a marker, 68
  clinical implications of, 92
  diagnosis of, 90

Lobular carcinoma in situ *(Cont.)*
    frequency of, 14
    involvement of ducts by, 90
    treatment of, 16–17
        bilateral total mastectomy, 17
        vs. DCIS, 92
Lobular carcinoma, invasive, mammography and, 15
Lobular hyperplasia, 72
    atypical, 90–91, 92–93
Local recurrence, prediction of, 170–171
Lumpectomy, 169
    for DCIS, 89
    local failure following, 170–171
Lymph node metastases, and ploidy, 143
Lymph node status, and treatment failure, 173
    5-year survival and, 167
    surgical pathology report and, 173–174
Lymphatic invasion, and tumor ploidy, 146
    by tumor, 172–173

Mammalian cell cycle, 140
Mammogram, preoperative, 26–27
Mammographic screening, effect of, on patient outcome, 16
    frequency of breast cancers and, 12–14
    size of breast cancers and, 14–16
Mammographically directed biopsies, reserving tissue from, 122–123
Mammography, **1–10**
    abnormal findings of, 24
    impact of, on size and frequency of breast cancers, **11–21**, 51–52
    mortality reduction and, 2
    positive predictive value of, 4
    technique of, 2
Mastectomy, for DCIS, 89
    for lobular carcinoma in situ, 17
    vs. lumpectomy, 176
Metastases, distant, and tumor ploidy, 143–144
    of invasive carcinoma, size of cancer and, 52
Methylene blue, in needle localization, 5, 7, 8–9
Microcalcifications, 24, 25, 26–27
    and soft-tissue densities, 30–31
    biopsies of, interpretive errors in evaluation of, 39–42
    localization of, 37, 39
Microglandular adenosis, 70, 72
Microinvasive tumor, 168
Micrometastasis, 173–174
Minimal breast cancer, 52
Minimally invasive, 168
Mitotic index, 155
Mitotic rate, 145
Monoclonal antibody reagents, for measuring steroid receptors, 103–104
Monoclonal histochemical receptor assays, 122–126

National Surgical Adjuvant Breast Project, 164
    grading scheme of, 165
NSABP grading scheme, 165
Needle localization, preoperative, of suspicious lesion, 4–7
    problems and pitfalls of, 7–8
    technique of, 5–6
Needle localization film, 32–33
Needle localization guided excisional biopsy, **1–10**
Neu oncogene, amplification of, 175
Nipple, adenoma of, 98
    florid papillomatosis of, 98
    Paget's disease of, 99–100
Nonproliferative fibrocystic change, 69
Novaldex Adjuvant Trial Organization, 107
Nuclear DNA analysis, touch preparations of tumor for, 56
Nuclear DNA histogram, 61
Nuclear DNA ploidy, 142–147
Nuclear grade, 145
    criteria for, 166
    prognostic value of, 166–167, 177

Occult malignancy of the breast, features of, 2–4
Outcome, of patients with small breast cancers, 52
    patient, mammographic screening and, 16

Pagetoid spread, in LCIS, 90, 94
Paget's disease of the nipple, 99–100
    clinical implications of, 100
Palliative therapy, steroid receptors and, 107–108
Papilloma, 96
    definition of, 98
    clinical implication of, 98–99
    intraductal, 96
        vs. intraductal papillary carcinoma, 96
Pathology report, essential pathologic features in, 162
    of breast biopsy, 42–45
        diagnosis, 45
        gross description, 42, 44
        microscopic description, 44
Photometry, in quantification of steroid receptor content, 118–119
Ploidy, 139, *See also* Tumor ploidy
    age/menopausal status and, 147
    nuclear DNA, correlation of, with prognostic variables, 142–147
        distant metastases and, 143–144
        lymph node metastases and, 143
        tumor size and, 142–143
    steroid receptor proteins and, 146–147
    tumor grade and, 144–145
    tumor necrosis and, 145–146
    tumor stage and, 144
    tumor type and, 144
Ploidy status, S-phase values and, 146

Postsurgical Treatment Pathological Classification, 168
Precursor lesion, 68
Preoperative mammogram, 26–27
Preoperative needle localization, of suspicious lesion, 4–7
Primary tumor, size of, 167–168
Progesterone receptors, 104–128
   See also Steroid receptors
   endocrine therapy and, 111
   in management of breast cancer, 104–108
      in situ carcinoma, 108
      prognosis, 104–105
      response to therapy, 105–106
      treatment decisions, 106–108
Progesterone receptor content, determination of, 111–112
Prognostic indicators, 53–54, 56–57, 155
   future directions and, 175–176
   in combination, 156
   in small invasive carcinoma, case study of, 57–62
   unfavorable, 63
Proliferation, cancer cell, measuring of, 140–141
Proliferative fibrocystic change, 69
Proliferative rate, correlation of, with prognostic variables, 147–150

Radiation therapy, value of, 176
Radical scar, 3
Radiography, *See also* Mammography
   specimen, 24
Receptor proteins, steroid, **103–134**
   See also Steroid receptor proteins
Relative risk, definition of, 66
   of invasive breast carcinoma, 66–67

Scarff-Bloom-Richardson grading scheme, 165
Sclerosing adenosis, 69–71
   vs. carcinoma, 70
Soft tissue abnormality, 25, 28–29
   biopsies of, interpretive errors in evaluation of, 42
Specimen radiogram, 8, 24, 34, 35, 37, 38
   intraoperative, interpretation of, 25–27
      documentation of, 25, 27
   of breast biopsy, 55
   of microcalcifications, 43–44
   processing of, **47–49**
S-phase fraction, 141–142
   as a prognostic indicator, 175–176
   preparation of biopsy specimen for, 56–57
   proliferative rate and, 151–152
Steroid hormone receptor assays,
   false negative, 124–125
   histochemical techniques for, 122–126
   indirect histochemical methods of, 120–121
   of small carcinomas, 123
   record-keeping and, 125–126
   reproducibility of, 110

Steroid hormone receptor assays *(Cont.)*
   reserving tissue for, 122–126
   role of, in differential diagnosis, 126–128
   small biopsies and, 123
   specimen for, 29
   timeliness and, 124–125
   usefulness of, in other neoplasms, 128
Steroid receptor proteins, **103–134**
   adjuvant therapy and, 106–107
   and tumor ploidy, 146–147
   computer-based photometry systems and, 118–119
   concentrations of, 109–110
   content of, 111–112
   cytosol assays of, 111–113
   dissociation constant of, 110
   DNA index and, 147
   grade of tumor and, 108
   growth fraction and, 108–109
   histologic type of tumor and, 108
   immunohistochemical demonstration of, 113–120
      quantification and, 117–119
      vs. cytosol assays, 113
   in other neoplasms, 127
   ploidy and, 108–109
Steroid receptor proteins, proportion of breast cancer specimens with, 109–110
   quantification of, 117–119
   specific activity of, 108
   status of, after treatment, 111
      over time, 110–111
Steroid receptor protein status, S-phase fraction values and, 149
   surgical pathology report and, 174–175
Surveillance, Epidemiology, and End Results (SEER) Program, 167
Swiss cheese disease, 98

Tamoxifen therapy, steroid receptors and, 106–107
Tetraploid breast cancers, 151, 156
Thymidine labeling index, 139, 141–142, 175
   proliferative rate and, 151–152
Touch preparations, for tumor nuclear DNA analysis, 56
Tumor cell proliferative rate, as a prognostic indicator, 139–142, 151–152, 154
   correlation of, with prognostic variables, 147–150
   distant metastases and, 148
   intraparenchymal lymphatic invasion and, 149
   lymph node status and, 147–148
   menopausal status and, 149
   steroid receptor proteins and, 149
   tumor grade and, 148
   tumor necrosis and, 148–149
   tumor size and, 147
   tumor stage and, 148
   tumor type and, 148

Tumor DNA content, as a prognostic indicator, 150–151
Tumor grade, and tumor ploidy, 144–145
  as a prognostic indicator, 137–138, 154–155
Tumor necrosis, and ploidy, 145–146
Tumor nuclear DNA content, and tumor proliferative rate, as a prognostic indicator, 152
  as a predictor, 154–155
Tumor ploidy, 175–176
  and survival, 151

Tumor ploidy *(Cont.)*
  chemotherapy and, 153–154
  endocrine therapy and, 152–153
Tumor size, and tumor ploidy, 142–143
  and proliferative rate, 147
  5-year survival and, 167
Tumor stage, and tumor ploidy, 144
Tumor type, and tumor ploidy, 144
Tylectomy, 169

Xeromammogram, 36

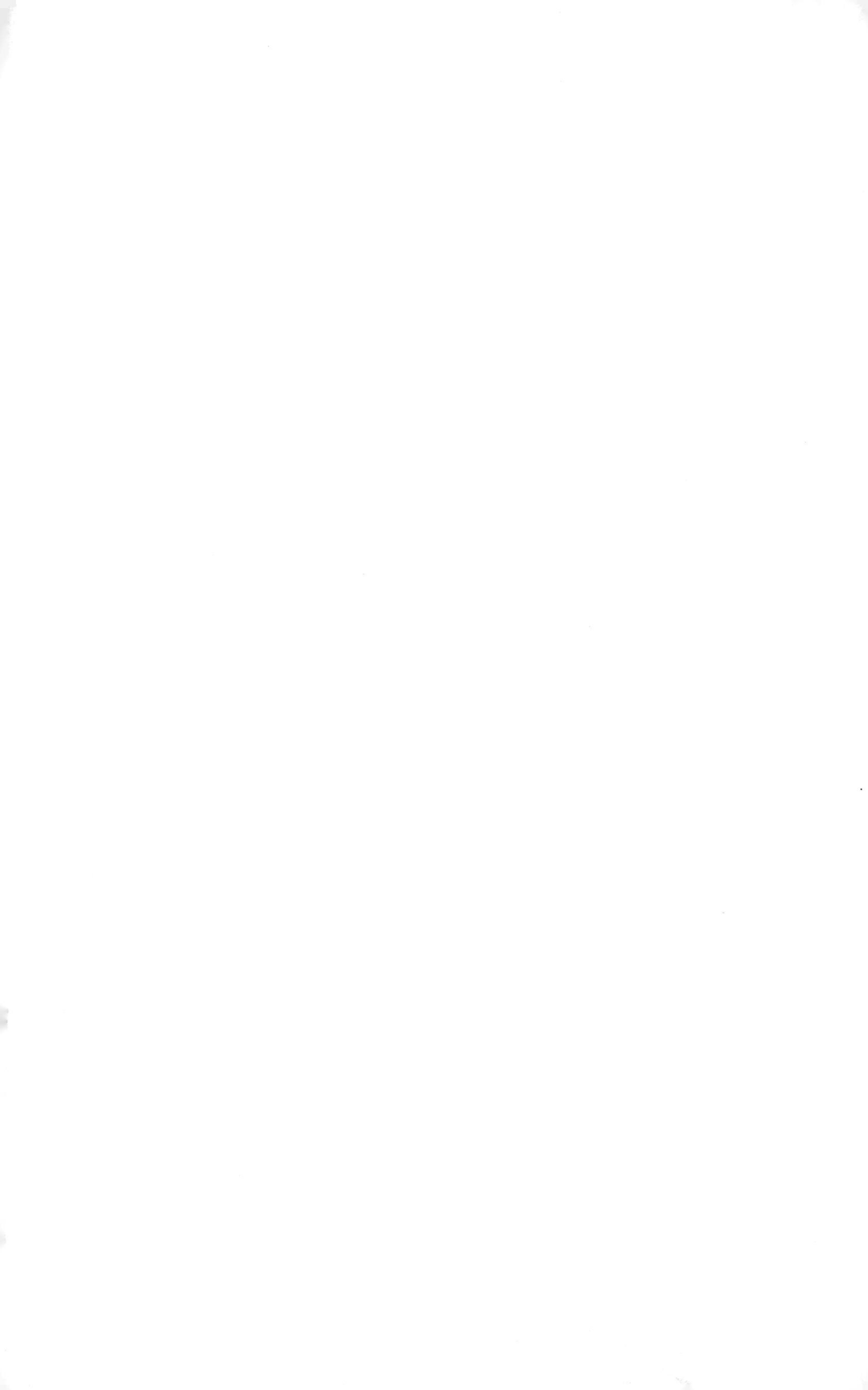